RIOTOUS FLESH

AMERICAN BEGINNINGS, 1500–1900
A Series Edited by Edward Gray, Stephen Mihm, and Mark Peterson

ALSO IN THE SERIES

Holy Nation: The Transatlantic Quaker Ministry in an Age of Revolution
by Sarah Crabtree

A Hercules in the Cradle: War, Money, and the American State, 1783–1867
by Max M. Edling

Frontier Seaport: Detroit's Transformation into an Atlantic Entrepôt
by Catherine Cangany

Beyond Redemption: Race, Violence, and the American South after the Civil War
by Carole Emberton

The Republic Afloat: Law, Honor, and Citizenship in Maritime America
by Matthew Taylor Raffety

Conceived in Doubt: Religion and Politics in the New American Nation
by Amanda Porterfield

RIOTOUS FLESH

Women, Physiology, and the Solitary Vice in
Nineteenth-Century America

APRIL R. HAYNES

THE UNIVERSITY OF CHICAGO PRESS
CHICAGO AND LONDON

APRIL R. HAYNES is assistant professor of history at the University of Oregon.

The University of Chicago Press, Chicago 60637
The University of Chicago Press, Ltd., London
© 2015 by The University of Chicago
All rights reserved. Published 2015.

24 23 22 21 20 19 18 17 16 15   1 2 3 4 5

ISBN-13: 978-0-226-28459-0 (cloth)
ISBN-13: 978-0-226-28462-0 (paper)
ISBN-13: 978-0-226-28476-7 (e-book)
DOI: 10.7208/chicago/9780226284767.001.0001

Library of Congress Cataloging-in-Publication Data

Haynes, April R., author.
  Riotous flesh : women, physiology, and the solitary vice in nineteenth-century America / April R. Haynes.
      pages cm
  Includes bibliographical references and index.
  ISBN 978-0-226-28459-0 (cloth : alkaline paper)—ISBN 978-0-226-28462-0 (paperback : alkaline paper)—ISBN 978-0-226-28476-7 (ebook) 1. Women—Sexual behavior—Social aspects—United States—History—19th century.
2. Female masturbation—Social aspects—United States—History—19th century.
3. Women—United States—Attitudes—History—19th century. 4. Feminism—United States—History—19th century.   I. Title.
  HQ29.H39 2015
  305.42097309′034—dc23
                                                             2015003802

FOR HEX

CONTENTS

	Introduction	1
1.	The Gender of Solitary Vice	26
2.	Licentiousness in All Its Forms	56
3.	Making the Conversation General	81
4.	A Philosophy of Amative Indulgence	107
5.	Flesh and Bones	132
	Epilogue	163
	Acknowledgments	179
	Notes	183
	Index	231

Introduction

"They used to say that masturbation would make you crazy—but I'd go crazy without it." In responding to Shere Hite's 1972 questionnaire on women's sexual practices, an anonymous member of the National Organization for Women acknowledged a profound historical change. The same behavior once deemed a perversion that caused insanity had come by the 1970s to represent, for many feminists, the healthiest of all sexual expressions. While Hite's respondent charted a clear reversal in attitudes about masturbation, she could not account for why so many Americans had ever believed that it "would make you crazy."[1]

What did seem clear to many feminists was that patriarchal definitions of female sexuality, not masturbation, had made women mad. Dell Williams, founder of the feminist bookstore Eve's Garden, announced that women who purchased vibrators liberated themselves from "the shame and guilt of centuries of oppression." The writer and activist Anne Koedt was more specific. Sigmund Freud and his popularizers, who had dominated American sexual thought since the 1920s, had pathologized women's natural sexual functioning in order to maintain male dominance. Freudians held that "vaginal orgasm," achieved exclusively through heterosexual intercourse, signified a woman's maturity. Women who "fixated" on the clitoris instead, particularly those who masturbated beyond the years of puberty, were described as infantile, neurotic, maladjusted, frigid, and mannish. Koedt denounced the vaginal orgasm as a "myth" that kept women fearful and sexually dependent upon men. Women's liberationists thus set out to demystify their bodies, to speak the "truth" about healthy female sexuality.[2]

To this end, feminists began to distribute two kinds of information: first, physiological studies, such as those conducted by William Masters and

Virginia Johnson, which traced the process of "female sexual response" directly to the clitoris; and second, women's testimony about their own experiences, such as those Alfred Kinsey had compiled in his landmark study *Sexual Behavior in the Human Female*. Kinsey's respondents testified again and again to the importance of clitoral sensation, and statistically speaking, female masturbation seemed perfectly average. Feminists cited Masters and Johnson and Kinsey in manifestos and self-help guides.[3]

By combining the facts of physiology with the evidence of experience, feminists such as Hite, Williams, and Koedt popularized a new norm of female sexuality, which centered on the clitoris and made masturbation, in the words of the Boston Women's Health Collective, "our sexual base." *Our Bodies, Ourselves* assumed that women shared a common socialization toward "guilt and repression" and therefore needed to be educated in the steps of masturbating to orgasm. Soon consciousness-raising groups throughout the country took up the subject of "liberating masturbation." Betty Dodson launched a series of self-help seminars in which women practiced masturbating together. They did so based on the belief that political and sexual maturity went hand in hand: "independent orgasms" would "lead to independent thoughts." By getting "in touch with their own sexuality, their own power," they would become able to "act in such a way as to change the world."[4] The act that had once threatened demise now heralded salvation.

The quest to liberate masturbation assumed, however, that *all* women had been oppressed through a set of sexual prescriptions—passivity, receptiveness, self-denial—that specifically structured white, middle-class femininity. African American women faced distinctive sexual constraints that had been historically constructed as counterpoints to the prescriptions of white femininity. In particular, black feminists confronted two intertwined stereotypes: the sexually voracious Jezebel and the castrating matriarch. Both functioned to deny their oppression by claiming that they already had (too much) sexual freedom and power in their families. Black feminists also built upon an ongoing tradition of activism in antiracist and working-class struggles and therefore seldom envisioned women's liberation in terms of a sudden awakening from passivity. As the black freedom struggle radicalized and faced violent repression, female masturbation hardly suggested itself as the bedrock of liberation.

A unique quest for self-definition—including, but not limited to, sexual politics—became a defining principle of black feminist thought.[5] For example, the black feminist Toni Cade Bambara rejected the sexual universalism expressed by white feminists such as Dodson and Williams as a "false romantic notion of *the liberated woman*," one who "must be freed to enjoy orgasm . . . and that is that." She pointed out the irony that "this new field of experts (white, female)" had replaced "the old field of (white, male) psychiatrists." Doubting "that our priorities are the same, that our concerns and methods are the same, or even similar enough," Bambara urged black women to look to one another for self-definition and to theorize "the whole area of sensuality, sex." As black feminists and other women of color organized throughout the early 1970s, many spurned "Western individualism" in order to grapple with issues of sexuality as one component of systemic transformation.[6] Autoeroticism did encourage self-definition and self-love. But few black feminists made masturbation quite the panacea it became for a time in white feminist spaces. Audre Lorde envisioned erotic power as a "self-connection" and "a longed-for bed which I enter gratefully and from which I rise up empowered."[7] Alice Walker later added, in reference to clitoral masturbation, that "the God of woman is autonomy."[8] Both Lorde and Walker, however, conceptualized women's sexuality as more pansexual and holistic than masturbatory. Relatedly, both insistently linked sexual liberation with the need for systemic change.

Many socialist feminists also wondered whether sexual liberation might become a new opium of the masses, a distraction that set middle-class women to "vulva-gazing" instead of fighting capitalist patriarchy. They especially critiqued the commodification of sexual liberation in the form of the vibrator. When the National Organization for Women invited Dell Williams to organize a 1974 Women's Sexuality Conference, one attendee complained that "again and again the vibrator . . . was presented as the messiah—everywoman's dream come true (only $19.95)." Lesbians and other radical feminists argued that sexual oppression must not be pitted against bread-and-butter issues, but such nuance attracted less publicity than flashy promises of sexual liberation on one end of the spectrum and sex-baiting on the other. In any case, radical lesbians also maintained that sex formed only one dimension of power. No sexual practice, nor any theory of sex, could in itself create social justice against the backdrop of patriarchal white supremacy and neocolonial capitalism.[9]

Similar debates occurred during the 1830s and 1840s. Then, too, large numbers of white, middle-class women dominated the conversation, asserting their equality with men of their own race and class in sexual terms. Unlike their feminist descendants, these women led the crusade *against* masturbation. But they did so precisely because they sought to challenge the sexual relations that structured patriarchy in their own time and to envision what sexual autonomy for women might look like in practice. Quite unknowingly, the Boston Women's Health Collective shared with evangelical white women of the 1830s a belief that subjectivity—the individual self-definition that made possible social agency—hinged on what women did (or didn't do) with their sexual bodies when all alone.

Between 1968 and the present, it has become hard to imagine how women could ever have believed that solitary sex was inherently pathological. Yet only through the efforts of antebellum female moral reformers did a majority of Americans come to consider it a deviant, crazy-making act. Like twentieth-century feminists, they believed that women could access the "truth" about sex by studying physiology and exchanging accounts of their own experiences. In doing so, they formulated a sexual politics independent of men and male desire. In both historical moments, a vocal cadre of white, middle-class women posited their particular construction of sexuality as *the* "prowoman line" on sex. However, in the nineteenth century, as in the twentieth, women of color strove for sexual self-definition. Black abolitionist women struggled primarily against legal and economic structures that codified black subjugation through sexual and reproductive coercion. In order to counter dehumanizing stereotypes that blamed black women for their own victimization, they engaged white women in a much broader debate over the nature of female sexuality, its relationship to social power, and divergent visions of autonomy. As part of that dialogue, they adapted white women's language to their own priorities. In this way, black abolitionist women also came to forswear "the solitary vice."

Riotous Flesh tells the story of how masturbation became a reviled sexual act charged with political meaning in the United States between 1830 and 1860. We will see that women—white and African American—led that process. They did so for disparate reasons and in various ways, yet they shared a strong desire to transform the contemporary politics of sexuality. Their thinking about gender, race, and sex thus forms a central topic of the book. At times, those discussions may seem unrelated to masturbation, yet it is precisely because a new argument against "the solitary vice" invited women into public sexual discourse that so many became concerned with the act. By the same token, women's capacious discussions of sexual politics deeply shaped, even drove, contemporary understandings of masturbation. Legions of relatively unknown women embraced the opportunity to proselytize friends, neighbors, family members, students, and coreligionists about sex, and they succeeded in creating a remarkable consensus. By the eve of the Civil War, Americans on all points of the political, religious, and cultural spectrum—people who could agree on nothing else—shared one certainty: masturbation would "make you crazy."

Women's centrality to the great masturbation phobia of the nineteenth century, an aspect of cultural history that has long been associated with "reforming men and manhood," may come as a surprise.[10] Yet in the United States, conflicts over femininity sparked widespread concern with this seemingly trivial behavior. Before 1830, only a handful of Americans thought seriously about masturbation, precisely because its critics supported colonial and early national forms of patriarchy. Health-based arguments against "onanism" (the spilling of semen) traveled from England to North America during the early eighteenth century, inspiring leaders such as Cotton Mather and Benjamin Rush to sporadically warn young men that "self-pollution" enervated the body and emasculated the will. They imagined the "effeminate" masturbator as unable to restrain his own passions, enslaved by his unruly flesh. If he could not master his own body, he certainly could not be trusted to govern his dependents. Because little about such advice elicited controversy, antimasturbation tracts faded into a sea of conduct manuals marketed to elite men.

Then, between 1833 and 1837, a lecturer named Sylvester Graham (1794–1851) ignited a controversy that suddenly drew a great deal of attention to masturbation. If modern Americans remember Graham at all, it is usually only as the namesake of the graham cracker. But during the 1830s, he inspired a cultural movement called *reform physiology*, which held that by following a set of "laws of life and health" culled from the Bible, women and men could prevent both individual and social ills.[11] Educated for the ministry at Amherst College, Graham embodied the evangelical spirit of the Second Great Awakening, the chain of Protestant revivals that spread across the Northeast between 1790 and 1840. Evangelicals believed that Jesus Christ would return to earth at the end of a millennium of social harmony. Christians should strive to convert nonbelievers, and each individual should strive for spiritual perfection. Sylvester Graham argued that *physical* perfection was equally important, that ordinary people could achieve such perfection on earth rather than waiting for the afterlife, and that the key to perfect health lay in the management of bodily desires. Those who kept their "flesh in subjection" would live for centuries—like the biblical Methuselah—then die painless deaths. After a short and unsuccessful career as a minister, Graham set out to evangelize all who would listen to his doctrine of health. His lectures provoked conversions similar to those experienced by church members, and converts called themselves Grahamites.¹²

Graham began by lecturing on the evils of alcohol but soon expanded his subject to include the physiological impact of diet, dress, and sex. Merging the science of physiology with the evangelical ideal of perfection, he argued that gluttony and vanity stimulated lust and disease by heating the blood. Graham insisted that the Bible forbade meat eating as well as drunkenness, citing Proverbs 23:20—"be not among wine-bibbers, among riotous eaters of flesh." French scientists had recently illuminated the process of digestion by vivisection, and Graham summarized their findings in ways that affirmed the connection between the indulgence of the appetite, nervous stimulation, and debility. Audience members hungered for advice they hoped would prevent illnesses that contemporary physicians could not cure.¹³ Cheap physiological lectures also held tremendous entertainment value for city dwellers and rural townsfolk alike. To people who had never seen a picture of the internal organs that sustained life, mock dissections of papier-mâché manikins offered a stunning form of "edutainment."¹⁴

The first step toward what would become a sweeping cultural obsession with masturbation began in 1833, when Graham advertised a lecture on sexual physiology to women only. In an earlier lecture to young men, he had framed the old warnings against onanism as the sexual standard of evangelical perfection: more than simply avoiding illicit sex, young men must control the urge most easily indulged. Now, promising details too explicit for mixed-gender audiences, he asserted that women needed exactly the same information—the same warnings against *onanism*, which Graham recast as the *solitary vice*—that advisors had long offered to men. He argued that women and men shared an identical sexual nature: both experienced desires that, when stimulated, might "kindle into passions." When he lectured to men on the topic of solitary vice, the streets remained silent. Yet each and every time Graham offered the "Lecture to Mothers," his announcements "produced an explosion": "men and boys" rioted in streets.¹⁵

Such drama helped to make Graham one of the most widely recognized figures in nineteenth-century America. Contemporaries held strong opinions about his "system," a bland diet intended to prevent individuals from succumbing to other "depraved appetites." It consisted of unseasoned vegetarian fare, whole-grain bread, and nothing but cold water to drink. The riots, however, focused particular attention on his sexual advice—especially his determination to warn women as well as men that masturbation caused illness, insanity, and death. This argument often strikes twenty-first-century readers as both laughably wrong and somewhat sad, the sign of a benighted past. But most early nineteenth-century people also found such prognostications ridiculous. Beyond a tight corps of physiological reformers, most Americans mocked Graham as a "humbug": a medical huckster who thrived on the public's credulity, a laughable caricature of the extremes to which reformers could go—or worse, a "male monster," whom enemies considered sexually ambiguous and therefore barely human.[16]

Why, then, did Graham enrage the "multitudes"? How did such a harmless, even laughable, figure provoke not one but *seven* recorded riots? Clearly, enemies targeted not only the lecturer but the women who listened to him, their male allies, and the ideas to which they subscribed. The lecture on chastity became inflammatory when delivered to women because it insisted that all bodies were subject to the *same set* of God-given "laws of life and health." In this way, reform physiology minimized the significance of physical differences such as sex and, implicitly, skin color.[17] Rioters perceived Graham's sexual universalism as challenging the basic hierarchies of gender and race that limited and defined Jacksonian democracy.

Two sexual ideologies—patriarchal governance and libertine republicanism—anchored those hierarchies in 1833. *Patriarchal governance* justified elite white men's social, political, and economic dominance on the grounds that only they possessed a capacity for true virtue. Patriarchs bore the responsibility for governing the unruly passions of their household dependents and social subordinates (including male slaves, servants, and apprentices).[18] The market revolution, combined with political and religious democratization, destabilized this logic. By the 1830s, growing numbers of propertyless and laboring men claimed equal entitlement to the privileges of white manhood in the Republic. *Libertine republicans* insisted that all white men, regardless of economic class, shared a special set of sexual liberties that distinguished them from people of color and white women. However unequal the economic conditions of white men's lives, they could take pleasure in libertinage and the sense of superiority that followed. Moreover, by aggressively asserting their sexual entitlement in newspapers, taverns, and city streets, they controlled public space. This, in turn, allowed them to police the boundaries of civil society and monopolize most forms of waged labor.[19]

Both patriarchy and libertinage bolstered white male supremacy by claiming that white men shared a basic sexual nature that justified their power. Patriarchs represented masculine sexuality as naturally passionate, yet subject to manly restraint. Libertines described it as explosive if not permitted free expression. Both considered the hydraulics of the male body to justify men's need for regular "release" (whether within marriage or outside it). Significantly, this physiological argument did not have the same resonance when applied to black men. Though also governed by hydraulics, they were subject to external restraints on their sexual freedom. Indeed, the hydraulic model of male sexuality helped to justify the gradual creation of a racially segregated northern public sphere, ostensibly to protect white women from the "eruptions" of black men. Imagining sexual violence as a natural consequence of explosive lust (rather than an expression of power) rationalized free black men's exclusion from civil society. It also obscured white men's use of sexual violence and harassment to maintain dominance.[20]

Patriarchs and libertines also contrasted masculine propensities from the dual sexual nature they ascribed to women. From either viewpoint, feminine sexuality revolved around a false dichotomy between virgins and whores. White women who passively submitted to the governance of patriarchs were, theoretically, rewarded with protection from sexual predation. Women outside the protected class—those who were enslaved or poor, those who refused to conform, and those "abandoned" by their designated protector—were deemed sexually accessible. Libertine republicans mainly consorted with women of the latter group, whom they designated whores. Nevertheless, in their view, *all* women secretly craved heterosexual intercourse; some just needed to be awakened to their desires. A libertine triumphed when he seduced a "virgin" and rendered her a "whore." In sum, patriarchs and libertines considered male sexuality essentially *active* (either questing or controlled) and female sexuality *passive* (either receptive or obedient).

Chapter 1, "The Gender of Solitary Vice," recounts the ways in which Graham provoked riots by attacking the underlying premise of sexual difference. Regarding sex, he argued, "human nature is radically the same everywhere."[21] He denied that men required periodic release in the form of sex on demand, as libertine republicans insisted. Nor were they inherently better able to govern their bodily urges than women, as patriarchs alleged. In physiological terms, earlier writers had warned that masturbation caused excessive seminal loss and harmed the male body in particular. By contrast, Graham told women that nervous stimuli, not the presence of a sexual partner, caused sexual arousal. *Over*stimulation caused blindness, epilepsy, and insanity. However, by ridding themselves of solitary vice, women could attain its opposite: *social virtue*. Those who faced and conquered their passions possessed the same virtue that prior advisors had enjoined on patriarchs. Reform physiology disaggregated virtue, the defining feature of republican citizenship, from manhood.[22] The women who embraced such advice asserted their individuality and capacity for sexual self-government: they neither needed patriarchal supervision nor lived to pleasure libertine republicans. In doing so, they threatened the contemporary gender order from both sides.

If rioters hoped to quell threats to the gender order by suppressing the women's lectures, their actions backfired. Observers with no prior interest in physiology (let alone the solitary vice) concluded that something important must be at stake since it provoked such violent backlash. Many began taking reform physiology seriously because the riots seemed to prove that republican liberty had lapsed into license. Rather than "eating flesh and drinking wine and rioting in every form of sensual pleasure," each individual must contribute to the rebuilding of an ethical society. "Ultras" (radical evangelicals) extended this logic still further: greed and self-indulgence caused not only disease but systematic poverty and prostitution, slavery, and war. They charged intimate acts and sexual ideas with political significance. Only by conquering one's base and selfish instincts—being "governed by principle rather than by appetite"—could a person contribute to "moral regeneration." By refusing alcohol, meat, and coffee and by committing to sexual restraint, ultras marked an activist subculture in opposition to the dominant society's self-indulgent values. Thus, the Christian anarchist Edmund Quincy abandoned "all riotous eating of flesh," declaring "the *chain of ultraism* is incomplete without this link."[23]

The riots especially piqued the interest of women involved in two emerging reform movements: *moral reform* (the evangelical campaign for a single standard of sexual morality for women and men) and *abolition* (the movement for an immediate end to slavery instead of colonization, a scheme that would force free blacks to move to Africa). Abolitionists and moral reformers condemned men who flaunted their power by forcing women, both free and enslaved, into "catering for vicious and depraved appetites." Powerful men benefited from "systematized licentiousness," institutions that maintained their sexual dominance as a means of asserting social, economic, and political power. In their eyes, the anti-Graham riots fit into a larger pattern of lawlessness: proslavery men mobbed abolitionists, libertines reveled in brothels. Such "licentious men" seemed themselves reduced to "slaves of their appetites and passions." Governed by riotous flesh, was it any wonder that the nation seemed to run riot?[24]

From the outset, the riots against Graham's universal theory of sexuality also targeted women who publicly challenged male sexual privilege. During the late 1830s, thousands vowed to eradicate the sexual double standard and joined the female moral reform movement, the first social movement led by women in United States history. Historians usually associate female moral reformers with crusades against prostitution and seduction. This scholarship attends to moral reformers' efforts to restrain everyone except themselves: licentious men, unregulated youth, and "abandoned females."[25] But the first public lectures on solitary vice gave them an opportunity to theorize their own sexual desire even as they evangelized their peers. Over time, moral reformers turned away from self-scrutiny and created mechanisms to control the sexuality of others. However, this outcome was neither inevitable nor foreseeable during the 1830s.

Chapters 2 and 3 trace the process by which diverse women took up the solitary vice as part of a more general effort to redefine sex in their own terms. While men rioted in the streets, ostensibly in the name of protecting innocent women from a sexual charlatan, female moral reformers refused the favor. They denounced it as *false delicacy*, a smoke screen that disguised the true conflict between men who wanted to preserve the sexual status quo and women who wanted to change it. While claiming to defend feminine delicacy, libertine republicans actually hoped suppress women's participation in public debates about sex—especially those that threatened male privilege or white supremacy. Next, moral reformers applied the concept of false delicacy to those who simply *refrained* from challenging the sexual double standard—women who refused to become activists or learn about their own bodies because they feared being perceived as salacious. Over time, false delicacy grew increasingly elastic and appealing. Advertisements of popular physiology lectures, for example, warned against false delicacy. The shorthand signaled that lifesaving warnings against the solitary vice would be imparted and established the pure motives of the reformers within, even as they tackled wide-ranging issues of sexual politics.

Chapter 2 argues that African American women applied false delicacy to defenders of slavery, authoring an important sexual counterdiscourse that bridged abolitionism with moral reform. Black abolitionist women familiar with the New York Female Moral Reform Society transformed its attack on "licentiousness in all its forms" into a targeted campaign against "the licentiousness of slavery."[26] They forged this alliance with white women in response to brutal race riots in the summer of 1834. Enraged by rumors of *amalgamation*, the antebellum pejorative for interracial intimacy, rioters attacked the meeting places of abolitionists and moral reformers, then turned on African Americans more generally, sacking their houses, churches, and schools. In the aftermath of the riots, women in the African Methodist Episcopal Zion Church, in conjunction with men such as David Ruggles, pointed out that amalgamation rioters had no qualms with interracial sex as long as it maintained white dominance. They also pressed white female moral reformers to rethink the racial terms of sexual discourse and to put their moral authority to work for black freedom. Despite the great risks of such an alliance, avoiding white women and refraining from sexual speech had not, thus far, protected black abolitionist women from racist violence. They therefore chose to participate actively in the female moral reform movement between 1835 and 1840.

Black moral reformers such as Sarah Mapps Douglass, Lavinia Hilton, Hetty Burr, and Nancy Gardner Prince made formative and lasting interventions in American sexual thought. Concerned with matters of sexual violence, harassment, and oppressive stereotypes, they said little at first about the solitary vice. However, their unique counterdiscourse created a necessary precondition for it to become a topic of interest to female moral reformers in general. African American women challenged the notion of white feminine *purity* and proposed instead a definition of *virtue* that transcended gender and race. Collapsed with whiteness and virginity, purity connoted a passive, fragile, bodily state. Virtue, on the other hand, indicated responsibility, intention, and active striving. Whereas purity could be "polluted" and thus lost forever, a virtuous individual could not be sullied by the actions of others. Reform physiology reinforced this conception of virtue by insisting that "human nature is radically the same everywhere."[27] No race or gender, as a group, could embody sexual purity or pollution.

This unique confluence—the physiological argument of nervous stimulation, the backlash against women's sex education, and African American women's strategic counterdiscourse—inspired a profound reconsideration of female sexuality. In this activist context, it became both possible and necessary for a few white women to question assumptions of their inherent purity. As they did so, they applied the language of solitary vice to their own lives. African American women, who comprised a noticeable presence at reform physiology lectures, also adopted solitary vice discourse. However, they did not share white female moral reformers' growing preoccupation with it. While black abolitionist women crafted a sexual politics aimed at uprooting slavery and white supremacy, growing numbers of white women became more interested than ever in individual sexual restraint.

Chapter 3, "Making the Conversation General," explains the collision of these trends. During the late 1830s, white moral reform women asserted their leadership of reform physiology. In Boston, a Ladies' Physiological Society formed, heralding a new and internally focused subculture among white activist women. They championed the lectures of Mary Gove and allowed the embattled Sylvester Graham to retire from the lecture circuit.

With Graham out of the picture, the riots abated. Gove's lessons inspired other women to become lecturers to ladies on anatomy and physiology. Their lectures contributed to the moral reform movement's growth and diffused the message about solitary vice throughout the countryside. Within their own small-town moral reform societies, thousands of white women learned to testify to their own experiences and to regard their peers as experts on female sexuality. Much like twentieth-century consciousness-raising groups, female moral reform societies linked female masturbation with other aspects of sexual politics. (They placed comparatively less emphasis on other aspects of reform physiology, such as vegetarianism.) Although women advised one another against *acting* upon their passions, the mere *recognition* of female desires that did not revolve around men broke radically from early national concepts of women's sexuality. If women did not need men to feel passion, they also did not need men to rein in their sexual behavior (whether through patriarchal governance or the sexual satisfaction that libertines promised). Some, such as Paulina Wright Davis, turned the logic of sexual citizenship into a direct argument for their civil rights. By constituting women as liberal individuals endowed with republican virtue, the campaign against solitary vice contributed to a very specific pursuit of "woman's rights."

The white moral reformers who turned inward failed to sustain the challenges to the racialized notions of purity and licentiousness that African Americans had initiated. Between 1840 and 1845, the movement fractured over the sexual politics of slavery and racism. Three factions emerged: black moral reformers, who pursued their own agenda mainly in separate institutions; white ultras, who gravitated toward the emergent women's rights movement; and white "guardians," who considered themselves stewards of the nation's sexual morality. The guardianship wing defined moral reform as a single-issue movement devoted solely to the "cause of purity." They wrested control of movement newspapers, petitioned to make seduction a crime, and built houses of refuge and industry. Moral guardians also continued to crusade against the solitary vice. Having established their own virtue, however, they turned antimasturbation discourse away from self-discipline and toward the discipline of young, poor, and colonized people. By midcentury, they had helped to make the fear of masturbation a cultural phenomenon. But the guardians disseminated a different set of warnings against "self-pollution" than had Grahamite women. Most interested in protecting the purity they deemed inherent to women similar to themselves, guardians deflected attention from the individual desires of adult white women. Although they challenged patriarchs and libertines in various ways, they shared with both one basic assumption: men lusted, women were conquered by lust. As a result, they revived the old association of "onanism" with male youth.

The final two chapters tell the stories of the women who left the female moral reform movement as it turned toward guardianship. Nascent feminists, both African American and white, continued to adapt reform physiology to their own purposes. Their actions during the 1840s and 1850s introduced ever greater numbers of people to the solitary vice.

Chapter 4, "A Philosophy of Amative Indulgence," traces white women's embrace of a new argument in favor of their right to healthy sexual pleasure. They claimed this right as consumers and activists within a changing context. As the female moral reform movement turned away from interracial solidarity and toward sexual guardianship, its terms lost their radical edge. Secular physicians, proprietary healers, and pornographers appropriated concepts such as false delicacy and the solitary vice. One such entrepreneur, Frederick Hollick, won the support of white feminists in Philadelphia during the mid-1840s by insisting that respectable women could and should find pleasure in "moderate" heterosexual intercourse. He distinguished healthy pleasure from the solitary vice, which, because it could be endlessly repeated, constituted an inherently *immoderate* sexual act. He also capitalized on the emergence of racial science in his sexual physiology lectures. Unlike Graham, Hollick located the propensity to sexual excess in the bodies of black women. Rather than objecting, white women's rights advocates bought his books, promoted his lectures, and helped him avoid an obscenity conviction. In the process, they explicitly linked Hollick's "philosophy of amative indulgence" to their own citizenship. Amid the booming medical marketplace of the 1840s and 1850s, the physiology of solitary vice helped to purify and whiten heterosexual pleasure.[28]

As greater numbers of white, middle-class Americans from across the political spectrum learned the dangers of the solitary vice, the campaign against it became institutionalized. Asylum reformers, teachers, and medical doctors further entrenched antimasturbation discourse. Others, such as alumnae of the New England Female Medical College (1848) and the Female Medical College of Pennsylvania (1850) institutionalized a two-pronged form of sex education. On the one hand, they argued that very young students must learn that healthy bodies, female as well as male, required solitary restraint. "Lunatic asylums abound through the prevalence of secret vice," argued one reformer; therefore, states would save the public funds spent on housing the insane by mandating physiological education. On the other, they deemed pleasurable, married intercourse as a physiological necessity. The first wave of female physicians disseminated both sides of this ideology through physiology lessons at normal schools and teaching institutes. Soon, teachers fanned out across the nation instilling children with reasons to avoid "a solitary, but fatal vice."[29] Reform physiology thus gave rise to the first wave of sex education in public schools. The Republic needed physiologically informed women to educate its future citizens and spouses.

Chapter 5, "Flesh and Bones," steps into the classroom of Sarah Mapps Douglass, the first recognized African American sex educator, in order to explore the racial and gender politics of early sex education. Douglass first became convinced of the importance of physiological education during the interracial moment in moral reform. She went on to lecture for decades to African American women on anatomy, physiology, and hygiene. In addition, Douglass offered a delicate, yet surprisingly explicit, sex education to her teenage students in the girls' department at Philadelphia's Institute for Colored Youth. These anatomy and physiology lessons never focused exclusively on sex; they also directly challenged the new racial science of craniology. While warning African American women not to allow false delicacy to prevent them from learning the laws of "womanly health," Douglass modeled for students an affirming and holistic counterdiscourse on black female embodiment.[30] At the same time, she warned women and girls to beware of the solitary vice, putting its cultural associations with virtue and scientific rationalism to her own use. In this way, Douglass participated in and extended the spread of antimasturbation discourse in ways that resonated with young black women for generations.

As a whole, this book addresses three key questions about the history of sexuality in the United States. First, how did a particular sexual prescription—one that may appear foolish and wrong in hindsight—become a cultural norm? Second, to what extent did nineteenth-century Americans truly believe that white, middle-class women were passionless? And third, how did free black women conceptualize sex, embedded as it was in systems of slavery, patriarchy, and white supremacy? Each of these questions concerns the ways in which ordinary people interpreted, challenged, or promoted particular sexual ideas at specific moments in time.

The solitary vice illuminates the historical processes by which one idea about sex could grow into a dominant discourse. Historians have analyzed the implications of the antimasturbation advice found in religious and medical texts.³¹ But what did those ideas mean to the people who read or heard them? And why, when British writers had written against "self-pollution" more than a century earlier, did this fear take so long to thoroughly grip the United States? We know much more about the *content* of sexual discourses than the circumstances in which large numbers of people encounter them, begin to take them seriously, and adapt or apply them to their own lives. This book narrates the creation of consensus about masturbation in the antebellum North.

White southerners, by and large, remained suspicious of reform physiology since they rightly associated it with abolitionism and women's rights. Those who bothered to notice Sylvester Graham considered his lectures part of a larger, sectional attack on southern civilization and deemed moral reformers "poor ignorant fanatics—the very fag end of society."³² More often, however, silence prevailed over denunciation of the solitary vice in public southern spaces. Social and political barriers obstructed the flow of northern reform literature in general, and the new physiology of solitary vice provoked as few responses in the South as had the prior century's literature on onanism. The fear of masturbatory insanity in particular spread across the North deterring thousands from the act between 1835 and 1860 but did not find similar purchase in the South. Northern asylums in Worcester, Massachusetts; Utica, New York; and Columbus, Ohio, regularly diagnosed patients with "moral insanity" or "mania" caused by masturbation, but the solitary vice was not listed among the causes of mental illness in Virginia's Eastern Lunatic Asylum or the New Orleans Charity Hospital for the insane during the same years.³³ Only after the Civil War did northern sex education—including antimasturbation physiology—make significant inroads in the South through the US Sanitary Commission, Freedmen's Schools, and Young Men's and Women's Christian Associations.³⁴

In describing the construction of the solitary vice, *Riotous Flesh* departs from scholarship on the medicalization of sexuality.³⁵ Prior to the advent of sexology, evangelical women—not medical doctors—established a normative discourse on sexuality. During the years of this study, physicians had little authority in the United States. In fact, doctors gained credibility after the Civil War only by deploying existing sexual conventions in order to persuade the public of their righteous leadership.³⁶ Skeptical of the popular lecturers who vied with them for prestige, antebellum doctors came relatively late to the belief that sex constituted a legitimate field of scientific study.³⁷

During the mid-1840s, medical doctors began to take seriously the physiological argument against masturbation. However, they framed it as a masculine problem best documented in medical case studies—not popular science lecturers.³⁸ Moreover, by this time, female moral guardians had infantilized masturbation in order to cast themselves as maternal agents of sexual discipline, rather than its liberal subjects. Medical writers who concentrated on male youth worked within this framework. They resurrected the older paradigm of seminal loss (diagnosed as spermatorrhea), thus placing boys and young men once again at the center of antimasturbation advice. However, the medical concern with onanism never completely displaced girls and women. Certainly, late nineteenth-century writers such as G. Stanley Hall defined "self-abuse" primarily as a peril to American manhood. Yet postbellum Social Purity advocates continued to warn young women against "solitary vice, or self-abuse" in a scientific idiom through the turn of the twentieth century. In addition, some doctors advocated radical interventions such as clitoridectomy to prevent female masturbation, which they associated with nymphomania.³⁹ Mid- and late nineteenth-century writers continued to pathologize masturbation in women as well as men. What had begun as an activist ideology became a cultural norm and *then* a medical diagnosis, so that physicians never completely determined the direction that the sexual discourse might take.

To be clear, the appearance of consensus did not prevent some people from masturbating. Administrative records suggest that sailors, students, prisoners, and asylum inmates did so in open defiance of institutional discipline. Yet their actions only strengthened the act's cultural association with marginality and deviance. Reports that these populations were the most likely to masturbate appeared in daily newspapers and religious tracts. Such publications implied that Americans must confirm their sanity, maturity, and freedom by distancing themselves from masturbation. In daily life, secrecy and denial became imperative. Beyond disciplinary institutions, no nineteenth-century person identified as an unreformed, unashamed masturbator. In this respect, antimasturbation discourse outdid the twentieth-century "American obsession" with homosexuality.⁴⁰

Moreover, the campaign against solitary vice helped to create a *foundation* for heteronormativity. Jonathan Ned Katz defines heterosexuality a "different-sex pleasure ethic," which sexologists "invented" at the end of the nineteenth century. More than merely pathologizing same-sex desire, they valorized the pleasure that men and women experienced together and sidelined reproduction as the main purpose of marriage. According to popular advisors, readers should actively pursue the *right* kind of pleasure in order to, in Christina Simmons's phrase, "make marriage modern." Marriage manuals promoted female pleasure in heterosexual intercourse as both a right and a duty, one that could prevent deviance. Feminist critics of the sexual revolution later critiqued this logic as a form of social control and a bulwark of male privilege.[41]

Because scholars of heteronormativity often prioritize sexological sources, they have not accounted for the long historical roots of these ideas. *Riotous Flesh* finds that antebellum writers legitimized the pleasures of normative sex between men and women through the antimasturbation discourse of the mid-nineteenth century. By the mid-1840s, marriage reformers described companionate heterosexual love as healthy, natural, and "pure"—everything "self-pollution" was not. Romanticized views of gender complementarity naturalized mutual pleasure between women and men, drawn together magnetically "like the needle and the loadstone." Some popular physiology lecturers suggested fertility-control techniques in order to equip women to enjoy heterosexual intercourse. Others coached men in techniques for stimulating their wives—and sold aphrodisiacs in case those methods failed. Many women of the 1840s relished the argument that they, too, should experience pleasure—even multiple orgasms—during heterosexual intercourse. At the same time, they learned to separate these orgasms from the dangerous "paroxysms" of solitary vice. As long as they did not descend into masturbatory deviance, their desire, pleasure, and passion were absolutely normal.[42]

Thus, *Riotous Flesh* also complicates historical notions of white, middle-class feminine purity and passionlessness. In 1966, Barbara Welter named "purity" as one of four pillars of an antebellum "Cult of True Womanhood" (the others were piety, submission, and domesticity). She explained that men and women subscribed to this ideology for different reasons. Men clung to the stability and dominance that it afforded them amid the changing, atomistic, "heartless world" of the market revolution and Second Great Awakening. Businesses failed, churches pronounced competing truths, but "a true woman was a true woman, wherever she was found." According to Welter, the women who participated in the cult of true womanhood used sexual purity to turn dependence and inferiority into "superiority and . . . power."[43] Welter's reasoning has proved tremendously influential. One of its more problematic legacies has been to frame discussions of female desire around the sex women had—or did not have—with men. This tendency bolsters an interpretation of the past that Jen Manion has recently named "historic heteroessentialism."[44]

During the 1970s, historians influenced by the sexual revolution and women's liberation debated the implications of feminine purity. Responding to Welter, G. J. Barker-Benfield objected that, due to the strength of nineteenth-century patriarchy, "women were in no position" to gain power over men by withholding sex. On the contrary, he argued, male physicians characterized the female body as inherently "sexless" in order to shore up patriarchal control over the women of their own class. Recognizing women's sexual power, they sought to defuse and deny it. The women who accepted prescriptions for purity therefore did so passively and against their own interests. Importantly, both Welter and Barker-Benfield contended that the doctrine of elite white feminine purity served specific ideological ends. Neither assumed that it accurately described women's sexual experiences, let alone their desires. Both scholars also argued that at least some historical actors—whether both men and women, or men alone—invoked it rhetorically. In the words of Carl Degler, the purity ideal prescribed "what ought to be," rather than describing "what was."[45]

Nancy Cott coined the influential term *passionlessness* in 1978 and further elaborated the social functions of this ideology. Acknowledging (as Barker-Benfield had not) that a culture of unrestrained sexual passion could also support patriarchy, she argued that women took up passionlessness as a strategy for their own empowerment. As women became more numerous than men among church members, ministers had an incentive to praise their spiritual strengths rather than castigating their somatic weaknesses. The Christian tradition had long defined women in primarily sexual terms that justified their subordination, and female congregants responded warmly to sermons on their "moral equality." Around the same time, however, the marriage market increasingly disadvantaged women in relation to men. Passionlessness furnished young white women with a reason to withhold sex until a suitor proposed. Once engaged, however, they suddenly discovered their passion, for premarital pregnancies boomed between 1760 and 1800. After marriage, wives once again asserted their right to say no to sex—this time to control their fertility.[46] (It should be noted that other arguments could also assert women's negative sexual rights: freethinkers from Mary Wollstonecraft to Fanny Wright insisted that female passion could coexist with bodily sovereignty.)[47] All in all, Cott suggested that women *deployed* passionlessness in order to garner moral worth, marital choice, and fertility control. Rather than passively absorbing it, they used it rhetorically to gain practical ends.

While passionlessness offered rewards, however, its adherents did not always wield it in calculating ways. According to Cott, they also wove it into the very fabric of their identities as "an important shared trait which distinguished them from men." To be a woman was to be different from a man, and that difference was constituted in large part through sexuality: men were lustful, women passionless. Here, Cott agreed with Carroll

Smith-Rosenberg's prior study of elite and middle-class white women's intimate relationships with one another. Smith-Rosenberg had suggested that romantic friendships thrived because neither the women involved nor their society considered them sexual or subversive in nature. These women had so thoroughly incorporated sexual purity into their sense of self that they experienced their *own* most intimate feelings as free of erotic desire.[48]

Historians have since debated the place of sex within women's romantic friendships, yet the underlying belief that white, middle-class women internalized passionlessness continues to shape the history of sexuality.[49] An example can be found in the continuing influence of Kathryn Kish Sklar's argument that women pursued hydrotherapy, or the nineteenth-century water cure, partly because it afforded an opportunity for "sexual release." Sklar reasoned that passionlessness encouraged men to believe that their wives needed no sexual gratification, and as a consequence most married women sorely lacked sexual fulfillment. At water cures, they could expect to receive "vaginal injections," which presumably produced orgasms. Like Smith-Rosenberg's romantic friends, Sklar's water-cure patients compartmentalized such "genital stimulation," distinguishing it from "overt masturbation."[50]

More recently, Rachel Maines has applied the same logic to the invention of the electric vibrator. According to Maines, women sought out medical therapies that included clitoral stimulation without ever considering themselves masturbators. This "social camouflage" evolved from what she calls an "androcentric definition of sex," which held that any form of contact with women's genitals other than penile-vaginal penetration did not count as sex.[51] Physicians therefore turned to the vibrator in order to meet their female patients' demands for therapies that medical men considered both onerous and beneath them—but not sexual. Variations on this theme have also appeared in novels and films, such as T. C. Boyle's *The Road to Wellville* and the 2011 film *Hysteria*. In this view, passionlessness circled back upon itself, driving a technological innovation that would eventually become a hallmark of liberation for a particular variety of feminists.[52]

Though seductive, this interpretation includes a certain amount of wishful thinking. With regard to the water cure, it is important to note that "vaginal injection" was only one of many therapies prescribed for women (and the genitals only one part of the body at which practitioners aimed streams of water). Patients seeking genital stimulation would have been disappointed to find themselves wrapped in wet sheets for hours at a time, day after day.[53] Moreover, hydrotherapy centered on *cold* water. An icy jet directed at the genitals likely produced strong sensations other than orgasm.

This does not rule out women's experiences of social, political, and even various kinds of physical pleasure in water cures, which historians have documented.[54] Nor does it deny that female patients have shaped medical treatments or that the marketers of vibrators have used certain forms of social camouflage. However, Maines assumed that men defined sex exclusively in terms of penile-vaginal intercourse because that definition served their own interests, while privileged women not only *appeared* to conform but also actually *accepted* those definitions. Otherwise, female patients would have recognized their behavior as masturbatory and been tormented by the specter of their own deviance. In this light, what may seem like a clever form of sexual agency actually reinforced androcentrism.

By contrast, *Riotous Flesh* argues that antebellum women *and* men understood that women experienced sexual passion and that clitoral stimulation was fundamental to female orgasm. Popular physiology lecturers captivated female audience members by telling them what they already knew: "The clitoris . . . appears to be the principal seat of venereal pleasure!"[55] Female moral reformers stated unequivocally that a great majority of women, even "ladies of the first respectability," did in fact become "addicted to the solitary vice" in just this way.[56] And when female patients solicited genital treatments, at least some physicians accused them of malingering "to gratify a morbid and prurient desire!"[57] Above all, this book contends that many women did not work within the androcentric definition of sex, but directly challenged it. While leading the charge against masturbation, they also claimed other, more permissible pleasures along the way. They constructed and reconstructed their own sexual definitions. In doing so, they powerfully—though not always admirably—shaped the nation's sexual culture.

Beyond the issue of sexual sensation, passionlessness also raised significant questions about the very category of "woman" in historical analysis. According to Cott, the notion that women *shared* passionlessness was an essential characteristic that did critical ideological work. On the one hand, it prompted many to reflect on their common "bonds," the circumstances and attributes that distinguished them as a class apart from men. In this way, passionlessness became a kind of precondition for feminism; it encouraged women to think of themselves as a group, theorize their common oppression, and begin to seek justice. On the other, it obscured class differences among women.[58]

During the 1980s and 1990s, historians of African American women added that passionlessness defined white womanhood in service to slavery and white supremacy. Angela Davis analyzed the dialectical relationship between notions of passionless white femininity and hypersexual black womanhood. The ban on the transatlantic slave trade exponentially increased slaveholders' incentive to profit from enslaved women's reproduction; at the same time, the emerging market economy increasingly devalued white women's domestic labor. In Davis's view, the cult of true womanhood arose to romanticize white women's dependence and mystify their lost economic power. The same ideology denied black women the compensatory protections of true womanhood: only in this way could a society that claimed to venerate purity and motherhood reconcile the rape of enslaved women and the selling of their children. Jacqueline Dowd Hall similarly noted the "symbiosis" between passionlessness and white supremacy. The ideology of white feminine purity masked the reality that rape functioned as a form of racial terror—not an expression of uncontrollable sexual passion. It recast raped black women as "breeders" and masked the violence perpetrated against free black men in the name of "protecting" white womanhood from eternally lustful "brutes."[59]

Two years later, Deborah Gray White further explored the gendered stereotypes rooted in slavery, such as the alleged temptress she named "Jezebel." This caricature deflected the reality of rape and coercion by representing black women as inviting any man's sexual advances. The equally exploitive archetype of "Mammy" was imagined as cheerfully vacant of all desires—including the desire for a family of her own—except to serve whites. Though passionless, the Mammy figure did not empower black women to leverage moral authority. Both Jezebel and Mammy did more than distort the brutality of slavery, according to White. They also placed black women beyond the pale of femininity. The ideology of passionlessness thus discounted women who did not share white women's bonds.[60]

Over the next two decades, Paula Giddings, Elsa Barkley Brown, and Nell Irvin Painter documented the implications of this entangled history for black women's lives, for feminist politics, and for the concept of gender itself. Across a variety of geographic and temporal studies, their works modeled a historical interpretation of gender as both *intersectional* and *relational*. Gender always intersected with race and class, these scholars argued, and those intersections were historically constituted in relationship to one another. As Brown put it, "Middle-class white women's lives are not just different from working-class white, Black, and Latina women's lives ... middle-class women live the lives they do precisely because working-class women live the lives they do."[61] These scholars also located sexuality at the very heart of racialized gender.[62] In this light, the doctrine of purity did not merely exclude women of color; it depended on their sexual debasement and effected their continued exploitation. By conflating womanhood with whiteness, passionlessness hid this reality and prevented its transformation.

Similarly, several important studies documented the ways in which the ideology of passionlessness helped both to constitute middle-class formation and to obscure class stratification as a fundamental facet of American society. Mary Ryan has argued that within smaller, more affectionate families, mothers instilled in their children the habits of sexual and financial restraint essential to maintaining middle-class status. Having fewer children also freed them from much of the domestic labor that their mothers had performed, and they used this time to participate in benevolence and reform. The ideology of passionlessness sanitized and justified their interest in public activities, particularly when they prescribed new behaviors for the men of their own class—husbands, rakes, and errant youth. Christine Stansell found that middle-class women promoted sexual restraint and domesticity in hopes of controlling working-class women and cleansing urban space. Poor women, however, rejected their sexual advice and continued to engage in occasional prostitution both as a survival strategy and as a gendered expression of class struggle. Lori Ginzberg interpreted the ideology of female moral authority as a screen that masked bourgeois hegemony. "This ideology about gender," she wrote, "contributed to a process of middle-class self-definition, to the notion that the United States itself was a middle-class society and that it was virtue, not wealth, that determined individuals'—and therefore the nation's—success." Each of these studies conceived of passionlessness as a rhetorical tool—one that historical actors often understood to hold advantages for some people and disadvantages for others, but not a neutral description of reality.[63]

Thus, passionlessness has never been innocent. *Riotous Flesh* contends that people in the past understood it as a power-laden concept and analyzes the ways in which diverse women interrogated, denaturalized, and transformed it. While sexual discourses convey power through subtle and intimate incitements, specific historic circumstances occasionally expose their inconsistencies, liabilities, vulnerabilities, and loopholes. During such moments of crisis, people have reevaluated the core terms of those discourses, sometimes ushering in widespread cultural changes. They have done so in unpredictable ways and with unanticipated consequences. The 1830s, a decade of seemingly chaotic change, intense activism, and social experimentation, should be seen as one such moment. Black women in the nominally free states seized upon the opportunities afforded by this context, limited as they were, to intervene in an oppressive sexual ideology. In challenging passionlessness, they coauthored a major nineteenth-century sexual discourse—albeit one that differed terribly from their original goals.

Therefore, this book's third major contribution is to account for African American women's constrained yet significant contributions to sexual thought. Because the vast majority of black women were enslaved between 1830 and 1860, historians have interpreted African American women's sexual agency primarily in terms of resistance to rape, coerced reproduction, the destruction of their families, and the ownership of their bodies.[64] Others have questioned whether the concept of sexual subjectivity holds any explanatory power when applied to a system that radically limited black women's ability to resist and caused untold psychic damage.[65] Northern black women, who were also constrained by labor exploitation and sexual harassment even after their states gradually eliminated slavery, involved themselves in mutual aid, abolitionism, and the creation of a black public sphere. Within literary societies, autobiographies, and lecture halls, they engaged in self-definition.[66] Yet little has been written about the sexual values, ideas, and experiences of black activist women in the antebellum North. This omission risks representing nineteenth-century African American women as reactive rather than creative historical actors—in Hortense Spillers's evocative phrase, "the beached whales of the sexual universe, unvoiced, misseen, not doing, awaiting *their* verb."[67]

Darlene Clark Hine's discovery of a "culture of dissemblance" among early twentieth-century black women raises the question: how explicitly could African American women afford to engage sexual discourse from within a culture that persistently hypersexualized them? Unable to change the ugly stereotypes that blamed them for their own victimization, Hine argued, black women survived with their sanity intact by shielding their inner lives from view.[68] The Jezebel stereotype, though a product of slavery, also pervaded northern sexual culture. Antebellum black women of all classes felt its effects in their everyday lives.[69] Unlike Hine's later subjects, however, antebellum black activists participated in a culture of *exposure*. Those who had experienced slavery wrote narratives that consistently described "the ever present threat and reality of rape." By testifying to their own experiences, women such as Sojourner Truth and Harriet Jacobs made sexual politics central to northern black protest and opened a discursive space for contemplating sex, gender, and power.[70] This culture of exposure actually began during the 1830s, nearly two decades before Truth and Jacobs would become famous among white abolitionists. During this period, as chapter 2 explains, free black women used the moral reform press to document cases of sexual harassment and exploitation in "free labor" contexts, especially domestic service. Their exposés elicited white women's solidarity in opposing powerful men and asserted their own sexual propriety.

By contrasting their own chastity with the licentiousness of powerful white men, it may appear that black abolitionist women participated in what Evelyn Brooks Higginbotham has called "the politics of respectability." Expanding on Hine's concept of dissemblance, Higginbotham argued that, during the late nineteenth and early twentieth centuries, the "female talented tenth" both embodied sexual restraint and inculcated working-class black women with the same ethos. Selectively educated by white Baptists in the wake of the Civil War, they advocated "sexual purity, child rearing, habits of cleanliness and order, and overall self-improvement." They also pursued policies that did *not* benefit white capitalists, such as organizing domestic workers. Working-class black women adopted the politics of respectability in order to "define themselves outside the parameters of prevailing racist discourses." Although they had very little power in Jim Crow America, they could at least control their own bodily habits. Yet respectability cut both ways: by emphasizing bodily conduct, it suggested that those who failed to conform were culpable for their own oppression. Overall, Higginbotham described respectability as "a deliberate, highly self-conscious concession to hegemonic values."[71] More recently, several historians have also applied the politics of respectability to African American women activists of the early nineteenth century.[72]

Riotous Flesh stresses a different aspect of black women's interest in moral reform. The African American women in this study did not become sexual activists in order to convince whites of their morality, nor did they receive incentives from whites to promote the doctrine of sexual restraint to other African Americans. To be sure, some antebellum blacks did aim to disrupt the racist stereotypes that "justified" their oppression by giving the lie with their behavior. And there were certainly times when white philanthropists condescendingly advised black men, women, and children to prove their morality. But black women participated in the interracial moment in moral reform because they chose to confront, not accommodate, hegemonic sexual values. In order to reveal the inconsistencies and dismantle the sexual logic of the racial order, they needed allies. They therefore finessed relationships with white moral reformers by strategically adopting their language and forums. However, they also *challenged* northern white women. Exposés of sexual harassment in northern white homes, for example, did not allow moral reformers to distance themselves from black women's oppression.

African American women understood that destroying the Jezebel stereotype required deeper ideological work than declarations of sisterhood. Because the myth of the voracious black woman existed in symbiosis with that of the passionless white lady, they insisted that the two archetypes must stand or fall together. Thus, black moral reformers pressed the critique of white feminine purity. Reform physiology seemed to be preparing a group of outspoken white women to question their own passionlessness—and to brave mobs of angry white men in the process. By seizing upon this specific opportunity, antebellum black women fundamentally changed the ways in which white women conceived of sex. Far from merely reacting to white racism, they had a formative influence on nineteenth-century sexual discourse.

At the same time, the outcomes of their intervention evince the real constraints on black women's ability to transform sexual thought in ways that challenged white supremacy. The need for white female allies to authorize and amplify their sexual politics should be seen as one such constraint. In times of crisis, most white women found it easier to turn toward selfhood than to maintain coalition. One such crisis occurred in 1840 when the antislavery movement fractured over the question of women's rights, prompting white moral reformers to distinguish their sexual campaign from abolitionism. Around this time, members of small, rural moral reform societies forswore the solitary vice with a vehemence disproportionate to its actual relationship to women's status. Those who would become champions of women's rights made it into a fetish—a powerful symbol of their more elusive goal of sexual autonomy—while moral guardians reasserted passionlessness with a vengeance. Within separate institutions such as the Institute for Colored Youth and the Moral Reform Retreat, African American women continued tailoring reform physiology to meet their own needs. Yet in the society at large, they lacked control over the ideological uses to which their vision might be put.

Based on a physiological model that has since been debunked, masturbation phobia may seem to hold little modern relevance. Yet this book offers a prehistory of heterosexuality and liberal feminism, significant aspects of contemporary American culture. It also tells the story of a path not taken, a forgotten moment during the 1830s during which African American and white women temporarily disrupted passionlessness—and the deliberate choices that closed off more transformative possibilities. This story cautions activists to build and invest deeply in functional, sustainable coalitions. Otherwise, our political and cultural interventions may have unpredictable consequences, including the creation of newly oppressive sexual norms.

CHAPTER ONE

The Gender of Solitary Vice

How cold Providence must have felt that afternoon in December 1833, when Sylvester Graham first saw an angry crowd collecting around the hall where he was scheduled to speak. Placards at the street corners summoned "those that wish to rid this city of one of the greatest nuisances that ever came along," to "Tar and Feather the Imposter Mr. Graham, and banish the villain from the city." News of the unrest traveled rapidly. As far away as New York, the image of a mob menacing "the author of the prison-fare system of dietetics" entertained skeptical omnivores. Sympathetic observers closer to the action described Providence as "filled with unfriendly excitement." Accustomed to editorial squibs, the reformer had never confronted real danger. But his appointed "Lecture to Mothers" on sexual physiology touched a nerve. During the lecture, he would show illustrations of genital anatomy and advise moderate sex even within marriage. He would also warn women not to indulge in the solitary vice. In effect, this extended to adult women the same logic of sexual virtue—temptation conquered by self-denial—formerly restricted to young men. By addressing women as passionate beings both capable of and responsible for restraint, Graham outraged patriarchs and libertines alike. Men from all points on the continuum participated in "mobs, frays, and scenes of confusion" each time he advertised the lecture to women during the next four years.[1]

As it happened, Graham's anonymous enemies failed to "banish" him from Providence. Local reformers shielded him from real violence, puffed his reputation, and raised "some four or five thousand dollars" in ticket sales. He abandoned the women's lecture but continued speaking in the city through the winter, prompting one critic to complain that having avoided the *tar*, he was not averse to *"feathering* . . . his own nest at other people's expense."[2]

The next summer, however, the conflict escalated considerably. At first, Graham successfully delivered a lecture "on chastity" to the young men of Portland, Maine. A subsequent course on diet and regimen for mixed-gender audiences also drew no fire. But two full-fledged riots erupted after Portland's *Daily Advertiser* informed local men that the itinerant stranger planned to meet with married women, barring their husbands, in order to freely discuss "reprehensible" subjects.[3] About thirty men and boys gathered outside the building and threw rocks until they broke up the lecture. A small group of women escorted Graham to safety, at which point constables persuaded the men to leave "without doing any material injury." But when the women reconvened the next evening, hundreds of men surrounded the lecture hall, calling for Graham "to pay forty shillings and be hanged—without judge or jury, nay without a hearing." The lecturer fled, disappointing the women who had braved the crowd to hear him speak. A month later, Graham tried once more to meet his obligations to ticket holders, only to face yet another riot of Portland men. He escaped unharmed but terrified by the men who reveled menacingly in the streets surrounding the lecture hall, declaring their control over public space and the women of their city. Graham identified the "Lecture to Mothers" as the source of his troubles and refused to repeat it for three full years.[4]

In 1837, Graham tried to lecture to women in Boston, and faced the largest and angriest crowds of men yet. He later claimed that he had only agreed to deliver the "Lecture to Mothers" because female organizers—"without consulting me, and without my knowledge"—had rented a hall, sold tickets, and advertised it. On March 2, 1837, a "miscellaneous multitude" of one thousand "men and boys" succeeded in suppressing the lecture. Local women arranged a second lecture, despite warnings from the mayor and police marshal that *"if the house is pulled down over your head, we cannot help it."* The women, aware of the risks and determined not to allow another of their meetings to be disbanded, placed themselves at the center of the conflict.[5]

On the day appointed for the second Boston lecture, three hundred onlookers gathered to "see the fun." Two youths bellowed "Riding on a Rail"—music to tar and feather by—and were arrested before the rough chorus could spread. Revelers turned to hiss the arrests of William Davis, a familiar "underling" of the nearby Lion Theatre, and his accomplice (called only "another boy" by witnesses). The hall's owner, a reformer named Willard Sears, seized this opportunity to slip into the momentarily unblocked doorway and implore the crowd not to demolish his property.[6] About two hundred women pushed their way "by great perseverance" to the front of the action, then streamed past Sears as if drawn into the building by a vacuum.

The mob scrambled to follow. "From that moment," synopsized the *Boston Post*, "all was confusion worse compounded." Those still outside "avowed an intention of maltreating Mr. G. should he fall into their hands," and the crowd grew to more than a thousand.

Inside the hall, male rioters and female reformers faced off, culminating some of the broader tensions that had lurked beneath the assaults on Graham ever since that gray day in Providence. Supporters hid the lecturer "locked up in a nice little room" and stood their ground. Once the rioters lacked a convenient male target, they directed their hostility toward the women who had planned to attend such a lecture. Henry F. Harrington, a ringleader of the crowd and the "little scurvey editor" of Boston's *Daily Herald*, claimed that "several females of infamous character" were present. If so, they shot back, "he alone seemed to be acquainted with them." A vocal reformer named Thankful Southwick stood on her chair, admonishing the men "on the spot." Others drowned out the mob's catcalls with "loud and repeated cries" and hisses of their own. One editor concluded that the conflict reflected "no credit on the *women*."[7] Nevertheless, they had triumphed in an important way. Boston's female reformers had not yielded their access to public space, nor had sexual slurs cowed them. Yet the trouble did not end there. The next day another, larger crowd burst into the Marlboro Hotel, reportedly "maltreating" Graham and forcing him to flee, "over a number of sheds and through Graphic court." By March 9, a full week after the women of Amory Hall first exchanged hisses with "lewd fellows of the baser sort," the city had "not yet resumed its quiet."[8] The next year, Graham retired permanently to Northampton, and Boston's reform women took leadership of reform physiology—including the campaign against solitary vice.

Such riots help to account for why Graham never *published* the "Lecture to Mothers," unlike his well-known *Lecture to Young Men* (1834). Just when he began to negotiate the publication of the women's lecture, the worst riot yet drove him from Boston and discouraged printers in neighboring cities from accepting a job that could result in the ransacking of their presses.[9] These events have left historians without a transcript of Graham's lecture to women. Lacking such a source, most have interpreted his sexual ideas as the basis for a new doctrine of manly restraint.[10] It is true that ultras critiqued patriarchal and libertine manhood, idealizing instead political passion, spiritual zeal, and a Spartan disdain for physical comforts. Like traditional patriarchs, Grahamite men praised the virility of those who battled their baser instincts. Unlike them, they shared the responsibility for restraint with women; some even considered sharing power with women a sign of true manhood. Libertine republicans found these values bizarre and ridiculous, the people who embodied them grotesque. Both Graham's assailants and his proponents pronounced firm and conflicting standards of masculinity, but neither side could foresee the outcome of this culture war.

Yet Graham was never *only* interested in remaking manhood; he believed that women and womanhood also needed reform. From an evangelical standpoint, each individual bore the stain of human depravity and must strive for purification before his or her God. Graham adhered to the doctrine that "there is neither male nor female: for ye are all one in Christ Jesus." The "Lecture to Mothers" offered various kinds of sexual information, but its argument against the solitary vice applied this biblical interpretation directly to sexual physiology. By igniting public battles over the gender of the solitary vice, it inspired large numbers of women to associate those arguments with challenges to the patriarchs and libertines who defined women in sexual terms that justified male dominance.[11] When Graham retired from public life, reform women launched a feminized, grassroots campaign that ultimately turned the physiological theory of a marginal lecturer into a mainstream obsession. Before women took their place at the center of these conflicts, few Americans paid attention to antimasturbation advice.

BEFORE THE RIOTS

The fear of masturbation hit England more than a century before it became an American obsession. The historian Thomas Laqueur has traced the origins of masturbation phobia to the 1712 publication of *Onania*. Presented as a religious tract, *Onania* first convinced many British readers that the sin of "self-pollution" wrought physical, as well as spiritual, damage. Ironically, its author, John Marten, contributed openly to the growing market in pornography and had little genuine interest in reforming readers' sexual practices.[12] An abridged version of *Onania* crossed the Atlantic during the eighteenth century, but it made little discernible impact and certainly did not stir riots. Nothing within the text or its subsequent imitators appeared controversial in colonial society. Eighteenth-century antimasturbation writers addressed men, focused on male sexuality, and explained how men could best maintain social power. This literature supported existing gender conventions and failed to spark the sort of public debate that might have attracted converts to a new way of thinking. Instead, the earliest antimasturbation publications to reach America blended seamlessly into the market in imported conduct manuals.

Laqueur argues that *Onania* "broke the gender barrier" by treating masturbation in women as well as men. Further, this "democratic" aspect helped to make it the signal vice of modernity.[13] Female masturbation per se had mattered little to premodern writers. When writing about sex, they tended to focus instead on women's adultery (which threatened the orderly transmission of property) or prostitution (which included a fantastic array of acts united in the purpose of pleasing men). Ancient satirists described women, especially courtesans, as humorously dependent on dildos when men were absent. These fantasies, produced by and for men, often depicted women masturbating in groups. Neither female masturbation nor lesbianism produced children to muddy patriarchal property transmission; therefore, writers treated them as comical and threatened no grave repercussions.[14] Early Christian texts similarly addressed adult men—scholars and monks, for example—and expressed little genuine fear of even their masturbation. By warning that masturbation harmed women as well as men, *Onania* departed from this literature.

However, it is simply not the case that *Onania* inaugurated a democratic pattern of thinking about sex. On the contrary, it set the tone for eighteenth-century antimasturbation discourse as a conversation among men in which women figured only marginally (women did not advise one another in print on this subject until more than a century had passed). It did this in three ways: first, by framing the physical consequences of masturbation in terms of seminal loss; second, by depicting female masturbation in humorous and prurient sidebars; and third, by arguing that married men must have unrestricted access to their wives' bodies in order to prevent masturbation and its ills. Marten's claim to address "self-pollution in both sexes" was as disingenuous as were his religious avowals.[15]

The very word *Onania* associated masturbation with "spilled" semen and thereby defined it as a masculine act. Marten's title referenced the Old Testament story of Onan. After Onan's brother died in battle, their father commanded him to father a child with the widow of the slain man. Onan had sex with her but, refusing to raise a child for his brother's lineage rather than his own, he "spilled his seed" so that she would not conceive. His crime was social rather than solitary in nature: he disobeyed his patriarch, placed selfish glory above filial duty, and took his pleasure from a woman under false pretenses. For these reasons, God struck him dead. The aspects of shirked duty, lechery, and wasted semen lurked in the word *onanism*, which, until the nineteenth century, named masturbation as a problem of manhood. "Women have no Seed," Marten admitted, yet "I could not think of any other word which would so well put the Reader in Mind both of the Sin and its Punishment at once." Promising such "punishments" as impotence, priapism, uncontrollable seminal loss, and gonorrhea, the text explicitly addressed "the MALE YOUTH of this Nation."[16]

Readers affirmed and amplified *Onania*'s focus on manhood. In testimonial letters, which were reprinted in each edition until they comprised more than half of the text, men confessed to having practiced onanism and recounted the sexual miseries that followed. By 1717 twenty-seven male testimonials appeared, compared with only three female cases. "The Supplement to the Onania," a cache of readers' responses appended to the main text, incorporated twenty-one new letters by "Men of Sense" but only five accounts of female masturbators. The female testimonials may also have been fabricated by Marten or by the network of male publishers and booksellers who profited from *Onania*. Contemporaries evidently doubted the authenticity of the women's letters, prompting the narrator to swear (somewhat defensively) that they were real.[17]

Because Marten primarily aimed to reach men, he alluded to female masturbators in light and entertaining ways before quickly dismissing them. *Onania*'s nubile girls frolicked together in masturbatory bliss, ignorant of the devastation to come. One woman, "Mrs. E.O.," described "being entic'd and shew'd the way" from other girls in her boarding school. Lesbian play, however, left her "vehement Desires" for men unsatisfied. She married the first man who made an offer, only to fatally exhaust him with "Delights of the Marriage-Bed." In desperation, the young widow returned to her "former wicked Practice, so often, and with so much Excess that I could hardly sometimes walk, or sit with ease, I was so sore."[18] Women made even spicier appearances in the *Supplement*. The account of "Mrs. E.N.," for example, invited readers to imagine her bedchamber, where, at age eleven, she had learned how to masturbate from her mother's twenty-year-old chambermaid. "So intimate were we in the Sin," she confessed, that "we, in short, pleasured one another, as well as each our selves." Overstimulation caused Mrs. E.N.'s clitoris to grow "to the exact likeness and size of a human Penis, erect." Her maid's body changed, too, allowing them to penetrate each other "by turns." Following the ancient tradition, Marten represented masturbating women who made do with each other but actually longed for penetration by a phallus. At the same time, he deemed onanism such a masculine practice that it might actually transform a clitoris into a penis. None of this addressed female readers with any seriousness. *Onania*'s female masturbator did not make "her own sexual destiny."[19] In eighteenth-century London, as in second-century Rome, she offered a titillating joke—the sugar that made the medicine go down—to offset young men's quest for self-mastery.

That mastery consisted of directing "Man's eruptibility" into one appropriate channel: the marital bed. In order to convince young men that marriage provided the correct outlet for their sexual urges, *Onania* equated masturbation with fornication, adultery, and sodomy. *Within* marriage, by contrast, male desire must be given free rein. Marten clarified this position in response to a "Lady's Letter" inserted in the fourth edition. The "Lady"—again, likely fabricated by the author—argued that all nonprocreative sex within marriage should be considered onanism of sorts, equally sinful and dangerous. Furthermore, *women* should be allowed to decide when marital sex should not take place, for while "the Man be at all Times capable of Generation . . . the Woman is not." Both on physiological and moral grounds, wives should be empowered to check "the Man's Brutality." Marten answered these arguments with eighteen pages of biblical exegesis, appropriating the sexual philosophy of the Protestant Reformation for his pornographic pamphlet. Protestants cited 1 Corinthians 7:3, "Let the husband render unto the wife due benevolence: and likewise also the wife unto the husband." From their perspective, sexual pleasure within marriage constituted both a positive good and a safeguard of social stability, whereas all pleasure derived from any partners other than one's spouse (including oneself) threatened moral and social chaos. Catholics also considered masturbation sinful, but they placed it on a continuum of sin in which all sex carried some degree of taint. Few were capable of true celibacy, but all should strive to be as chaste as they could. Protestants countered that abstinence drove men to rape and sodomy, women to fornication. *Onania* extended this argument to the notion of marital restraint, which "instead of rendering People more chaste, would serve rather to whet their Lust, and prompt them on to all manner of Uncleanness." Furthermore, the wife's duty to offer due benevolence mattered more than the husband's. If pregnant and menopausal women refused intercourse, any woman could "obstruct the nuptial Enjoyments" at any time by claiming to be in one of these states. Marten denied wives' sexual sovereignty and affirmed husbands' sexual privilege.[20]

The Boston publisher who brought out a colonial edition of *Onania* failed to inspire public debate. Possibly having learned that many considered John Marten an obscene writer, he purged the text of its most graphic sexual matter—a move which automatically reduced the market.[21] More important, the American *Onania* shared the London original's focus on male mastery. American writers also adopted *Onania*'s masculine emphasis. Cotton

Mather warned the young men of Massachusetts as early as 1723 not to "dishonor their on Bodies alone by themselves." Christian patriarchs must rule their own bodies if they were to govern unruly wives, children, and servants. Only "the Effeminate" allowed physical impulses to dictate their behavior. Every time a man masturbated, he invited an "unclean spirit" to "take possession of him." Both by allowing the flesh to rule the mind and by exhibiting a submissive and violable soul, the masturbator unmanned himself. Mather's advice, like *Onania*, failed to ignite widespread concern over masturbation in the colonies.[22]

This apathy persisted through the rest of the century. While intellectual and cultural historians have attributed new concerns over masturbation to political democratization and the secularization of morality, republican ideology does not in itself not explain the advent of masturbation phobia in the United States. The age of revolutions, these scholars argue, provoked fears that individual desires might wreak havoc on the commonweal and cause virtuous republics to crumble into licentious anarchies. By spurring individuals to embrace self-discipline, sexual advisors such as Jean-Jacques Rousseau and Samuel Auguste Tissot hoped to train citizens to manage liberty.[23] Yet in the United States, which also underwent political and religious transformation, the gender of onanism remained stable. Concern with it therefore remained limited, especially when compared with the pervasive discourse of the next century. Onanism's masculinity served the revolutionary gender order just as it had served colonial authorities such as Mather. The ostensibly universal "Man" of the Enlightenment, the virtuous citizen, required as much masculine self-control as had his predecessor, the ideal patriarch.

Eighteenth-century sexual writers masculinized onanism precisely because they strove to build manly citizens. Rousseau chose a male figure, *Émile*, to allegorize masturbation's evils. American pedagogues cited *Émile* to argue that boys needed discipline and instruction to prepare them for the responsibilities of republican manhood. Proponents of republican motherhood argued for women's education on the grounds that they could best instill moral discipline in the future citizenry—their sons. Few women had reason to consider *Émile*'s warnings against masturbation applicable to themselves or their daughters.[24] Samuel Tissot's treatise *L'Onanisme* elaborated on Rousseau's secularism but otherwise shared much with *Onania*. Tissot simply removed Marten's religious language in favor of a strictly physiological approach. The male body required ejaculation, he argued, but only when "when the *vesiculae seminales* are replete with a quantity of liquor." While all orgasms expended nervous energy, "unnatural" ejaculations (those produced by onanism) overtaxed the nervous system. As for female masturbators, "the sexual humor that they lose" was "not so elaborate as the sperm of man." Therefore, sexual excess did not cause nervous maladies in women. On the contrary, when deprived of regular intercourse with their husbands, some women became hysterical. Others stumbled upon "another kind of pollution, which may be called *clitorical*"—that is, lesbian friction, or tribadism.[25]

In 1812, the American physician Benjamin Rush followed Tissot's physiological explanation. Rush cited cases *only* "in young men." Ironically though, two aspects of his analysis unintentionally suggested the possibility that women's relationship to solitary sex might be as real and significant as men's. First, he argued that masturbation grew out of immoderate "passions," by which he meant "diseases of the mind." Onanism was therefore a problem of temperament and will, rather than genital hydraulics. Second, he used the phrase "the solitary vice of onanism," which Sylvester Graham later truncated to the gender-neutral "solitary vice." Still, Rush prescribed for men, and his book circulated in masculine milieus. It met as little fanfare as had Mather's sermon almost a century earlier.[26]

Despite roiling debates over the nature of citizenship, liberty, and license in the early American republic, no serious attacks on "the onanian mischief" spread throughout the populace. A few elite men sometimes wrestled privately with their own guilt.[27] But little evidence has survived to suggest that most eighteenth-century Americans embraced the advice against onanism. Popular humorists chalked it up to a malady of bachelorhood. Asylum administrators did not diagnose patients with masturbatory insanity in measurable numbers for another generation. Even popular healers who prescribed for the masturbatory ailments of the British failed to find a significant market in the United States before midcentury. Because European discussions of onanism supported the gender status quo, nothing about this imported sexual advice commanded widespread attention. All this changed in 1833, when women became central subjects rather than marginal characters in antimasturbation physiology.[28]

VICES SOCIAL AND SOLITARY

The solitary vice became an issue of major concern when Sylvester Graham began offering identical sexual advice to women and men. The editors who called a mob to ride Sylvester Graham out of Providence on a rail claimed that what had "annoyed and exasperated the multitude" was his decision to lecture to women only. The *Providence Patriot* demanded to know why he deemed it necessary to exclude men from a physiology lecture. Why would unchaperoned women want to listen to a strange man hold forth on bodily matters? In Portland and Boston, rioters responded to newspaper articles that claimed that Graham's lectures to women "turned husbands against wives, and children against fathers." Editors urged local men to protect the innocence of their wives and daughters. "If the proposed lectures contain nothing *indecent* or offensive to ladies, there can be no reason why gentlemen may not be present," reasoned one; but "if they *do* contain any thing of that character, they are not fit for ladies alone." It was only natural, they suggested, for men to explode in rage when an unknown man spoke to their wives about sex in their absence. As news of the lecture spread, however, the questions deepened. What exactly did he *say* to women? The title, "Lecture to Mothers," indicated subject matter parallel to his better-remembered "Lecture to Young Men on Chastity." Because the lecture to young men described the physical repercussions of the solitary vice, some listeners described it as having "descended lower" in its details "than many of his hearers wish[ed] to accompany him." Why did he think *"ladies"* needed to hear these same troubling details? Ultimately, the content of the lecture proved the more important catalyst.[29]

The lecture in question was actually only one among several in Graham's repertoire. For most of the 1830s, he delivered whole "courses" treating all aspects of human physiology. The decision to separate women and men for only one of these lectures—the one on sex—originated from his formative experiences as a paid lecturer while employed as an agent for the Pennsylvania Society for Discouraging the Use of Ardent Spirits in 1831. The agent's job was to travel around the state giving lectures, collecting donations, and forming temperance societies. In fulfilling these duties, however, Graham ran into trouble. Hoping to organize a female auxiliary in Harrisburg, he advertised a special lecture "exclusively to the ladies." In it, he departed from the usual script on drunkenness and identified "intemperance in dress" as a threat to women's health. Some local people thought that he had "outraged decency" by explaining that "the wearing of corsets injured the *breasts* and the *womb* &c &c."—words "which young ladies should only hear from their mothers." This accusation imperiled the reputations of those who listened to him. The women swore "that they heard nothing from Mr. G which savored in the least of indelicacy." But a few men, aggrieved by their exclusion, complained that he had set the date of his lecture to women "with the design of preventing their attendance on a dance which was held on that evening." He had disrupted these men's courtship plans by diverting local women's attention to himself, and they considered him a kind of verbal seducer.³⁰ The Pennsylvania Society responded by sending Graham to Philadelphia, to be supervised "on probation" by the philanthropic doctors John Bell and D. Francis Condie. He studied physiology under them and, in the interest of keeping his job, tried to restrict himself to mixed-gender lectures about the hazards of alcohol.³¹

Nevertheless, Graham seemed unable to stop alluding to the physiology of *all* "passions and appetites." Angelina Grimké—having recently left her slaveholding family in South Carolina, soon to begin a career as an abolitionist and women's rights advocate—heard him lecture at Philadelphia's Franklin Institute in late 1831. She described the content as a general appeal to "bring under the body and keep it in subjection." Striving to "crucify the flesh" meant total abstinence from *anything* consumed merely for pleasure. Self-indulgence was the wellspring of all vice, and overstimulation lay at the root of all illness. Grimké embraced these arguments and ever afterward aspired to self-discipline. Word traveled along the "chain of ultraism," and soon afterward, New York reformers invited Graham to lecture expressly on physiology. He gladly resigned his temperance agency to pursue "a better destiny, for which Divine Intelligence and Purpose had, all my life, been training me."³²

As a newly minted physiology lecturer, Graham revisited the possibility of sex-segregated lectures. Some women "recoiled" from attending them in mixed company; others warned that he was "vulgar" and "not decent to be heard" at all. But a "goodly array of females" sought out reform physiology. One listener proposed a solution: "Is there no way thou canst benefit the sexes individually," she implored, "without lessening thy influence collectively?"³³ Graham tested the waters by offering separate physiology courses to women in New York's Clinton Hall. No riots erupted yet. Remembering the Harrisburg incident, Graham held back from broaching sex in the early women's lectures but began to offer a segregated lecture to young men on chastity. Male audience members passed resolutions of support, thanking Graham for alerting them to the dangers of the solitary vice and recommending that he publish the lecture in order to save others like themselves. By the time he set out on the tour that would bring him to Providence, he had learned that separate men's and women's lectures on the physiology of sex could draw approving audiences. That development would in turn set off a chain reaction of riots and publicity battles over the gendered implications of his ideas.

Two social influences convinced Graham to offer the "Lecture to Mothers" in 1833. First, he met male leaders of the early moral reform movement and, by traveling with them, discovered that women in several cities demanded to be included in public discussions of sex. Second, he found himself in competition with freethinkers (secular utopians) whose physiology lectures struck him as morally and medically dangerous. Here again, large numbers of evangelical women would prove his greatest allies.

While still in New York, Graham became familiar with John R. McDowall, whose antiprostitution exposé called *The Magdalen Report* had stirred controversy and attracted a growing following. Graham parlayed McDowall's battle against the "social vice" of prostitution into a parallel crusade against the solitary vice. The complementary concepts of virtue and vice connected the two reforms. If virtue meant the rational subordination of one's own selfish desires in service to the greater good, vice meant endangering the community in the pursuit of personal gratification. For McDowall, no vice was "so ruinous . . . as lust." The votaries of lust broke the seventh commandment (thou shalt not commit adultery), treated "fallen" women as expendable, and exposed their own family members to syphilis and gonorrhea. His male followers called themselves the American Seventh Commandment Society. Graham convinced several of them that simply refraining from illicit sex with other people was insufficient in a society that catered to "depraved sensuality." Married people may be innocent of adultery and still indulge in excessive "connubials," for example. Even celibates might secretly "pollute" themselves. The virtue of restraint increased with its difficulty. In the words of a moral reform tract addressed to working men, "without temptation the virtue of self-denial would be unknown."[34] Requiring no partner, risking neither pregnancy nor disease, the solitary vice could potentially tempt anyone at any time. The *only* reason to avoid it was to cultivate bodily discipline, to strive after perfection—and this was the centerpiece of Graham's worldview.

Equally persuaded by each other's philosophies, McDowall and Graham joined forces in Providence during the fall of 1833. There, before mixed-gender audiences, McDowall denounced "social vice" in all its guises. Graham followed by connecting the social with the solitary by discussing "indulgences of the most dangerous kind." Though explicit, the "promiscuous" lectures provoked conversions, not riots. Local ultras Joseph Whitmarsh, J. N. Bolles, and T. T. Waterman organized Rhode Island's first moral reform society. Others formed a Graham Association in which members could assist one another in their pursuit of bodily virtue. The first of many physiological societies inspired by Graham's lectures, the Providence association was also the last to include women and men on the same terms.[35]

The mobbing of the "Lecture to Mothers" coincided with a profound shift in moral reform. During the months leading up to the first riot in 1833, some evangelical women began stridently insisting "that a double standard of morality would not be tolerated." As McDowall and Graham toured cities along the eastern seaboard, local reformers created a spate of societies in which women increasingly outnumbered men. In Providence, for example, two-thirds of moral reformers in 1833 were female; subsequent groups of women included no men at all. The New York Female Moral Reform Society formed in May 1834 partly to take charge of the spreading web of similar societies. They took over *McDowall's Journal* for that purpose, renaming it the *Advocate of Moral Reform* in 1835. By 1837, the rioters who surrounded Boston's "Lecture to Mothers" battled an organized corps of female moral reformers.[36]

These evangelical women embraced reform physiology because it stressed prevention rather than cure. Philanthropic men had created Magdalen Asylums decades earlier to "rescue" prostitutes by placing them in waged employment. McDowall, by contrast, stressed conversion over benevolence; by saving souls, he hoped to "prevent" both the supply of and demand for sexual commerce. Female moral reformers vastly enlarged the prevention strategy. They saw prostitution as a problem of power, not merely of sin. A powerful narrative of seduction and abandonment warned young women against suitors who tried to pressure them into having premarital sex. Those who succumbed, the story went, lost value in the eyes of their lovers and, once abandoned, slid inevitably into prostitution. Though hyperbolic, the story contained an element of truth: a woman who lost her marriage prospects had few options for supporting herself and any children she might have. Prostitution, when weighed against alternatives such as domestic service and factory work (both of which could also be refused to a woman deemed "of low character"), could seem like her best prospect. Moral reformers believed that this "systematized licentiousness" kept the brothels and city streets stocked with a permanent underclass of women doomed to cater to men's sexual demands.[37] The only way to prevent any more women from falling into such straits, they insisted, was to eliminate the double standard that maintained male dominance and female vulnerability. This required nothing short of cultural transformation, and reform physiology appeared a valuable means to that end. One moral reformer identifying herself only as "Helen" welcomed Graham to Portland because his lectures cut to the heart of "the heinous vice which we are contemplating"—that is, "the unhallowed indulgence of animal propensities."[38] Graham, for his part, tailored his messages to appeal to women such as Helen.

He also reacted against freethinkers, such as Robert Dale Owen and Fanny Wright, who invited women into public discourse on sexual physiology at this time. Graham denounced "infidels" because they celebrated pleasure and blamed Christian churches for forcing ignorance and repression upon a suffering public. The wealthy Scottish heiress Fanny Wright became one of the most despised women in the United States by arguing in public lectures that sexual passion was universal and that pleasure itself could be a positive force. She also denounced the sexual double standard, combining it with a critique of marriage as a form of state-sanctioned prostitution. Above all, Wright argued that people should discover their own moral laws through experience rather than relying on religious authorities (or, in women's case, husbands). The body would register whether a particular sexual act was harmful or healthy; sin meant nothing in this moral calculus.[39] Wright's comrade, Robert Dale Owen, agreed. In 1831 he published *Moral Physiology*, a pamphlet that described desire as a natural rise in temperature and orgasm as a necessary, self-regulating release of body heat. Owen's discussion of "onanism" followed *Onania* and Tissot: he considered it unhealthy, but inevitable as long as social conventions fettered (male) sexuality. Only perfect sexual liberty—not a blank check *within* marriage, but freedom *from* marriage—would prevent dangerous "substitutions" such as onanism, prostitution, and sodomy. To equip listeners to enjoy such freedom, he advocated coitus interruptus to prevent pregnancy.[40] Other freethinkers, such as Charles Knowlton and Russel Canfield, shared the same exuberant sexual philosophy and recommended douching as a contraceptive method. In both New York and Philadelphia, these freethinkers competed directly with evangelicals for audiences. The evangelical discourse on sex would eventually overwhelm that of the free-thought movement, but Graham had no means of predicting this outcome. He perceived himself as an underdog, even a victim, and blamed "atheists" for instigating the riots.[41]

Graham responded to freethinkers by giving a special lecture to both sexes, which appropriated Owen's title of "Moral Physiology." He objected to withdrawal, not simply because the "spilling of seed" harkened back to the story of Onan (although some moral reformers came to call it "the onanism of the married"), but because he objected to pleasure seeking for its own sake. The only physiologically sound means of fertility control, in his view, was to restrict "the frequency of connubial commerce." Those who sought sex without reproduction defiled marriage by using it to sanction their lust. In contrast to Owen, whose withdrawal method placed the power and responsibility for avoiding pregnancy entirely on men, Graham made sex a matter of negotiation between wives and husbands. He remarked that this part of his system—the one that most obviously confronted male sexual privilege within marriage—had caused "more offence than all the rest." One editor revealingly called it "an invasion of the rights of houses," an assault on husbands' entitlements. The argument surely appealed to many wives, who could use physiology to justify saying no to sex within marriage and avoid unwanted pregnancies.[42]

As important as women must have found Graham's case for periodic abstinence, it does not fully explain their interest in reform physiology. After all, they could also find arguments for fertility control and bodily sovereignty in Fanny Wright's propleasure physiological lectures. Yet freethinkers failed to attract large audiences, while reform physiology spread. In addition, the birthrate among white northerners had begun falling two generations earlier. Middling white women doubtless used periodic abstinence to control their fertility, but they did not wait for Sylvester Graham to authorize it. This aspect of his lecture merely confirmed their existing practices. It did, however, propose one novel argument. Middling white women of the 1790s and 1810s had chosen smaller families in order to enhance their families' financial welfare and affective bonds.[43] In the 1830s, they learned to abstain for the purposes of their own health and individual virtue. Graham innovated upon free-thought physiology by acknowledging the naturalness of female sexual passion and applying it to the moral reform campaign for a single standard of sexual restraint. He declared that "woman in all the laws of organic life is the same as man." Only "on account of her peculiar condition and circumstances in civilized life"—that is, the social construction of white femininity—did "woman" appear more delicate and less passionate than "man."[44] The conflicts between evangelicals and freethinkers both impelled Graham to discuss the solitary vice with women and attracted a great deal of attention to his intent to do so.

Lecture notes reveal that the classes returned again and again to the subject of solitary vice. In Maine, a female attendee noted that "blood drawn from meat is more stimulating, exciting, irritating." She added, "he might have here made remarks on the effect of such blood on the genital organs." On this point, Graham cited the case of McDonald Clark, a former audience member who had reported that when he "partook of coffee and beef steak," he "was broken down with nocturnal emissions &c." After attending the lecture to young men, he abandoned meat, coffee, and condiments. Clark found that, "when strict to the system," he experienced no emissions, but "whenever he indulged in coffee or flesh—3 a night."[45] Graham gave this young man's case to the women in his audiences because he lacked female testimonials about masturbation. For years, he begged female audience members such as Angelina Grimké and Cynthia Collins to supply him with the most intimate details of their individual "cases" for publication.[46] Most demurred, preferring instead to group together, pass general resolutions of support, and publish them in daily newspapers on their own account. Graham could only argue, as he did in the introduction to the *Lecture to Young Men*, that "all that is said in the following lecture concerning males is strictly true of females."[47] Individual women would later be more forthcoming with female lecturers, evidence that they interpreted cases such as Clark's as signs of overstimulation rather than simple seminal loss and applied an equivalent lesson to themselves. One anonymous woman lamented several years later that she had made herself ill through the solitary vice before hearing "that blessed man, Dr. Graham . . . speak on this subject." Only then did she stop "the wicked habit."[48] The content of the lecture and the responses it engendered challenged the doctrine of intrinsic passionlessness.

Despite relying at times on male examples, Graham did not advise women about the solitary vice solely to equip them to instill sexual discipline in sons and husbands. The title of the "Lecture to Mothers," on its surface, invoked republican motherhood and might be thought to suggest that women should be educated about sexual physiology in order to raise healthy, moral children. But while republican motherhood emphasized mothers' duty to raise virtuous *sons* (the future citizens and leaders of the nation), Graham made *daughters* the primary targets of maternal surveillance. "Every mother ought to know that if . . . her daughters should become so depraved as to practice self-pollution," they would suffer "the most calamitous evils." Daughters required, if anything, closer attention: "The vice which has now been described among boys, appears to be still more common among girls and produces similar symptoms." In his *Lecture to Young Men*, Graham described the case of a young woman who had damaged herself in this way. "Wantonness manifested itself in all her conduct, when in the company of males," he noted. "When she was alone with a gentleman, she would not only freely allow him to take any liberties with her, without the least restraint, but would even court his dalliance with her lascivious conduct."[49] Not because women lacked desire in comparison to men but because they understood the power of such temptations, mothers could guide their daughters away from vice. By imparting the same code of virtue to "mothers" that he did to "young men," Graham suggested that the two groups shared an equal capacity for citizenship.

Moreover, Graham never instructed women as mothers in a strictly literal sense. In fact, more than a third of the attendees who recorded their presence at one "Lecture to Mothers" had no children; many were also unmarried.[50] Addressing women as "mothers" implied that the intended audience would be both sexually experienced and dutifully feminine. Both Graham and his female attendees hoped to stave off riots by stressing the propriety of audience members. In Portland, for example, "nearly two hundred of as respectable ladies as are in that city" resolved that they learned "information, most important to mothers, the want of which, has ever been a fruitful source of disease and misery and death." Everyone understood the address "to mothers" to be rhetorical. Single women organized physiological societies, married and single neighbors canvassed together for signatures to these resolutions, and mothers brought their teenage daughters to hear the lecture firsthand. Women consumed reform physiology because it addressed them as individuals: rational beings capable of mastering their own passions and the equals of men.[51]

Women who attended the "Lecture to Mothers" also heard in its warnings against the solitary vice that their sexual desires existed quite apart from male partners, marriage, and reproduction. Occasionally, Graham departed from his overriding philosophy of universalism to make this point. For example, he quoted one author who suggested that women experienced stronger physical impulses than men, since "woman has a larger reproductive system than man." But even when Graham invoked this old assumption, he put it to new, egalitarian uses. According to the logic of republican virtue, the more intense the temptation, the greater the virtue obtained by disciplining it. If women experienced stronger urges than men, those who mastered their desires demonstrated not less passion but more fortitude. If they yielded, of course, the solitary vice could whet unpredictable desires: "Sappho indulged sexually with women," he noted. "So did the women of Lesbos, and the habits of Sappho are called Lesbian habits." Here Graham called forth the old trope that we saw in *Onania*. Unlike prior writers, however, he did so before an all-female audience and for a different purpose. Some of his female audience members may have heard in his Sapphic allusion a message separate from the warning he intended. The solitary vice so radically separated women's sexual bodies from their social roles that it raised the possibility of same-sex desire.[52]

Contemporaries wondered what all of this suggested about the women who attended the lecture. In Providence, enemies told of "a fashionable looking young lady who went to a bookseller and inquired in a *low voice* for 'Graham's address to Young Men,' taunting, "what could *she* want of

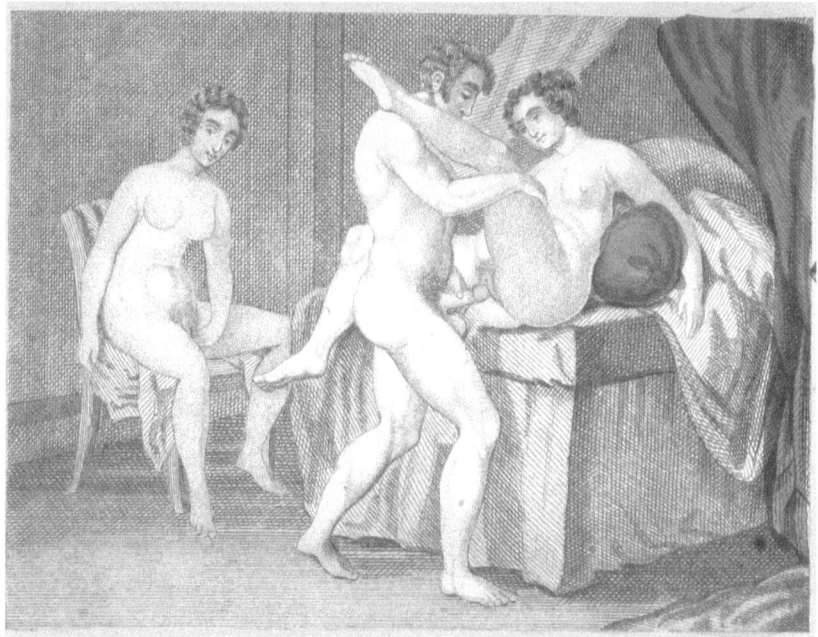

FIGURE 1. The pornographic masturbating woman invites the male viewer into the scene. Untitled hand-colored lithograph, figures likely by H. R. Robinson, pasted onto a preexisting background, ca. 1840s.
(*Source:* John Sweeney deposition, City and County of New York, June 27, 1850, American Antiquarian Society.)

such a book?" On the one hand, she might have spoken in a "low" voice in order not to be overheard buying a racy book; on the other, her voice might have been "low" because the lecture's sexual content had masculinized her, made her a Sapphist. Either way, the pun alluded to a whole bundle of unsavory associations. Sporting men knew that the booming market in erotic literature and images included titillating depictions of masturbating women disguised as antimasturbation advice.[53] Opponents called his lectures "indecent," then, with a measure of sincerity: they despised him for exposing the *wrong* women—mothers, not prostitutes—to scenes of Sapphism, nymphomania, and sexual commerce.

Indeed, female masturbation ranked among the top fetishes in eighteenth- and nineteenth-century pornography. The masturbating woman of contemporary sporting culture, however, was far from solitary. Instead, her craving for male attention drove her to the act. She usually appeared within group sex scenes, awaiting her turn in the action. At other times, she watched penetrative sex, longingly, through a secret window. Libertine republicans

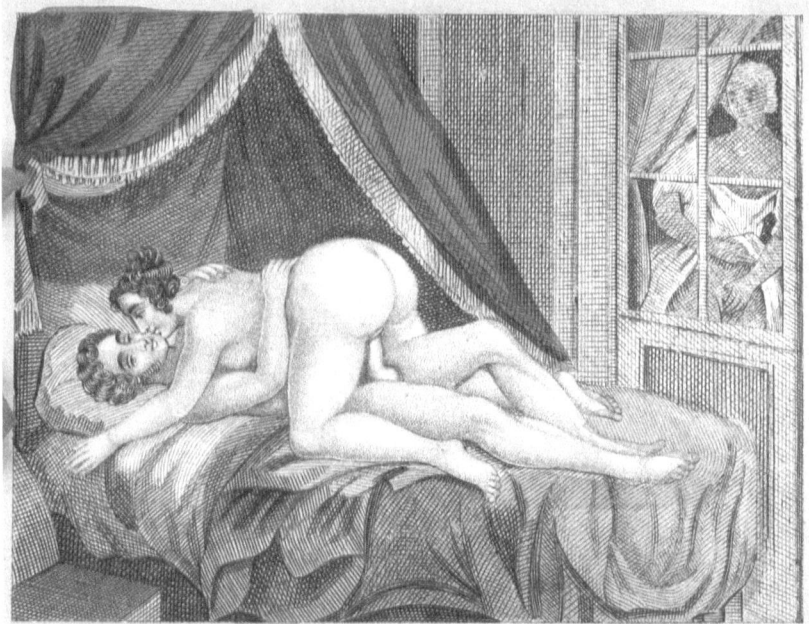

FIGURE 2. The pornographic masturbating women desires penetrative intercourse. The fantasy of the masturbating maidservant harkens back to *Onania* and subsequent erotica. European writers imagined her as the culprit who introduced vice into formerly virtuous households. Robinson may have shaded the servant's skin to represent her as a slave for American viewers. Untitled hand-colored lithograph, by H. R. Robinson, ca. 1840s.
(*Source:* John Sweeney deposition, City and County of New York,
June 27, 1850, American Antiquarian Society.)

fantasized about *this* masturbating woman, who longed for sex with them on their terms. Contemporary representations of the masturbating woman acknowledged female desire as natural, but only to the extent that it centered on men.

Such imagery suggested that it took male eyes, male bodies, and male will to *impassion* women, who knew not their own hunger. This was seduction itself: the thrilling fantasy that men possessed an irresistible power to turn any virgin into a whore. The harder edge of this fantasy played out in recriminations and violence against actual women who acted on their desires.[54] The "Lecture to Mothers" inspired riots by refashioning female masturbation from a pleasurable masculine fantasy into a challenge to male sexual prowess and privilege. Women attended the lectures in order to open a space for considering female desires and practices wholly separate from men. Turning onanism into solitary vice enabled them to contemplate their sexuality as individuals. Though proscriptive, this notion once called into being would not disappear.

LIBERTINE REPUBLICANS

On the streets and in the papers, men told themselves that they acted as righteous patriarchs in defending the women in their communities from obscenity. But problems with this rationale quickly surfaced. "Who are those who manifest so much alarm?" demanded a pro-Graham editor. "Are they individuals who have any right to control the actions of his auditors? Have *they* wives or sisters who listen to him? No, indeed, it is the wives and sisters of others whom they volunteer to PROTECT by *hissing, hooting, and yelping at as they pass through the streets!*" Women attested that their husbands and fathers were not among the rioters, nor did the behavior of "the mobocracy" square with the image of outraged virtue in the daily papers.[55]

Reformers described the typical anti-Graham rioter as "a street brawler, a bar-room swaggerer or a Billingsgate scribbler." The women who tried to attend the Boston lecture called their attackers a "riotous assembling of brutal, senseless, polluted, whiskey and wine-bibbing men." William Lloyd Garrison called them "lewd fellows of the baser sort."[56] Drawn from scripture—Acts 17:5—this phrase described a rowdy group of nonbelievers who persecuted a righteous man. It did not necessarily mark the economic class of rioters, for "gentlemen" and workingmen mingled in both physiology riots and lecture audiences.[57] Graham, for his part, named five specific men who "got up that mob" in Portland:

> Charles Mussey—a rich man—and infamous whore master—having a wife and child he is said and believed to have seduced two girls last winter.
> Henry H. Boody—a violent Jackson man—a bitter opposer of the temperance cause and is generally considered an Atheist—is City weigher & Gauger
> Randolph Augustus Lawrence Codman an infamous whore master shut out from society
> James F. Otis—an officious—conceited—contemptible and despised lawyer—who is reputed and believed to be the father to a mulatto bastard
> John D. Vainsman a lawyer—and the most respectable of the crew—member of the Congregationalist Church—but a conceited—self-important fellow.[58]

Informed by local reformers, these investigations yielded the very picture of vice. In addition to drunkards, corrupt lawyers, and lottery schemers, the mob's ringleaders included scoundrels of the specifically sexual kind: irreligious seducers, men who profited by prostitution, and at least one whose sin crossed the color line. Graham also smelled Democratic connections—the crew ranged from corrupt urban officials to "a violent Jackson man"—which he thought indicated a general hostility to reform. These sketches must be approached with caution: for example, the *Portland Daily Advertiser*, so active in drumming up hostility, was a Whig organ. The ideological freight of the allegations surely tilted Graham's perception of these men.[59]

James F. Otis (1808–67), a descendant of the brilliant and ill-fated revolutionary pamphleteer of the same name, provides a vexing example. The "scribbler" touched off a major riot by writing in the *Portland Advertiser* that Graham, having already insulted the city's wives, now hoped to lure "a new class of younger ladies." Otis quipped that "this *antiflesh* Dr. is not idle in the dissemination of his doctrines." It was a stretch to accuse Graham—champion of chastity—of outright lechery, but it made him a legitimate target for masculine rage. Otis clearly had a direct hand in "getting up" the Portland mob. But did he father a biracial child? Evidence to confirm or negate the claim proves elusive. The reformers who floated this rumor classed Otis with licentious slaveholders, who were known to father children by enslaved women and then hold or sell them as property. Ultras considered such behavior the antithesis of true manhood, and they had reasons to paint this northern editor with the same brush. After spending two years as a charter member of the New England Anti-slavery Society, he had denounced abolitionism when threatened by a proslavery mob. William Lloyd Garrison wrote in disgust that "Benedict Otis" lacked the moral vigor to stand by his beliefs. Instead, he fled in terror, "crying like a sick girl." Otis lacked the discipline and courage that defined ultra manhood. He spent the rest of his life writing theatrical gossip and other racy tidbits for sporting papers, the best known of which was the *Spirit of the Times*. Just as Otis fell out of favor with reformers, Graham impugned his misconduct in racial and sexual terms.[60]

While rumors clouded the biographical facts in this case, Graham's depiction of the other alleged conspirators can be confirmed. Randolph Codman (1796–1853), for example, did serve in the state legislature as a Democrat. Three years after Graham's tour he also went on to instigate another mob, this time targeting the Maine Anti-slavery Society. We shall see that the riots against abolitionists and reform physiology lectures became more directly linked over the course of the 1830s. Sources also bear out

Graham's depiction of Charles Mussey (1792–1876), whom neighbors *did* consider a seducer. Mussey's wife Elizabeth divorced him in 1839 for adultery, and he quickly married an already-pregnant woman, Susan, twenty years his junior. The men on Graham's list also shared shady business dealings. Mussey engaged in real estate speculation, organized a lottery that netted almost $122,000, and was sued twice for fraud. Codman and Boody also speculated on real estate under the auspices of negotiating railroad construction. It would not have been unusual for investors such as these to hold a particular financial stake in local brothels, which were fast becoming lucrative investment properties in multiple American cities.[61]

These men knew one another, were well connected in city politics, hated ultras, and shared both material and ideological investments in the pleasure culture. The list includes no butchers or bakers fearful that their businesses would suffer because of the Graham diet. Nor were the riots led by working-class radicals resisting a soon-to-be-hegemonic standard of bourgeois respectability. With average ages in their early forties, they also did not represent the unregulated youth who shocked so many urbanites. Portland's "street brawlers," at least, were *both* "lewd fellows of the baser sort" *and* "gentlemen of property and standing."[62]

Among anti-Graham rioters, we find self-appointed representatives of a masculine rake culture confronting a new doctrine of sexual restraint. As a point of pride, libertine republicanism united certain white men across classes and distinguished their privileges over women and men of color. The second group of anti-Graham rioters, the "billingsgate scribblers," expressed this philosophy in various ways. The editors of the Boston-based *New England Galaxy* provide a case in point. Throughout the 1830s, the *Galaxy*, though never acting alone, always had something to do with mobbing the "Lecture to Mothers." All three of its editors—William J. Snelling, John Neal, and Henry F. Harrington—ridiculed Graham's masculinity and sex reform in general. Snelling (deemed the "father of the flash press") explicitly argued that easy access to sexual pleasure was a masculine prerogative to which all white men were entitled.[63]

Both of Snelling's colleagues at the *Galaxy* shared this conviction. Neal cut his editorial teeth promoting the pleasures of bachelorhood before undergoing a personal transformation (he later became a well-known advocate for temperance and, eventually, women's rights). But during the late 1820s and early 1830s, Neal made his living by writing racy fiction for the *Boston Yankee* and the *Bachelor's Journal*. He printed seduction stories and ghostwrote lush letters in the voices of nubile young women who openly propositioned readers.[64] After these newspapers folded, he moved on to the *Galaxy*, in which he "crucified Dr. Graham" and helped to escalate the general unrest. When Neal left the *Galaxy*, Henry Harrington took up the charge, denouncing Graham along with the rest of "the Moral Reform folks," who demolished one masculine sexual privilege after another. He had "no more respect for these Vinegar-faced reformers, than for bears who overturn bee-hives and lap all the hoarded sweets there contained from the rightful proprietors." Sex was as natural and as sweet as honey, men its "rightful proprietors." Harrington, as we have seen, physically led the Boston mob.[65]

Ironically, libertines called Graham "totally obscene and diabolical." For all of his bluster against hoarding the "sweets" of sex, Harrington also feared that explicit lectures destroyed the very femininity that made women desirable, their natural "freedom from debasing passion." Here a libertine, *not a moral reformer*, argued that women were inherently passionless. Harrington's vacillation—condemning "debasing passion" on the one hand and demanding "the sweets of sex" on the other—captured the polarity between asexuality and hypersexuality (virgin/whore), that constrained women. But moral reformers, including Graham, strove to unhinge femininity from this dichotomy. They saw in the *shadow* of passionlessness a bleak world filled with fallen, ruined, murdered prostitutes. They proposed instead that women, like men, possessed both passion and reason. And so, in a kind of brothel riot in reverse, the rakes of Providence, Portland, and Boston fought back.[66]

MALE MONSTERS

The fact that the nature of female desire was equally at stake does not diminish the importance of masculinity as a field of conflict in the anti-Graham riots. Combatants expressed—both in words and in deeds—conflicting definitions of masculinity. What were men, if not women's guardians? What made a man a *man*, if not his difference from all that was feminine? How could masculinity remain stable when womanhood changed? These questions implied that other aspects of manhood and womanhood—characteristics that seemed correct, seamless, and universal on every other day—might be thrown off kilter just as easily. What did it *mean* for different definitions of gender to come into open conflict? The newspaper editors who instigated the anti-Graham mobs used emasculating humor against Graham and his allies, giving a sense of the rioters' gender politics. The vegetable diet provided endless material for reducing Graham's manhood in

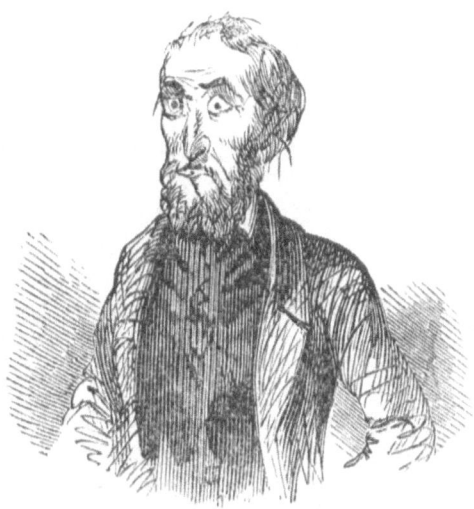

FIGURE 3. "The Inmate of a Vegetarian Boardinghouse." Wild-eyed with emotional intensity, the male Grahamite's translucent body fades into the atmosphere. (*Source:* Thomas Butler Gunn, *Physiology of New-York Boarding-Houses* [New York: Mason Brothers, 1857].)

bodily terms: "His face was so thin . . . that only one spectator could see it at a time," joked the *Providence Patriot*, "and his still small voice came forth without breath, like the gurgle of a town pump." These images dogged his male followers for years: wild-eyed men too emaciated to cast a shadow—a ghoulish "school of hypochondriacks and lantern-jawed disciples." They lisped Grahamite platitudes in "high-toned . . . branny voices." Any man who adopted the Graham system lacked substance, warned critics—and "we are not anxious to have the sun shine through us as we walk the streets." By contrast, the bodies of women who attended the "Lecture to Mothers" went oddly unremarked. Because corporeality was usually conflated with femininity, this silence underscored the association between Grahamism and emasculation. Food was a husband's perquisite, one that male reformers failed to command. Any husband who allowed his wife to attend these lectures deserved to be starved into "just such a long, lank weasel" as the lecturer himself.[67]

Jokes about the Graham diet domesticated and trivialized the sexual threat posed by the "Lecture to Mothers." Before Graham lectured to women in Boston, Charles Gordon Greene had actually promoted his lecture to men with sporting cheer. Greene told "the young bucks" of Boston that "all who think of making love" should wait until they heard it "lest they do things wrong." After Graham advertised his lecture to women, however, Greene questioned the manhood of his male followers. The lecturer had led them into a "sphere of the bigness of a wafer-box," he joked, where cookery and hygiene obsessed them. These effeminates could only "tramp and shout," from their limited sphere, that "the womb of events in the learned, the social, and the religious world is the seething cauldron of the household hearth."[68]

Still, a sexual thread ran through the problem of manly appetite. These women's husbands weren't just underfed, they were also sex starved—and they lacked the authority to do anything about it. Editors wished them "an appetite for your dinner," punning crudely: "You should have that sauce at least, for it seems you get no other." Female moral reformers might rage against the natural order of things, but the men who supported them were worse. What kind of man *yielded* his entitlements? Thus, a favorite way to emasculate Graham was to represent him as lacking all sexual desire for women. One notice of the "Lecture to Mothers" began: "No spinsters, or male monsters, except Mr. Graham, were admitted." Another, by contrast, deemed the audience of the Portland women's lecture an "antimatrimonial society." Gender ambiguity—coded as monstrosity—discredited both the lecturer and his listeners. The Portland women "unsexed" themselves by living beyond the pale of wife-and-motherhood. Only a man effete enough to forgo sex could match their androgyny.[69]

On the other hand, the fact that Graham spoke about sex to other men's wives led some critics to represent him as a mass seducer. This allegation—seemingly irrational, given his crusade for chastity—made sense in a culture that deemed sexually abstinent men perverts. From anti-Catholic screeds to the flash press, popular writers insisted that the tide of male sexuality could be channeled but not dammed. They used the phrase "male monsters" to describe sexually aberrant men who lived without women.[70] The *New England Galaxy* turned this logic against Graham by reporting that when "well-dressed women" thronged the streets, he never lusted over their "beauty or symmetry!" Graham had said so during one of his lectures, demanding to know why other men could not be as chaste. To the editors of the *Galaxy*, "There was never a more unfortunate question!"[71] The overwhelmingly male crowds who confronted the lecturer believed that chastity threatened manhood itself.

Other men who spoke against the solitary vice faced the same emasculating humor and, when they challenged the sexual double standard, similar mobs. For example, the Providence reformer Joseph Whitmarsh promoted ultra manhood and challenged male sexual privilege. In his eyes, the expectation that men's desires should always be fulfilled produced and reproduced the dual systems of prostitution and slavery that he abhorred. He gravitated to physiological reform in his early twenties and, shortly thereafter, became obsessed with eradicating the solitary vice. Whitmarsh helped to coordinate the McDowall-Graham lecture series and the men's moral reform society that published the *Lecture to Young Men* for a national audience. His newspaper, the *Illuminator*, enjoined readers to *"Strive, Quit Yourselves Like Men."* Citing Graham's *Lecture to Young Men*, he argued that under no circumstances was seminal emission necessary for health. Men could moderate their sexual urges to exactly the same degree expected of women. "Gentlemen rakes" responded by suing Whitmarsh for obscene libel and mobbing his office. But such martyrdom only fueled his vision of ultra masculinity. Surviving a burned press, physical assault, and incarceration, he declared, "I shall not be intimidated and put to silence, by threats of personal violence or by mobs." More than discipline for its own sake, abstinence would create hardy Christian soldiers capable of exhibiting fortitude even unto death.[72]

Whitmarsh found kindred spirits in J. N. Bolles and Daniel Colesworthy. In 1834, Bolles worked together with Whitmarsh in the Providence men's moral reform society before moving to New York. In 1834, he published *Solitary Vice Considered*, a cheap digest of Graham's *Lecture to Young Men*, William Andrus Alcott's *Young Man's Guide*, Samuel Tissot's *L'Onanisme* (1760), and Benjamin Rush's *Medical Inquiries upon Diseases of the Mind* (1812).[73] In Portland, Daniel C. Colesworthy critiqued dietary self-indulgence through his journal the *Juvenile Reformer*, which attempted to convince young readers that sugar and confections "strike us, if not destroy us" at the moral core. As a Grahamite, Colesworthy believed that sugar stimulated the genitals and led to solitary vice; as an abolitionist, he denounced it as a product of one of the most brutal industries built on slavery. Even free-produce sugar provided no solution, he argued. Men needed to learn to sacrifice and banish self-indulgence, rather than find new ways to cater to their bodily appetites. Though ostracized by moderate reformers, the *Juvenile Reformer* continued with unabated ultraism until Colesworthy was excommunicated in 1837.[74]

Colesworthy, Bolles, and Whitmarsh did not counsel abstemiousness for its own sake. Rather, they manipulated cultural symbols of men's entitlement to pleasure in hopes of remaking contemporary power relationships. According to Stephanie Camp, enslaved people resisted chattel status by stealing pleasure through dance, dress, and play.⁷⁵ This cohort of northern white ultras enacted the same principle in reverse: they rejected the privileged access to pleasure that their whiteness and maleness unjustly guaranteed. In itself, such conspicuous display of restraint posed no material threat to slavery or patriarchy. However, they did craft an alternative, antioppressive form of masculinity, which suggested that small, everyday actions—micropolitics—could transform their culture. Those who embraced ultra masculinity expressed, through their bodily practices, membership in a community of protest. Given the violent ostracism that met white men who departed from dominant masculinity, this counterculture appears to have struck contemporaries as threatening the social order.

If the new restraint seemed especially *important* for men to master based on the sexual license that male privilege afforded, ultras did not presume that men possessed more or less *ability* to discipline their bodies than did women. When Graham suspended his lectures to women during 1835 and 1836, Whitmarsh took it upon himself to address women throughout the New England countryside about, among other things, the solitary vice. Like Graham, he faced "a mob of gentlemen and whoremongers" for doing so. And, like the defiant women at Boston's Marlboro Hotel, local women became further motivated to take control of the moral reform movement. Female moral reformers in Holliston, Pawtucket, and Lowell donated generously to keep Whitmarsh's *Illuminator* afloat; at the end of 1837, Boston women took over the newspaper altogether. Dismissing activist women as "freaks," conservative editors continued to dress down male ultras through emasculating humor. Graham had made Whitmarsh into a eunuch, jabbed one editor, charged with minding his "seraglio."⁷⁶

LADIES AND CITIZENS

The suggestion that men and women did not have different, let alone opposite, physiological passions appealed to many more women than men. Since women lacked formal political tools other than the petition, they relied heavily on publicity battles to politicize their support for reform physiology. They learned to stage spectacular actions to attract the attention of the press, then to identify their assailants and denounce the rioters' charge of indecency as "false delicacy." Grahamites borrowed this phrase from moral reformers, who used it to admonish "Christians and persons of pure morals" to confront licentiousness. According to John R. McDowall, mistaken or overblown notions of delicacy led to passive silence and only encouraged libertines "to roar louder and louder."⁷⁷ Ironically, "false delicacy" originated in an older European tradition of libertinage, where it described courtship games in which libertines pushed for sex and women repelled them. A man who persuaded a woman to "yield" her modesty without the promise of marriage was considered to have conquered her. In this culture, "false delicacy" referred to unconquered women, those who pretended to be too delicate to give in to sex when in fact they hoped to ensnare bachelors into marriage proposals—such were *their* conquests. Libertines presumed a battle of the sexes and denied the possibility that a woman might truly be uninterested in sex with a particular man.[78] Moral reformers turned false delicacy into a critique of Christians of either sex who preferred to *appear* pious rather than honestly face their moral obligations.

In the context of the physiology riots, female moral reformers further transformed the meanings of false and true delicacy. Noting that local men hoped to silence activist women by branding them "indelicate," they redefined false delicacy as a hypocritical effort on the part of the guilty to suppress open discussion of "licentiousness, the crying evil of our land." One reform woman denied that these "pests—(they deserve not the name of men)" had any authentic interest in defending chastity.[79] Silence did not protect female innocence; it kept women from confronting male sexual privilege.

An inherently flexible concept, false delicacy grew into one of the most durable weapons in the moral reform arsenal. Opposition, even apathy, could be condemned as false delicacy. *True* virtue required reformers to speak openly about vices both social and solitary. Thus, the Providence Ladies Moral Reform Association declared that "it is the prerogative of virtue to contemn vice; it is the highest honor of delicacy to expose and guard against indelicacy." In Portland, Mary C. Porter presided over 160 women who had attended the "Lecture to Mothers." They voted to draft resolutions for publication, testifying that the lecture contained nothing "which could offend or alarm the most fastidious delicacy." Another Portland woman added that only those guilty of "a vice which is sapping the foundation of all that is valuable and dear on earth" would mob a lecturer who counseled honest women against it.[80]

Elizabeth Oakes Smith, who later became a women's rights activist and marriage reformer, started her career in reform in the midst of this tumult. Having attended the "Lecture to Mothers," she thought the riots "must have been gotten up by some suspicious old husband, who was denied admission to the lectures." Her own husband, Seba Smith, edited the *Portland Courier*. When "the whole city seemed to be boiling over with agitation," most editors feared that the mobs would turn against their presses if they printed Mary Porter's resolutions of support. But Elizabeth convinced Seba that such censorship was unrepublican and saw to it that the *Courier* published the women's resolutions. By naming the "Lecture to Mothers" as truly delicate and its enemies as hypocrites, female moral reformers shuttled the solitary vice subtly but effectively into women's appropriate domain.[81]

Boston women pushed this connection even further. In language echoing women's testimony from Harrisburg to Portland, they certified that no woman who attended the 1837 "Lecture to Mothers" had witnessed anything that would "wound the delicacy of the most fastidious." The hypocrisy of someone like Henry Harrington summoning "libertines, whoremongers, drunkards and theatre frequenters" in a riot "to protect the virtue of respectable married females" struck a deep nerve.[82] Whereas in 1834, only five Portland women had published their names, three years later, more than half of the Boston audience went public. By that time, women's activism in the city surged, converging in female antislavery and moral reform societies. Of 118 Graham defenders, 34 were active members of the Boston Female Moral Reform Society, and many more were affiliated with an antislavery society. Half testimonial, half petition, the Boston document reflected its signers' activist experience. No mere disciples of a male celebrity, they actively solicited the lecture and took responsibility for its content. While Graham framed them as mothers, these women identified as "ladies and citizens."[83]

CONCLUSION

At first, only the tiniest corps of radicals embraced reform physiology. With a reputation for "*ultra* ultraism" and a "screw-anger" lecture style, Sylvester Graham struck most commentators as "fanatical."[84] But in the eyes of female moral reformers, his position appeared more rational than that of riotous men who violently clung to the status quo. Hostile editors ridiculed them along with Graham in gendered terms, aiming to diminish their sexual politics. But the crowds of men who raged against the "Lecture to Mothers" belied such levity. Their defensiveness suggested that the new ideas about sex might destabilize social hierarchies.

Female moral reformers organized to shift the public's focus away from the superficial conflict among men over "indecency" and "protection" and draw attention instead to the power dynamics at work. Placing their own ideas and bodies at the center of the action, they goaded rioters into revealing that the male lecturer was little more than a symbolic target: rioters cared less about Graham than about maintaining their sexual dominance over women and control of public space. While laying bare these motives, diverse women also subscribed to reform physiology and vested it with political potential. After the smoke cleared, Graham thanked the women who had mobilized in his defense, but even he saw something larger at stake. "No efforts of my whole life, and perhaps none that I am capable of making," he wrote, equaled the "Lecture to Mothers" in importance. As rioters drove Graham out of the field, it would be women who carried on the campaign against solitary vice.[85]

Reform physiology asserted two fundamentally new principles, both of which departed profoundly from prior sexual advice and struck at the core of the sexual double standard. First, men neither physically needed nor were morally entitled to sex on demand, even within marriage. Second, physiology did not render women sexually passive or reliant on men. Possessing sexual desires all their own, only they—not husbands, fathers, or even seducers—could control their morals and behaviors. The riots only strengthened female moral reformers' conviction that mastering their physical bodies held political significance. They came to see the solitary vice as a symbol of female sexual autonomy. The obstacles to changing women's *institutional* subordination, such as marital law, overwhelmed all but the most determined reformers during the 1830s.[86] But *culturally*, large numbers of women insisted that they could at least govern their own flesh.

Reform physiology disputed the natural basis of divergent norms of sexual behavior—a contention that could destabilize racial, as well as gender, discourses. For if, as Graham stated, human nature was radically the same everywhere, then African Americans and whites shared the same capacity for virtue. When editors labeled Graham a "male monster," they suggested that he encouraged racial amalgamation as well as gender upheaval. A Providence paper claimed, for example, that he especially relished speaking to black women about sex, comparing him to "the ourang outang, celebrated for his attention to the Negresses of Central Africa."[87] African American women responded to such dehumanizing claims by asserting their own dignity, bridging abolitionism with female moral reform, and further problematizing the doctrine of white feminine passionlessness. In the process, they strategically adopted particular tenets of reform physiology. Their skepticism about white women's essential purity imbued the female moral reform movement with an intersectional sexual politics as it spread throughout the Northeast. Initially, it drew some white women into antislavery activism. But the more lasting effect of the antebellum critique of purity was to encourage white female moral reformers to spread the word against the solitary vice.

CHAPTER TWO

Licentiousness in All Its Forms

Amid the final physiology riots in March 1837, a fifteen-year-old named Lucia Weston wrote to her older sister with breathless excitement. "There was a mob in Boston," she reported, but "not *we* that were mobbed, but *Graham*, for lecturing to the Ladies *alone* and not even their husbands admitted!!!" By "we," Lucia meant abolitionists. The letter's recipient, Deborah Weston, had experienced a similar mob in Boston on October 21, 1835, "the day when 5,000 men mobbed 45 women" of the Boston Female Anti-slavery Society. Coming of age in an abolitionist family, Lucia had heard her sister's account of the proslavery riot initiated by "gentlemen of property and standing" as an object lesson in adhering to one's principles. The gender ratio was less egregious in 1837: two hundred women confronted "about one thousand mobbers." Still, the women fought back, Lucia proudly informed Deborah, until the mayor arrived to disperse the crowd.[1]

Despite Lucia Weston's perception that rioters targeted Graham rather than antislavery women, the Boston Female Anti-slavery Society had in fact made a strong showing at the lecture that day. A biracial cohort of abolitionists joined leaders in the Boston Female Moral Reform Society in resisting the mob. Relatively unknown black women such as Hannah C. Cutler, Louisa Drummond, Elizabeth White, and Mrs. Lewis York made up about a tenth of Graham's Boston audience. They entered the historical record by signing a defense of the "Lecture to Mothers," in which they too claimed rights as "ladies and citizens." Boston's black abolitionists also invited Graham to lecture at the Adelphic Union, a peer-education institution. Although his lectures on the science of human life had never excluded African Americans, many preferred to meet in black-defined spaces associated with what Carla Peterson has called "the community sphere."[2] The demand for the physiology course so overwhelmed the Adelphic Union's normal facilities that the audience had to move to the larger Belknap Street meetinghouse. However, Graham did not deliver the "Lecture to Mothers" at the Adelphic Union. Black women who wished to attend the lecture on sexual physiology would have to brave the majority-white women's lecture. Some did so in explicit protest against social segregation. Whatever their motives, African American women who gathered to discuss sex across the color line risked violence. Newspapermen named Graham's attendees "females of the abolition faith," drawing particular attention to the presence of "twenty-six ladies of *colour*." The specter of *amalgamation*, an offensive term for interracial intimacy, was meant to suppress the women's lecture once and for all.[3]

Amalgamation riots occurred with increasing frequency during the 1830s and often followed a recognizable pattern. Newspaper editors who opposed the immediate abolition of slavery, such as William L. Stone of the *New York Commercial Advertiser* and James Watson Webb of the *Courier and Enquirer*, floated rumors of amalgamation in order to encourage white male readers to attack antislavery meetings. The threat of mob action usually convinced elite men who owned lecture halls to ban antislavery meetings on their property. When antislavery societies did meet, speakers often found themselves pelted with rotten eggs or stones. City authorities and volunteer firefighters claimed that they could not stop rioters from burning buildings, destroying printing presses, and wounding—or even murdering—activists. In this way, racially and sexually charged symbols bred violence that rationalized a set of institutional barriers against abolitionist organizing. Historian Leslie Harris describes this nexus of power relations as "amalgamation discourse."[4]

Not coincidentally, some of the same editors also encouraged readers to strike at the "Lecture to Mothers," citing both gender disorder and amalgamation. John Neal, for example, who summoned Portlanders to suppress Graham's lecture to women, also helped to instigate at least one amalgamation riot.[5] And William Stone, a major instigator of amalgamation riots, wrote disingenuously: "Now we are opposed to riots in general, but if Mr. Graham has been instructing the wives and mothers of Portland to cram any of his bread down the throats of their husbands and children, we don't wonder at the excitement." Like Graham's doctrine of universal sexuality, racial amalgamation threatened "the rights of houses"—that is, white men's exclusive access to white women. Stone blamed male moral reformers such as Graham and McDowall for exposing white women to indecent images *and* encouraging them to mingle with African Americans. They represented the abolitionist quest for "social equality" as nothing more than a desire for intermarriage, particularly between black men and white women. Libertine republicans suggested that the mere presence of African Americans threatened white women's purity. One described Graham's audience as "a motley collection of white and black on the subject of the 'duties of women,'" which only proved "on anatomical principles, that in the dark all cats are gray." This ugly play on the long-standing feline metaphor for female genitalia suggested that the women would be sexually available (and interchangeable) to any man groping in the darkened lecture hall. Innuendo merged here with a threat: women who attended such a lecture invited sexual harassment.[6]

Although amalgamation rioters claimed to protect white feminine *innocence*, in practice they targeted women's interracial *activism*. For example, an 1840 mob threat drove a large group of abolitionists "of all colors and sexes, and some"—to hostile eyes—"of no sex at all," from their appointed meeting place in New York's fourth ward. They reconvened at a Grahamite boardinghouse. Rioters followed them, smashed the windows, dragged out an Ohio abolitionist, and "severely injured him." They reacted to a newspaper report that one of the abolitionists, "a very pretty white girl," had made a show of approaching another, an African American man, flirtatiously reaching into his pocket and taking "his watch out of his fob, to get the time o'day."[7] The black man was portrayed passively in this account, presumed to automatically desire physical contact with any white woman. The white woman, meanwhile, having "unsexed" herself through *political* activism, had also become *sexually* aggressive. If antislavery women, like "male monsters," had "no sex at all," they too became fair game for rioters' rage. Those who disobeyed the rules of white patriarchy lost its privileges and protections. In this context, many abolitionists denied any interest in sexual amalgamation. However, a few replied that the entire discourse of amalgamation rested on "false delicacy."

This chapter argues that black abolitionists adopted the language of female moral reformers in cautious hopes of bridging the two movements. In addition to appropriating *false delicacy*, they applied *licentiousness* to slavery and racist exploitation in the North. Female moral reformers promised to abolish "licentiousness in all its forms," and African Americans held them to this promise. Reversing stereotypes of black sexuality, they conceived of licentiousness in terms of not merely sexual excess but also excessive sexual *power*—the social *license* that permitted white men to take sexual liberties.[8]

During this brief but significant interracial moment in moral reform—roughly, 1835 to 1840—black abolitionist women within the African Methodist Episcopal Zion Church, the Boston Female Anti-slavery Society, and the Philadelphia Female Anti-slavery Society transformed the campaign against licentiousness into a protest against slavery and white supremacy. African American women's moral reform efforts should not be seen as a bid for respectability in the eyes of whites. Instead, they challenged white moral reform women to confront the racialized dimensions of the sexual double standard. In the process, they redefined virtue in terms of activism—"moral accountability"—rather than passive chastity. As a result of the careful bridge leadership of black women such as Grace and Sarah Mapps Douglass, a few white radicals such Sarah and Angelina Grimké popularized this standard of morality for *all* women. They went further than had Sylvester Graham in destabilizing white feminine purity. Yet they, too, insisted that women demonstrated virtue not by denying sexual feeling, but rather by acknowledging that they shared—with one another and with men—both physical passions and moral responsibilities. These arguments initially drew white moral reformers into antislavery activism but ultimately devolved into a more pervasive campaign against the solitary vice. The women's rights movement, which originated at the crossroads of abolitionism and moral reform, would bear the impress of this sexual politics.

ZION FEMALE MORAL REFORM SOCIETY

During the three decades before the Civil War, amalgamation discourse targeted all activists who challenged the racial status quo. However, African Americans experienced the brunt of the political repression, cultural backlash, and physical violence it engendered. Given these dangers, why would black abolitionist women consciously chance an alliance with white moral reformers? And why would even a few white women risk their privileges and protections by sexual politicking with women of color? In order to answer these questions, it is necessary to examine the first stirrings of interest in biracial coalition, forged in response to one of the earliest and most destructive amalgamation riots of the 1830s.

In 1834, a July Fourth celebration at Chatham Chapel in New York's Five Points neighborhood, where white women sang in a choir alongside African American men and women, triggered more than a week of the worst race rioting the city had ever seen. Stone's *Commercial Advertiser* and Webb's *Courier & Enquirer* emphasized the physical closeness of white women to black men in the church and the mingling of their voices in the choir. As it happened, Chatham Chapel stood at the intersection of abolitionism and female moral reform. The wealthy reformer Lewis Tappan had purchased it in 1832 as a home for Charles Grandison Finney's Presbyterian congregation, and soon afterward the church became a conspicuous site of antislavery organizing. Rumors that "the colored people and the whites have mixed promiscuously in the abolition assemblies convened in Chatham street chapel" became overtly sexualized when white women organized the New York Female Moral Reform Society at the chapel in May 1834.[9] Moral reformers chose a site in the Five Points neighborhood largely because it was a hub of sexual commerce. By vowing to eliminate prostitution, these women infuriated both libertine republicans who presumed to control the neighborhood's streets and real estate speculators who profited from brothel ownership.[10] The combination of interracial antislavery organizing and women's attacks on male sexual license created a powder keg that exploded in amalgamation riots. The mobs attacked buildings—"Mr. McDowall's Journal, the Chatham street Chapel, the African churches"—which symbolized these connections.[11]

The most severely damaged "African churches" were St. Philips African Episcopal and African Methodist Episcopal Zion, institutions of worship, education, and protest situated only a few blocks from Chatham Chapel. Both churches cultivated sexual propriety among members within a context of racism and sexual stigma. But beyond moral reform, they took different approaches to activism. St. Philips remained under the purview of the white Episcopal hierarchy and stressed personal holiness over activism. Its leader, Rev. Peter Williams Jr., joined the American Anti-slavery Society at its founding. Enemies targeted him in July 1834 by gossiping that he had performed a wedding ceremony between a white woman and a black man. Amalgamation rioters sacked his church. Afterward, Williams denied that he had ever conducted such a ceremony. Under duress from white church superiors, he resigned his antislavery office. By contrast, A.M.E. Zion had formed in 1796 in direct response to racism. Congregants forfeited the abundant resources of the white Methodist Episcopal Church in order to preserve their autonomy and pursue social justice without the threat of discipline. Zion, associated with separatism rather than integration, sustained only superficial vandalism amid the amalgamation riots of 1834. Nevertheless, the riots radicalized its female congregants. Their neighborhood was in shambles, members had been beaten and friends left homeless, their children's schools razed—all in the name of preventing amalgamation.[12] Something new had to be tried.

Zion women knew of white female moral reformers' new campaign against licentiousness, but before 1834 it meant little to most of them. One member, Isabella van Wagenen (who would later take the name Sojourner Truth), had preached to prostitutes alongside John R. McDowall but left the church before the New York Female Moral Reform Society formed. Although her coreligionists were aware of her activities, very few other African Americans risked a connection with white moral reformers.[13] Throughout the 1830s, the New York society dispersed white female "missionaries" throughout the neighborhood who did not appear to care to work together with black residents. Moreover, a movement built around public discussions of sex held particular dangers for black women and men. Stereotypes of black lasciviousness justified rape and vigilantism in the antebellum North just as they undergirded southern slavery. In addition, while white female moral reform efforts were highly controversial and relatively new, many African American women participated in an ongoing campaign within black churches to police sexual sin. Those who considered sexual behavior in need of reform could therefore work within black-defined spaces, away from white scrutiny and strictly for the salvation of African Americans.[14]

Chatham Chapel's white moral reformers may also have initially alienated black women by acting with dangerous naïveté about the racial dimensions of sexual oppression. Only two days after the formation of the New York Female Moral Reform Society, the church hosted a display of 395 "indecent pictures of various kinds collected from different sources."[15] The "exhibition" was meant to critique sexual commerce in all its variety. But James Watson Webb twisted this intent, insisting that the Christian women of the Five Points neighborhood were, like its prostitutes, "praying to be looked at." Such sexualized attention especially affected African American women in the neighborhood. When Zion congregants advertised an exhibition of their own—a fair selling handcrafts for the benefit of fugitive slaves—the *Free Enquirer* punned on the idea of "a Female Exhibition," suggesting that organizers Sarah Willets and Janet Mumford would publicly strip in their church for money.[16] This hypersexualization had real consequences: increased vulnerability to sexual harassment and assault. Sensing that white moral reform women might add fuel to this fire, African Americans remained guarded in May 1834.

However, six months after the riots, the women of Zion reached out to the New York Female Moral Reform Society. Congregants Eliza Coker and Mary Johnson initiated extensive discussion of "the efforts being then made among our white friends for the prevention of licentiousness." Coker and Johnson argued for some kind of "combined effort," and the church voted to form an auxiliary, the Zion Female Moral Reform Society. Within months, they more than doubled their numbers, counting a membership of 138 African American women and becoming one of the largest female moral reform societies in the country.[17]

By forming an auxiliary to the New York Female Moral Reform Society, Zion women aligned themselves with the flagship society of a growing movement while also holding separate meetings. This arm's-length alliance tasked them, rather than white moral reformers, with surveying "the state of morals among our colored brethren."[18] By sheltering their "colored brethren" from the prying eyes of white women, Zion women moved to deflect racist stereotyping. But this guardedness should not be conflated with the "culture of dissemblance" that Darlene Clark Hine has found among African American women around the turn of the twentieth century.[19] What is remarkable about Zion Female Moral Reform Society is not its members' hesitation but their *willingness* to enter into a fraught biracial alliance in 1835. Had respectability been of primary importance, Zion women would have avoided the New York Female Moral Reform Society at all costs. White female moral reformers hardly suggested themselves as respectable allies. They were maligned in the press, disowned by families and churches, and physically assaulted when they proselytized brothels.[20] Perhaps the shared experience of having been targeted by rioters contributed to a new sense of camaraderie and lent credibility to the white evangelical presence in the neighborhood. But a more important factor may have been the New York Female Moral Reform Society's new access to publicity. It had taken over *McDowall's Journal* and renamed it the *Advocate of Moral Reform*. Beginning in 1835, the newspaper persuaded a growing readership of white women to address the politics of sexuality. By declaring war on *systematized* licentiousness, the *Advocate* confronted white men in startling new ways. The Zion Female Moral Reform Society chose to campaign openly alongside white evangelical women against white men's sexual license and hypocrisy.

THE LICENTIOUSNESS OF SLAVERY

The root *license* gave licentiousness important political connotations, making it an ideal weapon for confronting powerful men in particular. Republican political discourse marked license as the outer limit of legitimate freedom. In the words of a Lynn reformer, "Rational liberty is one thing—licentiousness, or the abuse of liberty is another." When liberty was excessive, misused, or ungoverned, it could demolish the nation in a storm of anarchic or despotic violence. Members of the New York Female Moral Reform Society feared that unless they could "tear licentious men from the vitals of the republic, all our boasted liberties are gone forever." In "the existing state of licentiousness," men already possessed greater sexual liberty than did women. When they devised "machinations" to *take* liberties, they committed not merely lewd, but rather *licentious*, acts. Other newspapers across the political spectrum quoted this language, whether to endorse or, more commonly, to mock female moral reform. Regardless of intent, this process made *licentiousness* a household word, one that politicized the sexual arena.[21]

Republican ideology also defined license against liberty through an implicit reference to slavery. If liberty devolved into license, the next stop for the nation as a whole could well be slavery—whether in the form of tyranny or "mobocracy." White moral reformers often used slavery as a metaphor for sexual sin: those who succumbed to temptation were "enslaved by the flesh," and made "slaves of unbridled passion." Only the "liberty of the gospel" could free souls from such bondage. By conquering temptations rather than indulging them, individual Christians could replace "slavery to the flesh" with virtuous "self-government."[22] However, not all Americans thought about slavery, liberty, and licentiousness in such abstract terms.

Slavery certainly did not strike the women of Zion as metaphorical. Like most black abolitionists, they had ongoing contact with recently enslaved people and fresh memories of slavery in New York itself.[23] These experiences, as well as the amalgamation riots, profoundly shaped their sexual politics. The *Advocate*, which both expanded the meanings of licentiousness and popularized it as a movement buzzword, presented a potentially valuable resource in the concrete struggle against slavery and racism. In order to influence its direction, Zion women needed to build bridges. They did so by inviting several notable male moral reformers, including John McDowall himself, to address them in early 1835.[24] These high-profile lecturers would affirm the importance of the new organization to white *Advocate* readers.

Some of the men who lectured to Zion women published their addresses, producing in the process a documentary record of the sexual counterdiscourse that was developing within otherwise closed meetings. David Ruggles, a radical black abolitionist and founder of the Committee of Vigilance (an organization that defended self-emancipated blacks), published the most important of these lectures. Ruggles had initially approached Zion women in order to solicit funds for his Vigilance efforts and for the antislavery press. The outcome was mutually instructive: Zion organized a Female Vigilance Committee; Ruggles picked up the moral reform idiom. He became a member of the Seventh Commandment Society, a group of male McDowall supporters committed to the biblical injunction "Thou shalt not commit adultery." Adapting moral reform principles to the antislavery struggle, he titled his lecture "The Abrogation of the Seventh Commandment by the American Churches." In it, he named the *licentiousness of slavery*, pointing out the ways in which sexual power sustained the institution.[25]

Abrogation adopted and redeployed the female moral reformers' language. It described the "licentiousness of intercourse between the sexes, constant, incestuous, and universal," that characterized slavery. Ruggles also asserted that the licentiousness of slavery "from false delicacy, or an improper squeamishness, has never been presented in palpable form." Further, he argued that the fear of amalgamation amounted to nothing more than false delicacy. "Amalgamation is never disowned except when the woman is free," he observed, "because the offspring of the licentious intercourse cannot be grasped and sold as property."[26] Rioters were not moved by moral indignation, nor even by racist disgust. Instead, like the libertine republicans who mobbed moral reformers, they clung violently to power and privilege. The real goal of amalgamation rioters was to weaken the antislavery movement.

As agent of the *Emancipator* and owner of a bookstore, Ruggles had access to a printing press, which he used to publish *Abrogation* for circulation as a pamphlet addressed to "northern ladies." He used these resources to convey a challenge from the women of Zion to members of the New York Female Moral Reform Society—and all white women who claimed to oppose licentiousness. Moral reformers drew attention to the social conventions that quietly tolerated male improprieties. Ruggles added that "false delicacy" abetted white Christians in refusing to see slavery as a system rooted in the sexual exploitation of black women. Just as the double standard exonerated male seducers while unduly condemning their female victims, slavery rewarded rather than punished slaveholders for their predations.[27] *Abrogation* insisted that truly delicate women must sever ties with slaveholders and openly condemn them, despite their power and status, especially within churches. Otherwise, "ladies," too, were licentious—welcoming slaveholders into church membership made Christian women complicitous in rape.[28]

The licentiousness of slavery quickly become a watchword of the interracial abolitionist movement. Because white northerners wove it into their building sense of sectional superiority over "the erotic South," historians have attributed the licentiousness of slavery to opportunistic and prurient whites.[29] This literature overlooks long-standing African and African-American protests against the "violent depredations on the chastity of female slaves." Those who knew slavery firsthand testified earliest to the sexual violence that sustained it. Olaudah Equiano, who joined the British antislavery movement after securing his freedom, denounced slaveholders who raped enslaved women in 1789. In doing so, however, he wrote of sinful "abominations," not unrepublican licentiousness.[30] Similarly, Maria W. Stewart pleaded "the cause of virtue and the pure principles of morality" when she addressed all-black audiences in 1831. Like Equiano, she demanded sexual safety and dignity for black women without invoking licentiousness. Only after female moral reformers named license as an issue of sexual power did black women and men take up this language—and only in the interest of strategic alliance.

As a political slogan, the licentiousness of slavery addressed northern white women in terms calculated to make them accountable for cooperating. After 1834, the licentiousness of slavery became a staple of interracial dialogue.[31] James Forten used it in his address to the Philadelphia Female Anti-slavery Society, for example, as did William Wells Brown when he met with the Salem Female Anti-slavery Society. Over the next ten years, black and white abolitionists pressured moral reformers to publish the words of "our suffering colored sisters." Moral reform had become a women's movement, and the time had come to "recognize them as *women*." More than two decades after Eliza Coker and Mary Johnson approached the New York Female Moral Reform Society, Harriet Jacobs recorded her own experiences of sexual coercion in *Incidents in the Life of a Slave Girl*. Situated within Rochester's biracial community of antislavery women, Jacobs could be sure that white female readers would respond to her indictment of slavery as "an atmosphere of licentiousness and fear," a system built by "cunning" slaveholders who devised laws to ensure "that licentiousness shall not interfere with avarice."[32] In the meantime, black women argued that the licentiousness of slavery still did not capture the power dynamics of licentiousness in *all* its forms. Having coalesced in response to northern amalgamation riots, black moral reformers exposed the sexual dimensions of the northern race hierarchy. As one interracial society pointed out, fears for white women's purity rarely surfaced when they interacted with people of color "in the capacity of *servants*."[33] Such critiques made moral reform relevant to working-class African Americans in several northeastern cities.

NORTHERN LICENTIOUSNESS

Between 1835 and 1840, black women coauthored the moral reform movement's emerging sexual platform. Their counterdiscourse quickly surpassed the sexual critique of slavery to address local concerns. In the pages of the moral reform press, African American women testified to the ways in which sexual harassment by licentious white men endangered their safety, limited their mobility, and impacted their ability to earn a living. Some described the terror of being stalked through city streets by "respectable-looking white men," who presumed that they were prostitutes or, in any case, sexually available. One anonymous African American woman described a "father and son"—both "licentious men"—who, despite their "spirited indignation against the abolitionists for endeavoring to promote as they assert, 'amalgamation,'" were known for "following and insulting *coloured* females." Recounting her own experience with the harassers, she recalled telling one of them that "she was not of the character he wished." He responded "'that color made no difference,' and persisted in following her until she arrived at her home." *Advocate* editor Sarah Towne Smith, a white abolitionist, denounced "such amalgamation as this"—a sarcastic commentary on the hypocrisy of amalgamation rioters.[34]

The white women who controlled the moral reform press published these accounts of sexual harassment for ideological reasons. Many white abolitionists denounced the licentiousness of slavery in self-congratulatory praise of wage labor.[35] Female moral reformers, however, considered the labor market with more ambivalence. On the one hand, they criticized women's factory labor and valorized domestic "habits of industry, to which daughters were formerly trained, but which are fast disappearing from our land." As greater numbers of young women migrated to cities in search of jobs, moral reformers feared that urban anonymity, combined with low wages and precarious employment, would tempt working "girls" away from "the path of virtue."[36] On the other hand, they deemed paid domestic labor ennobling, particularly when compared to prostitution. As employers of servants, elite and middle-class women benefitted from this construction. In 1838, the New York Female Moral Reform Society created an Office of Direction for Female Domestics, on the grounds that placing single women in service "shielded them from the paths of the destroyer."[37] Having become brokers in the market for domestic labor, female moral reformers felt newly responsible for protecting serving women from licentious heads of household. These tensions in moral reformers' labor ideology created an opportunity for African American women to protest sexual exploitation as a regular feature of domestic service through the pages the *Advocate*.

Take, for example, the case of a black woman who anonymously reported that two "gentlemen" had assaulted her under the pretext of hiring her as a "servant." When she came to their house for an interview, they began by "offering her fruit, nuts, and wine, promising great wages, and many presents" if she would work for them. Next, they commented that her children "were *very light*," and "that if she should have others that were *light*, nothing would be thought of it, as they would be alike in that respect." Understanding the implied proposition, she refused. One of the men then "attempted to lay hands upon her," but she fought back and escaped, vowing to expose him. The episode followed a familiar script. Historian Sharon Block argues that by "placing forced sexual acts into a setting of voluntary social relations," elite white men "could recreate rape as consensual sex." According to Hannah Rosen, white men who raped black women often began by propositioning them, becoming violent only after a woman asserted that she was not available for casual sex. In doing so, they denied that black women—free or enslaved, married or single—possessed sexual boundaries worth observing. When this narrator publicized her attack in the moral reform press, she resisted the "gentlemen's" efforts to cast her as a prostitute and showed white moral reformers how the stereotype of promiscuity both incited and masked white-on-black sexual violence. She testified not only to her strength and resistance, but also to her vulnerability and suffering. She died of her injuries six months later.[38]

Such accounts made the moral reform movement meaningful to greater numbers of black working women. The reporters concealed their own identities for reasons of safety and job security, but felt it a "justice which we owe each other, to expose [the] names" of the powerful white men who had harassed or assaulted cooks, laundresses, or cleaners in their homes. The moral reform press alerted black women to the whereabouts of dangerous employers, citing, for example "wealthy merchants in Pearl street" known to target women of color. These descriptions served explicitly as a "Warning to Domestics."[39] Drawing attention to sexual harassment could not, in itself, transform the racial hierarchy of the labor market, which restricted the majority of black women to domestic work in the first place.[40] However, African American moral reformers used the available tools to shed light on the classed and raced dimensions of sexual exploitation in the North. In doing so, they further expanded the politics of licentiousness.

African American women in other cities, particularly those with active black abolitionist communities, also took greater interest in moral reform. In Cincinnati, for example, one white moral reformer marveled that the only efforts being made "to stop the progress of licentiousness, are those made among the colored people."[41] In New Haven, a "Colored Congregation" resolved to "do all in our power to reclaim the vicious and profligate."[42] Such intraracial activities are often interpreted as strategies for uplift. But in other cities, such as Boston and Philadelphia, black moral reformers followed the precedent set by Zion, cautiously engaging white women about the politics of licentiousness. Since abolitionists in those cities had integrated their female antislavery societies, they were more willing than Zion members to become members of interracial moral reform societies.

For example, black women took early leadership positions in the Boston Female Moral Reform Society and imbued it with their perspectives on the politics of licentiousness. Like their New York counterparts, Boston's black abolitionist women joined moral reform in the context of amalgamation riots. The most notorious of these, the 1835 mob of "gentlemen of property and standing," brought the Boston Female Moral Reform Society together with the Boston Female Anti-slavery Society. The original target of the riot had been George Thompson, a British abolitionist scheduled to address antislavery women. Newspaper editors had described "the handsome Mr. Thompson" as having an unseemly hold over "the *females*, who disgrace themselves by running after him." Such rhetoric represented Thompson as a mass seducer, just as editors elsewhere portrayed Sylvester Graham. The crowd's organizers therefore assumed that the same sort of women must be involved. Unable to find Thompson, they concluded that the moral reformers—a group of women who gathered to discuss sex and would therefore be receptive to the blandishments of an attractive foreigner—must have hidden him. "The meeting of the Ladies Moral Reform Society was thus broken up," even though the female antislavery society had been the original target.[43] Thereafter, Boston's female moral reform and female antislavery societies merged, and it was in this context that members became interested in the solitary vice.

Two activists, Lavinia Hilton, a black abolitionist, and Lydia Fuller, a white reformer, represent the interracial moment in moral reform. Having braved the 1835 riot and the 1837 mobbing of Sylvester Graham's "Lecture to Mothers," the two women joined the Boston Female Moral Reform Society's board of managers with the avowed intent of making the licentiousness of slavery an issue of concern to all women. Hilton and Fuller advocated for enslaved women within the national conventions of 1837 and 1838.[44] They also challenged amalgamation discourse by campaigning together for the repeal of Massachusetts's law against interracial marriage. Rather than expressing "natural repugnance" for interracial sex, they insisted, the "law of caste" maintained white supremacy and silenced dissenters.[45] Many white moral reformers joined the repeal efforts in 1839 because they believed that the law forced young women and men who would otherwise choose marriage into lawless licentiousness. Amalgamation rhetoric focused much more on the specter of courtship and marriage between white women and black men than on the reality of interracial sex in the brothels of New York, Boston, and Philadelphia, which catered primarily to white men. Prostitutes maximized their earning potential by manipulating and flattering, as well as physically pleasuring, their clients. Women deployed these tactics to negotiate the sexual marketplace, yet doing so necessarily reinforced white men's sexual power.[46] Female moral reformers pointed out that the same "licentious and polluted" rioters who attacked abolitionists also patronized the city's interracial brothels. Fuller and Hilton did not object to interracial unions per se; rather, they protested the social and legal processes that positioned black female sexuality as inherently illicit and available. While rejecting amalgamation discourse, they complained that northern white men sought out black women as mistresses.[47]

Other African Americans also found moral reform arguments useful, whether or not they formally joined the Boston Female Moral Reform Society. Nancy Gardner Prince, a black abolitionist best remembered for her extensive travels, spent most of her youth in domestic labor for various white New England families. She later married Nero Prince, a footman in the Russian imperial court, and went with him to Russia. After returning to the United States in 1833, she became a member of the Boston Female Antislavery Society. There she interacted with moral reformers, such as Lavinia Hilton, who introduced her to the politics of licentiousness.[48]

Prince's *Narrative* shows how African American women used moral reform language to critique race and class relations among women. Like the *Advocate*'s anonymous contributors, Prince challenged white moral reformers' glorification of domestic service. She recalled performing arduous work for low wages and experiencing severe physical abuse. Yet lacking better alternatives, she also placed her sister, Sylvia Gardner, in service "as a nursery girl." So miserable were the conditions of service, however, that Sylvia left to work in a brothel. The *Narrative* reversed white female moral reformers' assumption that placement in service would prevent a young woman from selling sex. The racially stratified market in domestic labor had itself precipitated Sylvia's "fall."[49]

In language echoing John R. McDowall's, Prince recounted how she had valiantly "rescued my lost sister." Yet rather than blaming a male seducer, Prince described a woman—"the mother of harlots"—who had "deluded" Sylvia into prostitution and then used violence to keep her from leaving.[50] Women, too, could wield corrupt sexual power over women: some employers abused domestic workers, others extracted profit from compulsory sexual labor. Prince had learned this from white housekeepers as well as her

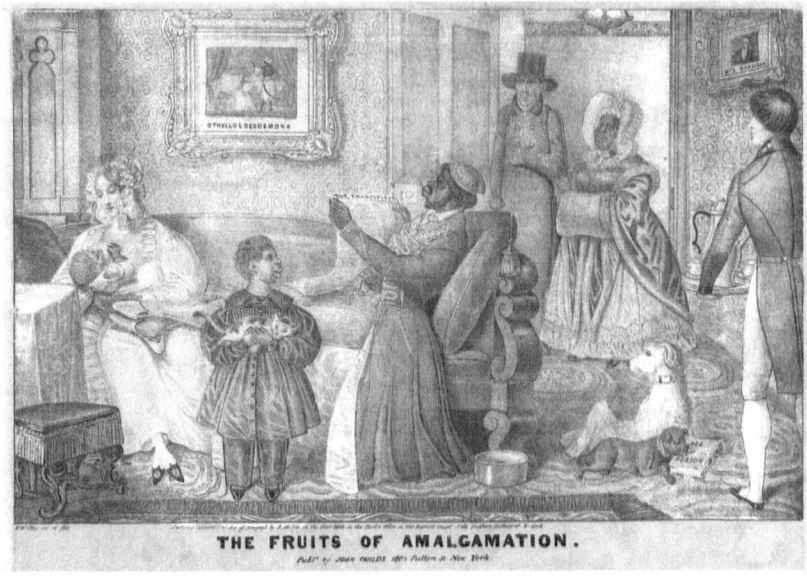

FIGURE 4. "The Fruits of Amalgamation," an Edward Clay cartoon (1839), portrayed a generic black husband as usurper, laying claim to a white wife as one of many middle-class possessions. In this domestic dystopia, a young white man has been reduced to domestic servitude. By contrast, the husband's African American mother enjoys mock refinement, the fruit of her new family connections. All told, the cartoon inverted the power dynamics of sexual commerce, which maintained white men's public and sexual dominance. (Courtesy of the American Antiquarian Society.)

sister's brothelkeeper. She redirected a common antislavery argument, that the licentiousness of slavery perverted mistresses' domestic authority into sadistic rage, toward northern white women.[51]

Above all, Nancy Prince's *Narrative* queried the concept of sexual purity itself. A devout Congregationalist, Prince objected to any breach of the seventh commandment on moral grounds. However, as Hazel Carby has argued, she did not consider her sister permanently lost because she had sold sex; rather, she welcomed Sylvia back into the family.[52] White female moral reformers, for their part, struggled with the issue of purity. The New York Female Moral Reform Society had made the "prevention, rather than remedy" of licentiousness a founding principle in 1834. Some believed that the first taste of sexual sin opened the floodgates to a "tide of pollution."[53] The emphasis on prevention assumed that this "pollution" could be checked only by defending "purity" at all costs. By contrast, Prince denied that the loss of sexual innocence forever debased a woman. Instead of purity, she and other black abolitionist women promoted *virtue*: an active, lifelong pursuit of righteousness and justice.

VIRTUE VERSUS PURITY

Nancy Prince was not the only African American moral reformer to distinguish virtue from purity. On the contrary, this idea permeated interracial moral reform networks during the late 1830s. Collapsed with whiteness and virginity, purity connoted a passive, fragile, bodily state. Virtue, on the other hand, indicated responsibility, intention, and active striving. Whereas purity could be "polluted" and thus lost forever, a virtuous individual could not be sullied by the actions of others. As the licentiousness of slavery became a pervasive theme in interracial abolitionism, it became necessary to emphasize that black women who experienced sexual coercion were not impure "Jezebels."[54] Rather, they demonstrated virtue by struggling to free themselves from systematized licentiousness and asserting their own dignity.

During the interracial moment in moral reform, the activist construction of female virtue took a radical turn. African American women convinced some of their white counterparts that modest—even virginal—white "ladies" might remain *pure* without ever becoming *virtuous*. Those who selfishly turned away from their "suffering colored sisters" were no "friends of virtue." By basking in the comforts of a privileged status rather than defending the bodily integrity of all women, they implicated themselves in systematized licentiousness. One southern politician frankly acknowledged that white women's purity hinged on the existence of a "class of females who . . . afford easy gratification to the hot passions of men."[55] From the black abolitionist perspective, until white women risked the protections and rewards that came with their reputation for purity, this system would proceed undisturbed. Because they had been trained to passivity, white women had to be convinced of their own moral accountability. Rather than embodying purity, white women needed to enact the politicized standard of virtue.

The white abolitionist Sarah M. Grimké became the most famous advocate of this reformulation. She forcefully argued that as "morally accountable beings," women must fight slavery though all available means. "Can any American woman look at these scenes of shocking licentiousness and cruelty, and fold her hands in apathy and say, 'I have nothing to do with slavery'?" she asked. *"She cannot and be guiltless."* Citing a woman who refused to sign antislavery petitions because "my husband does not approve of it," Grimké called the posture of wifely submission "a pretext to shield themselves from the performance of duty." Those who failed to stand up against slavery disobeyed God, "our Lawgiver, our King and our Judge," in order to please men. Placing the esteem of men above duty to God was idolatry, not righteous obedience. Thus, "with regard to all moral reformations, men and women have the same duties and the same rights."[56]

Historians have celebrated the ingenuity with which Grimké turned the argument for women's moral equality into a strong case for social, economic, and intellectual rights. Since "men and women were CREATED EQUAL," she argued, "whatever is *right* for man to do, is *right* for woman." Her sister, Angelina, made similar statements during her career as an antislavery lecturer. By linking women's moral duties to their rights, the Grimké sisters mobilized large numbers of white women even as they encountered fierce opposition. In a widely published "Pastoral Letter," conservative ministers condemned the sisters' public speaking as a departure from feminine modesty. They insisted that white women could best represent purity by shielding themselves from public debates. Women who strove for civic virtue only masculinized themselves. The division between champions of women's rights and defenders of male clerical authority split the antislavery movement in 1840.[57]

While the Grimké sisters certainly took heroic risks by arguing for women's moral equality, they should not be given sole credit for stirring women's consciousness. As we have seen, black moral reformers had insisted on white women's moral accountability since at least 1835. African Americans such as Grace Douglass, Sarah Mapps Douglass, Hetty Reckless, William Whipper, Hetty Burr, Robert Purvis, and Sarah Forten profoundly shaped the sisters' thinking about gender and sexuality. Angelina, the first sister to become an abolitionist, originally considered herself more a victim than a participant in oppression. While living with her slaveholding family in South Carolina, she felt slavery "a heavy burden to *my* heart" and groaned under "the evil *I* daily endure from Slavery." Her move north was not at first an antislavery mission but an "escape." Having observed her mother's violence against enslaved women and men, she concluded that "a Carolina Mistress was literally a Slave driver. . . . I tho't it degrading to the female character." By distancing herself from a corrupt system, she had protected her own feminine purity. When the American Anti-slavery Society formed in her adopted city, Angelina was busily touring seminaries, dispensing charity, debating theology, and contemplating marriage. Several months later, she concluded that it was not enough to be glad that she had freed herself from slaveholding and joined the biracial Philadelphia Female Anti-slavery Society.[58]

Sarah Grimké, who came to abolitionism later than Angelina, arrived at a more thorough understanding of black abolitionist women's sexual politics. She did so through earnest dialogue with Sarah Mapps Douglass, with whom she shared an unusually intimate and reciprocal interracial friendship. Having met Douglass through the Society of Friends before ever joining the Philadelphia Female Anti-slavery Society, Grimké struck up a "delicate dance of friendship" with her as early as 1835. Douglass had good reason to be cautious about befriending white abolitionist women. Her Quaker faith had long brought her into frequent contact with whites, but these interactions were often shallow and degrading. Philadelphia's Arch Street meeting relegated African Americans to a "bench for colored persons." In a New York meeting, a white Friend assumed that Sarah and Grace Douglass must be housekeepers accompanying their mistress. When they explained that they "did not live with anyone" as domestic workers, she told them to sit in a segregated balcony—had they been servants, they would have been seated with white women. Douglass also recalled bitterly that when her mother attended the funeral of a white Friend, she had not been allowed to ride in the carriage with other women (including white servants) but was made to walk behind with the men.[59]

Sarah and Grace Douglass introduced the Grimkés to Philadelphia's American Moral Reform Society, a black-led organization that pushed their thinking about the "licentiousness of slavery" and the meaning of sexual virtue. William Whipper and James Forten had conceived of the society while attending a Colored Convention in New York's Chatham Chapel in June 1834—just after the formation of the New York Female Moral Reform Society and before the amalgamation riots. This context convinced Whipper and Forten to refuse on principle to "recognize either nation or complexional distinctions." Their commitment to universal morality rather than black politics alienated other leaders, such as Samuel Cornish. However, many black women embraced Whipper's expansive vision and helped to launch auxiliaries in Harrisburg, Gettysburg, Cranberry, and Wilkes-Barre, Pennsylvania; Burlington, Salem, and Woodbury, New Jersey; Troy and Buffalo, New York; Providence, Rhode Island; and Washington, DC. Within the auxiliaries, African American women brought sexual politics to the fore, making "the transgression of the seventh commandment" a central agenda item. The parent society registered the influence of female moral reformers when it resolved that "licentious men should be held in the same disrepute as licentious women."⁶⁰ The phrase "licentious women" rejected inherent feminine purity and made virtue a universal pursuit.

It was within the meetings of the American Moral Reform Society that Sarah Grimké learned to distinguish "chastity" from virtue. Chastity involved mere "abstinence from . . . lust and indecency," which according to Whipper was an important but inadequate goal. Those sincerely concerned with "female virtue" must strive to "overthrow the accursed system of slavery," since it denied moral choice, as well as protection, to those enslaved.⁶¹ Some white abolitionist women (including Lucretia Mott, Mary Earle, and Anna Larcombe) formed a Philadelphia auxiliary to the New York Female Moral Reform Society, yet the Grimké sisters preferred to attend meetings of the American Moral Reform Society. Only there could they stretch their moral logic beyond the boundaries of their own experience.⁶² By 1837, Sarah Grimké considered it her duty to convince other white women that true morality meant something other than passive purity and denied the existence of "such a thing as male & female virtue."⁶³

Grimké began this undertaking at the First Antislavery Convention of American Women in New York, May 9–12, 1837, which Dorothy Sterling has called "the first interracial gathering of any consequence" in the United States. Angelina wrote to Boston and Philadelphia, pleading with the female antislavery societies to send African American delegates. Those who came, she assured, would experience respectful hospitality and exercise equal voting rights.⁶⁴ Moreover, the sisters took responsibility for confronting white women in New York about their "sinful prejudice." Angelina addressed the Ladies' Anti-slavery Society board of officers, calling prejudice "a canker worm among them" that "paralyzes every effort." The speech "was hard work," she reported, "but some were reached, I do believe, for tears were shed."⁶⁵

Meanwhile, Sarah Grimké brought the same analysis to the New York Female Moral Reform Society, adding the distinction between virtue and purity that grew out of her conversations with Douglass and other black abolitionist women. Those currently "sunk in misery & vice," she told white reformers, were not polluted or lost; they, too, could wear "the beautiful garments of virtue." As a result, the *Advocate of Moral Reform* published a retrospective of moral reform within the African Methodist Episcopal church and seated Zion delegates as equal participants in that year's national meeting. Only upon learning of these steps did Douglass begin to express a sense of ownership in the women's conventions.⁶⁶

Equally important, Grimké persuaded moral reformers to coordinate their regional meeting with the antislavery convention so the sisters could address both groups. On May 11, they would speak in the antislavery women's convention at New York's Third Free Church, then rush to Chatham Chapel, a few blocks away, and address the quarterly meeting of the New York Female Moral Reform Society. When the women's antislavery convention met, over a quarter of its delegates also held offices in their local female moral reform societies.[67]

African American women used the overlapping meetings of May 1837 to forge connections among themselves. At Chatham Chapel, Zion delegates Eliza Coker and Mary Johnson would have met Grace and Sarah Douglass and their friend Amy Matilda Cassey, the daughter of the Reverend Peter Williams. Boston reformers sent an interracial contingent that included Lydia Fuller and Julia Williams to both meetings. If Cassey, Coker, and Johnson recalled the profound impact of the 1834 riots, the Boston women would have been able to report their own experiences as targets of amalgamation rioters at the "Lecture to Mothers."[68]

Through one of the convention's publications, *The Appeal to the Women of the Nominally Free States*, a national readership of reform women learned the sexual counterdiscourse that black women had been formulating for the past two years. The *Appeal* is often attributed to Angelina Grimké, but Grace Douglass and Lydia Maria Child collaborated with her, and Sarah Douglass helped finance its publication.[69] This biracial cohort invoked licentiousness to persuade northern women that they had a moral duty to combat slavery and argued that "licentiousness is a crying sin at the North as well as at the South." Above all, the *Appeal* stressed white women's moral accountability. Combining the old rhetoric of male licentiousness with the new argument for female responsibility, the *Appeal* struck a nerve among white female moral reformers.[70]

In this context, Sarah Grimké worked the concept of moral accountability into a critique of sexual purity. Challenging "the distinction now so much insisted upon between male and female virtues," she argued that women could be just as licentious as men. Passive women colluded in a double standard that enabled male "license" yet demanded female "modesty and delicacy." While female moral reformers deplored the sexual double standard, even they sometimes fell into its trap. "We habitually speak of the crime of licentiousness, as if man were the aggressor, and as if his sin was far greater than that of woman; but where be the proof of this?" Grimké demanded. Quite convinced that women and men possessed a similar "sensual appetite," she rejected the idea that a male seducer must be responsible for any woman's own descent into licentiousness. To presume "licentious men most to blame" was to admit that men inherently possessed "more of that spirit which enables us to resist temptation." In sexual life as in activism, *resistance*—not *passionlessness*—determined virtue.[71]

Just as virtue knew no sex, according to Grimké, it also knew no color. All women possessed an equal capacity for virtue, if not the same freedom to exercise it. Caught in systematized licentiousness, the enslaved woman who "desires to preserve her virtue unsullied," who "dares resist her seducer," risked her life. Grimké bitterly contrasted enslaved women's virtue amid these constraints against the putative "moral purity" of southern white women. A woman of the slaveholding class, she pointed out, learned to witness "the virtue of her enslaved sister sacrificed without hesitancy or remorse." In the eyes of God, however, it was the slaveholding woman who "bartered away her virtue"—not the enslaved woman "who resists every attempt at seduction but who falls an unwilling victim to brutal lust." Left without recourse, she remained "unsullied in the sight of the Searcher of hearts . . . as innocent as if no act of violence had been perpetrated upon her."[72] Enslaved or free, no woman could be "robbed of her virtue." By privileging moral virtue over physical purity, Grimké not only argued for gender equality, she directly challenged the Jezebel stereotype that specifically harmed black women.

This intervention earned black moral reformers' respect. When the sisters traveled across New England in the summer of 1837, African American members of the Seaman's Moral Reform Society met them for tea, prayer, and discussion.[73] Nancy Prince, who likely encountered Sarah Grimké in Boston that year, endorsed her reading of Genesis: "He made man in his own image, in the image of God, created he him, male and female."[74] In Philadelphia, William Whipper invited the sisters to address the American Moral Reform Society three times and affirmed the sisters' principle that "what is morally right for a man to do, is morally right for women."[75] Not all black abolitionists supported women's rights; Samuel Cornish and Jehiel C. Beman, for example, disapproved.[76] But among those specifically committed to changing the dominant sexual culture, the Grimké sisters proved valuable allies.

White moral reform women, for their part, grappled openly with the new interpretations of licentiousness and virtue. The *Advocate* printed exchanges between Sarah Grimké and her male and female critics, and the *Friend of Virtue*, organ of the Boston Female Moral Reform Society, ran a series of critical letters interspersed with statements of support for the *Letters on the Equality of the Sexes*.[77] Ultimately, the distinction between virtue and purity proved more unsettling to female moral reformers than did Grimké's feminism. While they shared outrage against masculine license, they debated whether moral superiority and sexual passionlessness defined white womanhood. Having staked their ability to lead a social movement on what many considered a special relationship to morality, white women now had to consider whether they actually shared their cherished moral sense not only with men but also with women of color. Dealing directly with their own accountability also proved much more daunting than merely protesting shared victimization.

Female moral reform societies considered whether women such as themselves might be culpable in licentiousness, as Ruggles and Grimké had argued. In the first issue of the *Advocate*, Sarah Towne Smith had used the word *licentious* to describe sexually erring women as well as male seducers. Her colleague Sarah R. Ingraham scratched out the word *licentious* again and again in her copy, suggesting *profligate* instead when describing both genders.[78] Her discomfort intensified when the word directly described female behavior. Where Smith had written "woman cannot *be licentious* and still retain her standing in respectable society," Ingraham proposed, "woman cannot *sell her virtue* and still retain her standing in respectable society." Thereafter, Ingraham and Smith reached a détente: the *Advocate* generally described men as licentious in recognition of the power imbalance between the sexes.

But Sarah Grimké raised the question of female sexual responsibility for wider discussion. Could women—white, Christian women—be licentious? Did blaming men actually "increase the evils which moral reform societies are intended to lessen?" As tiny female moral reform societies formed across the Northeast, they drafted new constitutions and reports querying white women's moral and sexual accountability. New converts increasingly categorized "the licentious" by sexual behavior rather than by gender. Rural auxiliaries openly considered the possibility that women such as themselves might be licentious. One wondered, "Might not this appalling ruin have included even *yourselves*?—for Christianity teaches the humbling doctrine that . . . the purest are, *in no wise*, no better than the vile."[79] Another disowned "persons of either sex, known to be licentious," while still others put "the licentious of both sexes on a level." Virtue did not come automatically: both sexes struggled to keep their "flesh in subjection." Eventually, the New York Female Moral Reform Society adopted its national members' language of "placing licentious men on a level with licentious women." Recognizing "our own responsibilities," they asked male supporters to concede "no superiority, but only equality."[80]

Following this logic, rural societies wrote their constitutions around pledges, modeled on those of temperance societies, that explicitly required respectable merchants for employ, has found himself the object of so much public displeasure, that he has been obliged to leave the city. Now, all we want is, to bring public sentiment, stripped of its false delicacy, to bear upon the licentious, and they will be driven from all society but their own, and the mark of Cain will be put on them wherever they go. It will be one object we shall have in view to strengthen and extend this correct public sentiment, and bring it to bear in all its weight upon the head of the guilty.

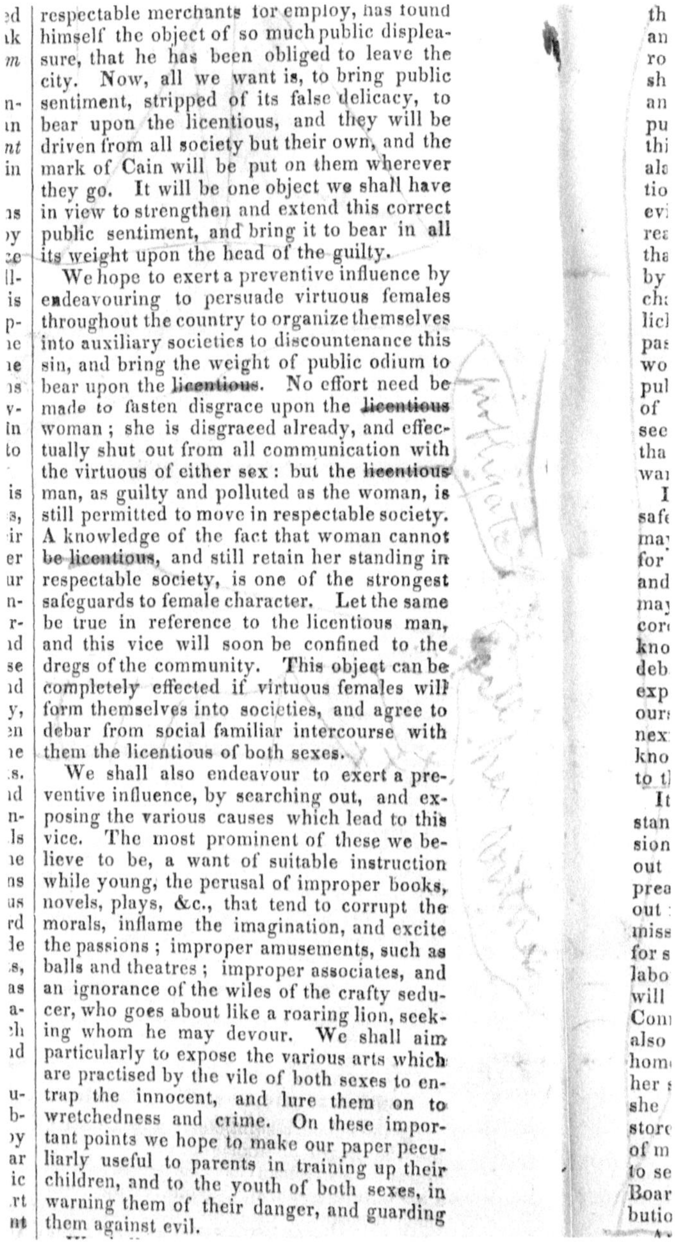

We hope to exert a preventive influence by endeavouring to persuade virtuous females throughout the country to organize themselves into auxiliary societies to discountenance this sin, and bring the weight of public odium to bear upon the licentious. No effort need be made to fasten disgrace upon the licentious woman; she is disgraced already, and effectually shut out from all communication with the virtuous of either sex: but the licentious man, as guilty and polluted as the woman, is still permitted to move in respectable society. A knowledge of the fact that woman cannot be licentious, and still retain her standing in respectable society, is one of the strongest safeguards to female character. Let the same be true in reference to the licentious man, and this vice will soon be confined to the dregs of the community. This object can be completely effected if virtuous females will form themselves into societies, and agree to debar from social familiar intercourse with them the licentious of both sexes.

We shall also endeavour to exert a preventive influence, by searching out, and exposing the various causes which lead to this vice. The most prominent of these we believe to be, a want of suitable instruction while young, the perusal of improper books, novels, plays, &c., that tend to corrupt the morals, inflame the imagination, and excite the passions; improper amusements, such as balls and theatres; improper associates, and an ignorance of the wiles of the crafty seducer, who goes about like a roaring lion, seeking whom he may devour. We shall aim particularly to expose the various arts which are practised by the vile of both sexes to entrap the innocent, and lure them on to wretchedness and crime. On these important points we hope to make our paper peculiarly useful to parents in training up their children, and to the youth of both sexes, in warning them of their danger, and guarding them against evil.

FIGURE 5. Sarah Ingraham's markup of the first volume of the *Advocate of Moral Reform*. (Courtesy of the American Antiquarian Society.)

members to monitor their own behavior and that of their peers. "We must strive to divest our minds from all indelicate, lewd and unprofitable thoughts," promised Grafton reformers, for "impurity of thought is the secret channel to the ocean of licentiousness." Women in Peterboro, New York, pledged "ourselves to refrain from all licentious conversation." Moral reformers in Rindge, New Hampshire, concluded that the success of the entire movement depended on whether "those now engaged will only keep the heart *pure* (difficult but possible)." By 1840, most moral reformers held that, like men, they themselves were equally prone to licentiousness or virtue.[81] This fundamental transformation in women's sexual politics spread with the growth of female moral reform societies and female antislavery societies throughout the countryside. It proved as powerful as Sylvester Graham's physiology in preparing large numbers of white women to apply the logic of solitary vice to their own lives.

CONCLUSION

African American women joined the female moral reform movement while it was still in its infancy. Together with male supporters such as David Ruggles, William Whipper, and James Forten, they profoundly shaped the movement's sexual politics. Their signal counterdiscourse, the licentiousness of slavery, blended the language of moral reform with the goals of black abolitionists so effectively that it exceeded the movement and took on a life of its own. The results were mixed. On the one hand, female antislavery societies and petition drives gained personnel and resources by persuading thousands of white women that the battle against licentiousness must also be a struggle against slavery. On the other hand, the images of enslaved women as victims of sexual abuse overshadowed other aspects of black women's oppression and, at times, reinforced stereotypes.

Meanwhile, many white moral reformers rethought their own relationship to morality. As accountable beings, they learned to strive for active virtue rather than to passively embody sexual purity. When Sarah Grimké withdrew from lecturing to help her newly married sister manage her health and household, others picked up her message. For example, Sarah Towne Smith described enslaved women as "our sisters—'bone of our bone, and flesh of our flesh.'" White women who crusaded against licentiousness must become accountable for the abolition of slavery. "The whole sex has been insulted and degraded in their persons, and she who turns coldly away from their bitter cry, is a traitor to the holy cause of female honor and virtue." Similarly, Mary Ann Brown argued that northern white women owed recompense for "the blood of the suffering slave—the price of virtue lost . . . because they have dwelt so long at ease in the midst of these abominations, and have even sustained them by precept and example."[82]

However, the demand for white female accountability shaded into an exaggerated sense of leadership. As white moral reformers increasingly identified themselves as protectors and defenders of all women from sexual predation, they reasserted a privileged relationship to virtue. The female moral reform society of Gardner, Massachusetts, lamented that "the poor victims of slavery are compelled to be impure by unprincipled and licentious masters," adding, "Can we remain inactive?"[83] Though able to see themselves as moral agents, they paid more attention to enslaved women's victimization than to the activism of free women of color. The distinction between purity and virtue also eluded many white women when it came to slavery. The constant refrain "our colored sisters in bonds, who have no legal protection for their virtue," harkened back to the belief that virtue could be lost—that it was a fragile, corporeal state.[84] White women's privileged claim to sexual morality, whether framed in terms of passive purity or active virtue, depended on black women's debasement.

It did not take long for this dynamic to shake African American women's faith in the potential benefits of this coalition. As the interracial moment in moral reform drew to a close, white women turned inward, applying the notion of active virtue primarily to their own capacity for sexual self-control. The next chapter documents white female moral reformers' campaign against the solitary vice. Black women continued to connect virtue to political activism by launching separate moral reform institutions in which they mobilized against slavery, in defense of northern fugitives, and for an improved quality of life. As we shall see, some invoked the solitary vice to justify and camouflage intraracial discussions of fertility control and sexual pleasure. Having encountered the discourse on solitary vice in lectures they attended during the interracial moment in moral reform, they used it to mask their own daring explorations of sexual subjectivity.

CHAPTER THREE

Making the Conversation General

"Great caution is needed to preserve true delicacy," lectured Mary Gove, "but false delicacy will do no good, but much hurt."[1] By 1838, when Gove lectured throughout New England on physiology, she imagined the falsely delicate as a group much larger than libertines and slaveholders. Rural white women, even moral reformers themselves—the supposed exemplars of passionlessness—exhibited false delicacy when they blamed men for rampant licentiousness but avoided confronting their own sexual desires. If these women were to conquer that "morbid" delicacy, they must not only be willing to speak about sexual politics, as abolitionists had demanded for the past several years. They must also learn about the physiological basis of their sexual feelings so that they could honestly confront their passions. Only after having been thus trained for true virtue could they embody both individuality and self-governance. A shiver of shared guilt and pleasure must have coursed through Gove's audience, for they responded with enthusiasm.

During the 1830s and 1840s, the growing female moral reform network—increasingly composed of white, rural women—helped to move the solitary vice from the margins of reform to the center of nineteenth-century culture. By midcentury, it would become America's dominant sexual obsession. A full generation before most medical doctors concerned themselves seriously with masturbation, thousands of evangelical women disseminated proscriptions against solitary vice through reform physiology. The trend began when the Ladies' Physiological Society of Boston (1837–41) decided to sidestep the riots that hampered their attempts to hear Sylvester Graham's "Lecture to Mothers." Instead of relying on a single male celebrity, they encouraged women to spread the word. They sponsored Mary Gove as "Graham in Petticoats" and helped make the "lecture to ladies on anatomy and physiology" a pervasive part of popular culture. Society members learned the precepts of reform physiology and the practice of public speaking, then followed in Gove's footsteps. Meanwhile, rural women formed hundreds of female moral reform societies throughout New England and upstate New York. Around fifty thousand women joined these societies between 1835 and 1840—just in time to learn that "where social licentiousness has slain its thousands . . . solitary vice has slain its tens of thousands." As female physiological lecturers traveled from one rural moral reform society to the next, women throughout the Northeast grew convinced that "to the moral reformer, Solitary Vice is a subject of deep and thrilling interest." Cities seethed with licentiousness, as everyone knew, but "this hydra sin" thrived even in the countryside. Members embraced the new physiology not because it seemed to demonstrate women's inherent purity, but because renouncing the solitary vice empowered every individual to govern her own flesh. Because this argument entered so many small-town societies during their formation, it struck many moral reform converts as a foundational tenet.[2]

Small-town female moral reform societies remade their meetings into confessional spaces in which members could rigorously pursue self-discipline, their new measure of *true* delicacy. An individual confessed her prior sexual errors, and after she demonstrated her personal reform, the group affirmed her moral worth. This process of abjection—of ridding oneself of the solitary vice—rewarded white women with a new sense of themselves as powerful individuals. In this way, they made the solitary vice into a dominant discourse, a compulsory precondition for legitimizing any kind of sexual speech.

At the same time, the crusade against the solitary vice gave rise to an ideology of sexual citizenship that powerfully shaped the nineteenth-century women's rights movement. Just as physiology provided a scientific argument for sexual equality, antimasturbation discourse provided a safe template for asserting women's equal capacity for virtue or vice. Without calling themselves Grahamites or becoming vegetarians, thousands of white women adopted the sexual principles of reform physiology. Aiming "to make the conversation general," they loudly shunned the solitary vice as a sign of their knowledge, virtue, and civil worth.[3] Thousands of ordinary white women both spread antimasturbation discourse and transformed its meanings along the way. The framework of sexual citizenship demanded sexual conformity as proof of civic virtue.

The crucible of opposition that had forged a radical critique of white feminine purity during the 1830s cooled over the next decade. Without a male scapegoat to target, libertine republicans stopped rioting. Female moral reformers lost their urgent need to challenge the very root of libertine republicanism. White women turned away from deep questioning of racialized sexual ideologies, such as licentiousness and purity. As the voices of rural white women grew louder and increasingly turned to issues of sexual selfhood, those of African Americans—whose ability to organize was concentrated in cities—were nearly drowned out in the moral reform journals. In 1840, a conflict over the priorities of the movement alienated the small but vocal minority of African American women who had been so influential in transforming the ideology of female virtue. The interracial moment in moral reform drew to a close. Black women redirected their energies to separate institutions where they continued to struggle against racial and gender oppression while also envisioning alternative models of sexual health and morality. As black women moved into separate campaigns and institutions, white moral reformers embraced the pleasures of belonging in intimate groups that rewarded sexual conformity.

In 1845, a second fracture alienated white abolitionists and women's rights advocates, leaving behind a movement whose "sole object" was "the promotion of moral purity."[4] Leaders such as Sarah Ingraham and Catherine Kilton declared themselves "guardians" of the nation's purity. First, they reinstated the "rescue" model in national moral reform organizations by building houses of refuge and industry. Second, they channeled what remained of the "prevention" philosophy toward petitioning states to criminalize seduction.[5] Those laws, originally framed as assaults on the sexual double standard, came to represent a shift back toward assumptions of white feminine passionlessness. If would-be seducers faced prosecution, the theory went, young and innocent (white) women would be protected from their first fall. Moral guardians gradually distanced themselves from the solitary vice. Rather than battling their own sexual desires, they struggled to instill discipline in unruly others: young, poor, and colonized people. The guardians wrested control of the national moral reform societies and journals. As a result, they have eclipsed their former colleagues in historical memory.

First in a united moral reform movement, then in separate campaigns for women's rights and moral guardianship, northern white women made themselves the nation's foremost purveyors of antimasturbation physiology between 1837 and 1845.

THE LADIES' PHYSIOLOGICAL SOCIETY OF BOSTON

The Ladies' Physiological Society of Boston, which organized to promote popular physiological education for women on a large scale, also brought the crusade against solitary vice into rural female moral reform societies and modeled how women ought to engage with this subject.[6] The society formed in response to the anti-Graham riots at Boston's "Lecture to Mothers" in March 1837. Rather than forming a mere "Graham association," leading reform women of Boston chose to dispense with Sylvester Graham as a figurehead and to take the helm of reform physiology.

Having repeatedly faced off with rioters, female reformers had learned by 1837 that they would need to organize in order to effectively counter their attackers. A small group of experienced activists—Susan Sears, Abigail White, Sylvia Cambell, and Louisa Purdy—met at the Marlboro Hotel and coordinated their plan of action during the predicted riot. Among other tactics, they chose physical confrontation with rioters. They knew that the spectacle of women fighting back against the crowd attracted newspapermen. Editors, interested in selling papers, recounted the "parley" between rakes and reformers. This gave women a valuable opportunity to name the rioters and expose their false delicacy to the readers of all the daily papers. After Graham arrived and the mob sent him into hiding, the organizers reconvened. Although rioters had succeeded in stopping the lecture, the women sensed that they had turned the tide of publicity. They "came to a conclusion that it would be profitable to meet as often as once a month" and formed a Ladies' Physiological Society for that purpose.

Like the New York Female Moral Reform Society, the Ladies' Physiological Society began as an auxiliary of an all-male organization but quickly sparked a broader, feminized movement. The male American Physiological Society formed after Graham delivered his "Lecture to Young Men" in Boston. William Andrus Alcott, a Yale-educated physician and cousin of A. Bronson Alcott, became its first president and guiding spirit. Alcott had also warned young men against solitary vice in his 1833 *Young Man's Guide* and nursed a priority dispute with Graham over the topic. He hoped to make reform physiology more empirical and to lead a following of his own. Alcott did not subscribe to the model of ultra manhood that aimed to share power with women. He acknowledged the Ladies' Physiological Society's "habit" of meeting separately each month but considered it auxiliary and subordinate. The American Physiological Society's constitution made "provision for the admission of female members"—but only as "mothers and housewives." Women were "indispensable" to reform, for it was they who baked bread, that singularly Grahamite "staff of life."[7]

Women, meanwhile, considered their physiological society independent, instituted with distinctive bylaws, elected officers, and auxiliaries of its own. Members demonstrated again and again that they embraced reform physiology not as an extension of "the household hearth" but to satisfy individual curiosity, religious conviction, and political allegiance. Although Alcott referred to the Ladies' Physiological Society as the wives and mothers of his male disciples, members were more likely to be *single* than to be married to a man in the American Physiological Society. A large majority knew one another through work, activism, or neighborhood connections. Women joined the Ladies' Physiological Society to network and organize with other women in their lives, not merely to improve their housewifery.[8]

The conditions under which the Ladies' Physiological Society formed gave its members an outlook different from that of male Grahamites. Public venues remained open to the American Physiological Society's lectures. On the same day that John Codman barred Graham from giving the "Lecture to Mothers" in Amory Hall, he opened its doors to the American Physiological Society and even became a member of that organization. Codman would host male physiological meetings for the next three years at Amory Hall, while the women (including his wife, Rebecca Codman) found it necessary—due to riots and exclusion, not a preference for domesticity—to meet in members' homes.[9] Though spatially constrained, women found themselves free within those spaces to openly discuss physiology and sexual health in protected, intimate settings.

Rather than continuing to defend Sylvester Graham's embattled lecture career, the Ladies' Physiological Society concentrated on peer education in women-only meetings. Placing themselves at the center of reform physiology's utopian potential, they created a support network and disciplinary regimen in which members could cultivate virtue through bodily management. This intimate, confessional peer education model proved alluring.

Boston women made frank, confessional discussions central to physiological reform. Shortly after the society formed, members voted to pass three strict bylaws that required each woman to testify aloud before the group to her past failings and current struggles. First, "The names of all the ladies belonging to the society" would "be arranged in Alphabetical order and called upon in order to give some account of their health before and since adopting the Graham system." Second, "Any lady shall feel privileged to ask the speaker such questions as concern the cause we serve." Finally, "No lady [shall] feel at liberty to refuse when called upon."[10] This arrangement defined the work of the society primarily in terms of supporting those who feared that their own path to physiological righteousness would be pitted with temptations and who sought the discipline of the group as an aid to reform. In addition, the Ladies appointed a "visiting committee whose duty it shall be to visit the absent members of the Society and enquire the cause of nonattendance if absent more than one meeting." Once a woman signed on, she could only opt out of the group's surveillance with great effort.

The men of the American Physiological Society neither shared nor understood the women's intense introspection. Although men also delivered testimonials, they did so as carefully crafted public performances. For example, Simeon Collins, a bookseller and founding member, reported his "experience in the Graham System" at a meeting of "not less than from three to four hundred." Sylvester Graham visited him beforehand and directed him to prepare a statement that could be heard by women as well as men. Collins testified that, having abstained from meat and coffee for four years, he experienced perfect health, happiness, and activity. He also incorporated his family's experiences into his own account: "At the time of entering upon this system I had a wife and five children, the youngest eight years of age, they all soon entered upon the same course of living with myself, and were soon all benefitted in health." Because white male bodies already signaled individuality and self-control in the dominant society, American Physiological Society members spent little time proving their self-mastery. Instead, Collins represented himself as a benevolent patriarch who led the dependents in his family into health as seamlessly as if they were appendages of his own body.[11]

Women, on the other hand, treasured their testimonial culture precisely because it enabled them to separate their own bodily needs and experiences from those of their husbands and children. Significantly, they did not testify at the behest of male authorities. On the contrary, Simeon's wife, Cynthia, declined Graham's request that she record her experiences of pregnancy and childbirth for a mass audience. Moreover, she resisted her husband's pressure to comply, even though her account would have strengthened the "Lecture to Mothers," which Simeon hoped to publish at a large profit.[12] Health reform women did not shun publicity from a sense of feminine propriety. As we have seen, they intentionally drew reporters' attention during the riots, circulated petitions, and published their own resolutions. Instead, women such as Cynthia Collins preferred to testify to their individual physiological reform in intimate, all-female spaces. Like the consciousness-raising groups of the 1970s, these meetings encouraged members to identify common experiences and interrogate the power relationships they reflected. Their discussions of physiology took place against the backdrop of the critique of male license. Testimonial meeting culture undoubtedly politicized members' perceptions of sexual vice and virtue.

Perhaps for this reason, some men in the American Physiological Society wished that women would spend less time testifying and more time reading physiology books written by credible authorities. John Kilton, secretary of the American Physiological Society, argued that "the thirst for information" contained in books should "not be less intense than it is for information by conversation and lectures." William Alcott, for his part, condemned women who addressed even all-female groups. Though a supporter of moral reform, he ridiculed women "figuring away in public," and believed that they should keep silent in the churches. Nevertheless, the Ladies' Physiological Society voted down such directives. Instead of reading, they would continue "to make [meetings] interesting without books."[13] Their intimate, interactive meeting culture worked because it was—in a word—stimulating.

The testimonials also trained women to "stand and speak" about physiology and paved the way for some to lecture on sexual matters. In July of 1838, a rising star named Mary Gove contacted the Boston society to propose a course of physiological "Lectures to Ladies" by one of their own. Male physiological reformers may have underestimated the Ladies' Physiological Society, but Gove recognized its members as key power brokers in Boston's reform culture. She submitted her syllabus for their review—"subject to amendment and alterations which may occur to the Society." The lectures would include "physiological facts of a delicate nature . . . which many Ladies married and single cannot bring themselves to hear from a gentleman."[14]

Graham had argued that solitary vice "is not confined to males," and Gove agreed: "Woman is by nature *no* more chaste than man." But because rioters repeatedly suppressed the "Lecture to Mothers," it would take a female lecturer to persuade them. The *Graham Journal* accepted that solitary vice, the "canker worm of death," threatened women as much as men. "But how to introduce it to all the world of both sexes, is the query?" Boston's whole physiological subculture saw that the "Lecture to Ladies" would meet this need. Even William Alcott threw his support behind Gove. If backed by the Ladies, Gove would secure a public venue in which women could discuss sex without a troublesome male speaker behind the lectern. She would convince greater numbers of women than ever that solitary vice was as much a "sin against nature" as "a sin against heaven." And, knowing her audience, Gove guaranteed that "a faithful exposition of these abuses will be given."[15]

The offer of juicy testimonials hit its mark. The Ladies' Physiological Society appointed a committee of arrangements to promote Gove's course. Sylvia Cambell led the committee, advertising tickets through her husband David's *Graham Journal* and selling them out of the *Zion's Herald* office.

As for "alterations" to the original lecture plan, Ladies' Physiological Society officers requested *more* detail, not less. Gove obliged them by adding a completely new lecture. The "Lectures to Ladies" proved a smashing success. Graham had had been unable to collect intimate testimonials from women, but the women in Gove's audiences were primed by their experiences as members of the Ladies' Physiological Society. Testifiers declared that, compelled by overheated systems, they had practiced the solitary vice while ignorant of the physical and moral harm it wrought. Now, they suffered disease as a consequence. The lack of such intimate information had prevented Sylvester Graham from publishing the "Lecture to Mothers." Now women came forward to help Mary Gove compile her own *Lectures to Ladies on Anatomy and Physiology*. Announcing that they no longer required a male authority to guide them away from sexual vice, female reformers launched a woman-run, woman-centered lecture circuit that lasted for more than two decades.

Soon, the demand for physiology lectures proved greater than Gove could satisfy. Two members of the Ladies' Physiological Society's visiting committee, Rebecca Eaton and Abigail Ordway, extended their travels into nearby towns to inform curious but unconverted women about physiological reform. Mary Ann Johnson, a manager in the Ladies' Physiological Society, also became a lecturer in her own right. All three women introduced listeners, who had never heard Sylvester Graham lecture, to the consequences of solitary vice. The turn inward appealed strongly to more women than ever before. Women in Worcester, Millbury, Lynn, Holliston, and Bangor formed auxiliaries to the Ladies' Physiological Society. By the time the Boston women elected Susan Sears "to write to the various health societies as soon as she is furnished with their addresses," physiological societies ranged from Maine to Ohio. New York reformers saw "the Female Physiological Society of Boston" as "the sheet anchor of the cause in that city.'"[16]

As women attained adherents on the physiological lecture circuit, male Grahamites toasted "Woman, the hope of our cause," with pure cold water. But members of the Ladies' Physiological Society were not content with lip service. They asserted their equality with—and autonomy from—male reformers. In 1839, "a Female member of the Society," demanded, "What is the duty assigned to woman as a member of the American Physiological Society?" Were the Ladies an independent society? If so, they expected freedom from the men's impositions. Or were men ready to fuse the two groups? In that case, they would expect to vote in the general meetings, including for female officers. Either way, the time had come to bury the women's auxiliary image. The men debated this question at "some length," before voting to recognize women's "equal rights, according to the Constitution."[17]

Six days after men voted for inclusion, about sixty women "literally packed" Sarah Perry's boardinghouse to articulate their vision for the new, cogendered American Physiological Society. Delegates traveled from ladies' physiological societies in New York and Worcester to have their say at this critical gathering. The first order of business, now that women could vote in the American Physiological Society, would be "to send up a remonstrance" against the constitution's "clause relating to making bread." They appointed a committee consisting of Rebecca Codman, Sylvia Cambell, Susan Sears, Susan Fitz, Nancy Hobart Prince, and Mehitable Blasland for that purpose.[18]

Yet despite this apparent unity, a few members of the original women's group resisted the push for organizational equality. A serious division within the Boston Female Anti-slavery Society over women's rights spilled over into the Ladies' Physiological Society. The health reformers most committed to "abridging the constitution so as to make it more convenient for the use of the ladies of the society" tended to agitate for women's equal membership within the antislavery movement as well. Garrisonian abolitionists such as Mary Ann Johnson, Helen Garrison, Lydia Fuller, and Abigail Ordway promoted physiology from an incipient feminist standpoint. However, the Ladies' Physiological Society also included clerical abolitionists—those who deferred to their ministers and preferred complementary, rather than equal, roles with men—including Lucy and Eliza Parker, Clarissa Leavitt, and Lydia Lathrop. One of the clerical abolitionists, Catherine Kilton, moved to reconsider amending the constitution. Kilton prided herself on her housewifery and, rather than agitating for women's rights, looked forward to the day when "the whole earth shall become willing subjects to the laws of God."[19] With neither side able to capture a majority, "the subject was indefinitely postponed." The Ladies' Physiological Society never regained the momentum it had enjoyed immediately prior to the antislavery split. Secretary Rebecca Codman recorded her final entry into the record book of the society on July 14, 1840. Strongly held political convictions had incited women to organize the Ladies' Physiological Society; the same convictions, when conflicting, also caused its demise.[20]

With the dissolution of the American Physiological Society in 1841, female physiological reformers moved in different directions. Secretary Rebecca Codman opened a Grahamite boardinghouse in Newton, Massachusetts. Sylvia Cambell went west to Oberlin with her husband, David, where they administered the Graham system to students at the nation's first college to admit African Americans and white women. Mary Ann Johnson moved to Providence with her abolitionist husband, Oliver. She continued to educate herself on recent physiological research and in 1850 cofounded with Paulina Wright Davis the Providence Physiological Society, a peer-education group that advocated for women's rights. In the meantime, Rebecca Eaton and Abigail Ordway continued to spread reform physiology and the campaign against the solitary vice through the female moral reform societies of the rural Northeast.

INTO THE HINTERLANDS

As early as 1833, rural women formed small societies dedicated to purging their communities of licentiousness. When the New York Female Moral Reform Society formed, rural women immediately addressed it as their "parent society." "Although we live in a country retired from the commotions of a populous city," wrote reformers in Gustavus, Ohio, "we considered it our duty to associate." Remote from "that *system* of iniquity which abounds in your city," rural women tended to emphasize personal improvement. In the process, they discovered "appalling facts among ourselves."[21]

Such communications encouraged the New York Female Moral Reform Society to envision itself as the director of a national women's movement. It hired lecturing agents to meet with rural women and encourage them to write local constitutions based on that of the New York society. Auxiliaries helped to fund operations by purchasing "life memberships" for one or more local officers in the parent society. They also purchased bulk subscriptions to the *Advocate*, using the paper to initiate conversations about sex within their communities. The annual reports of these societies crowded the pages of the newspaper, inspiring women in neighboring towns to form groups of their own and shaping the messages transmitted via the national network. They overwhelmingly endorsed physiological reform in general and Mary Gove's lectures in particular.

Auxiliaries, which proliferated at exactly the same time that Mary Gove, Rebecca Eaton, and Abigail Ordway began to popularize physiology among reform women, shaped the direction of the female moral reform movement. The Boston Female Moral Reform Society proved especially important in the early years, for many of its officers had experienced anti-Graham riots or attended Ladies' Physiological Society meetings. They resolved that "a knowledge of physiology and anatomy, is eminently calculated to aid in the cause of Moral Reform" and urged every society "to make special efforts to avail themselves" of physiological lectures. In 1838, Boston women launched the *Friend of Virtue* as a regional organ, and physiology melded further with moral reform. Every editor of the *Friend* from 1838 until 1851 took part in the Ladies' Physiological Society. Meanwhile, the physiological lecturers who traveled into the hinterlands played a formative role in creating ever more moral reform societies. As they had done in their own city, they encouraged women who attended the lectures to testify to their experiences of ill health caused by sexual and dietary excess. New auxiliaries replicated the intimate meeting culture of the Ladies' Physiological Society in town after town.[22]

For their part, rural women expressed an acute interest in physiology through newspapers, at lectures, and in intimate testimonial meetings. Because most towns lacked the libraries, bookstores, and lecture halls enjoyed by reformers in Boston and New York, they approached the *Advocate* and the *Friend* as sources of physiological education. Members frequently shared a few subscriptions among themselves, reading them aloud in meetings to inspire reflection and debate. In this way, they could break the monotony of life in villages such as Sheffield, Ohio—depressingly remote from active battlefields such as New York's Five Points district or Boston's Tremont Theater. Members trekked several miles simply to "read on the subject" and pray together.[23] Slogging through the snow to attend meeting after meeting, rural women prized the all-female spaces they were creating.

During the long months between visitors, the members of small societies met primarily to exchange their own accounts of illness, conversion, and recovery. The Grafton Female Moral Reform Society, with twenty-eight members in 1842, typified this intimate subculture. One member, Abigail Read, described the power of testimonials. Prior to her conversion, Read had fallen terribly ill. Thankfully, "an angel of mercy embodied in a female friend appeared" to her and imparted the "physiological truths" that had inspired her own conversion. Read's initiation into moral reform culture convinced her that accounts of the "recuperative agency" of reform physiology "ought not in justice to be withheld" from other women. These revelations converted others and transformed an austere regimen into a practice that felt "almost recreative." Rural moral reformers soon considered their individual efforts equal to the flashier campaigns conducted by "those dear sisters who are laboring in the city." In Grafton, Massachusetts, reformers argued that by cultivating their own virtue, they stemmed the tide of young women who moved to cities and sold sex, for "as is the mother so is the daughter."[24]

Physiological reform included temperance, dietetic restraint, and the abandonment of tightly laced corsets. But readers of the *Advocate* and the

Friend particularly craved information about the consequences of sexual mismanagement—in themselves as well as in licentious men and errant youth. For this reason, both moral reform journals published Mary Gove's serialized article on solitary vice, "To Parents, Guardians, and Those Who Have the Care of Children."[25] Like Sylvester Graham's "Lecture to Mothers," the title had rhetorical power, but actual motherhood did not in itself account for the appeal of physiology in the female moral reform societies. Gove's most vocal proponents were unabashedly not mothers. Take, for example, Maria Lincoln, a thirty-eight-year-old unmarried white woman. Lincoln made special arrangements for unmarried women to attend Gove's separate lectures on sex and the solitary vice. She lived with her brother Noah, sister-in-law Abby, and their three children. It was not the mother in this family who followed Gove's career, but the spinster—Abby never attended. In Grafton, Millbury, and other smaller societies, single women likewise carried disproportionate leadership duties. Widows (who were presumed to be sexually inactive) and mothers of grown children also led rural societies.[26] By denouncing the solitary vice, female moral reformers theorized their sexuality in a new way: desire could exist separately from marriage, pregnancy, and motherhood.

Women who attended physiological lectures focused more intensely on their own sexuality than that of rakes or prostitutes. Sharing a sense of struggle against "all the morbid passions" of the body, moral reform meetings turned inward. Mary Gove did more than male lecturers such as Graham and Whitmarsh to make this possible: after each lecture, Gove's listeners eagerly confessed their physiological errors, complained of their sufferings, and exulted in redemptive healing.

In the absence of a lecturer, rural women circulated moral reform pamphlets and read them aloud. At first, they could access only male-authored tracts that referred to the solitary vice, such as McDowall's *Memoir*, Graham's *Lecture to Young Men on Chastity*, Woodward's *Hints to the Young*, and so forth.[27] Then, in 1839, Mary Gove's *Solitary Vice* became available in pamphlet form. Three years later, female moral reformers could buy her book *Lectures to Ladies* to read aloud in hopes of stimulating testimonial confessions.

Lectures to Ladies provided a template for confronting the solitary vice out loud in all-female groups. Gove had gleaned cases from the women who made up her audiences, assuring readers that she had received testimonials only from "the most conscientious and worthy" and "ladies of the first respectability." In so doing, she stressed the pervasiveness of the solitary vice among white, Christian women who projected a false image of purity by denying their own lust. When these women confessed and reformed, she cited their stories as evidence that most women masturbated—and that all who did must stop. This hall of mirrors amplified rural white women's growing sense of importance. They *must* take power over their own sexuality by denouncing the solitary vice. In so doing, they would model sexual virtue to others.

One "lady of great worth and intelligence" testified that she "became addicted to solitary vice about the age of nine years." Her mental and physical health failed within three years, and her parents fruitlessly pursued aggressive medical treatments because they did not know the underlying cause. "During all this time," she recalled, "I was practicing solitary vice to a great extent. My conscience often told me it was wrong, but the force of habit prevailed." Contrary to the male fantasies of female masturbation prevalent in *Onania* and the sporting press, she "was never taught the vice" but had instead begun due to an overstimulating diet and bad parenting. Though "social licentiousness was alluded to as a very shameful thing" in her childhood home, "solitary vice was never mentioned." Framing the narrative in this way suggested that white girls experienced natural urges for sexual gratification. Rather than passionless virgins who "fell" as a result of seduction, they intrinsically needed to learn how to manage their desire.[28]

The typical testimonial blamed a woman's ignorance of physiology for her fall into vice and stressed the hidden guilt of other women in her social network. A "pious young woman" told Mary Gove that her "dear and intimate friend was a victim of this vice, though considered a pattern of loveliness by those who knew her." She herself had also practiced it, "though not to any great extent." After learning the cause of her suffering from "a Moral Reform paper that represented the evil in its true light," she "left the habit with loathing and abhorrence."[29] A moral reformer who heard such testimony became responsible for warning each woman in her own circle against the solitary vice. False delicacy kept women ignorant of their own physiology, and that ignorance proved lethal.

Thus, Gove enumerated both gender-neutral and female "diseases which are caused by this habit." Among her list of grim consequences were

> Dyspepsia, spinal disease, headache, epilepsy . . . impaired eye-sight, palpitation of the heart, pain in the side, and bleeding in the lungs, spasm in the heart and lungs, and sometimes sudden death, are caused by indulgence in this vice. Diabetes, or incontinence of urine, flour albus, or whites, and inflammation of the urinary organs, are induced by indulgence in this practice.

If women wanted to avoid yeast infections, urinary tract infections, or "sudden death," they must refrain from masturbating. Hyperbole aside, the effect was to redirect listeners' focus from the behavior of others, even cherished children, onto themselves.[30]

Not all moral reformers were prepared for this subject; some still preferred to focus on licentious men. "Madam," complained one woman to the *Friend*, "The lectures, delivered in this town . . . have suggested ideas which ought never to be alluded to—false, I fear, and certainly premature." Rebecca Eaton named "Solitary Vice" as the topic of concern and countered that this writer had probably "heard no part of the lectures." If she had listened and still took offense at the lecturer's "language of studied delicacy," then the delicacy that she affected must be false.[31]

But most rural women absorbed lectures against solitary vice—and with them the feminized argument against false delicacy—with enthusiasm. Grafton women sought out Rebecca Eaton's six-lecture course on "Moral Purity," which reserved an entire class for the "Solitary Vice." The Winchendon Female Moral Reform Society invited Abigail Ordway to lecture on social and solitary licentiousness, but complained that false delicacy in their town stunted their efforts to evangelize afterward. On the other hand, a rural physician testified that at least two of his patients had been "induced to abandon habits ruinous to life and health" by the female moral reformers' campaign against the solitary vice—and "there may be many more."[32]

Individual testimonials may seem inconsequential. But a flood tide of them powerfully shaped the sexual discourse of moral reform between 1835 and 1840. The *Advocate* and the *Friend* publicized the activities of even the tiniest of auxiliaries. Accounts of intimate meetings proved more influential than the sporadic lectures of Graham, Gove, or other authorities on the solitary vice. Through them, rural white women pushed the moral reform movement further away from its original, external gaze and toward internal scrutiny. Moral reformers relished what Eve Kosofsky Sedgwick called "the spectacle of the Girl Being Taught a Lesson." Renouncing solitary vice could be almost as pleasurable—and solipsistic—as masturbation itself.[33] It engendered a shared notion of white female sexuality, characterized by both individual desire and virtuous restraint.

MORAL REFORM IN BLACK AND WHITE

The interracial moment in moral reform had made such discussions possible by problematizing the convention of white feminine purity. But as growing numbers of white women substituted self-government for activism, black abolitionists lost interest in white moral reformers' sexual politics. Some groups, such as the Ladies' Physiological Society, still saw a natural affinity between moral reform and the abolition of slavery. In fact, a greater number of their members belonged to antislavery societies than to moral reform groups—a striking comparison in light of the connections between Grahamites and moral reformers. Members were also more likely to be abolitionists than they were to be politically inactive. On the other hand, the growing contingent of physiological lecturers visiting small-town moral reform societies tended to emphasize sexual restraint above all else. They helped to convince many white women that to remake the sexual culture, they must first cultivate and model their own virtue. Such internal focus alienated black abolitionists and obscured the distinction between purity and virtue they had introduced to moral reform discourse.

The antislavery schism that divided the Ladies' Physiological Society also reverberated throughout the national moral reform movement after 1840. In the all-white societies of rural New England, the division affected sexual ideology more than the racial composition of the groups. With the movement's geographic spread and numeric growth, moral reform newspapers connected formerly isolated groups of white women and brought them under the umbrella of either the New York or the Boston society. Within and across these groups, white women shared a common language of licentiousness, virtue, and false delicacy. However, these concepts had become elastic enough to mask underlying disagreements. Did licentiousness describe a power relation or merely a set of bad sexual habits? Did all professing Christians have a duty to "come out" of churches that countenanced slavery and its violations of the seventh commandment? Those who agreed with Sarah Grimké left such churches in protest, earning the title "come-outers." But many other women, clerical abolitionists such as Catherine Kilton and Margaret Dye, had gained status in their churches through their moral reform efforts and refused to come out of them under any circumstances.

The antislavery crisis brought tensions around such questions into the open. Many female moral reform societies felt strong allegiance to their ministers and resented the anticlericalism they associated with William Lloyd Garrison's faction of ultra abolitionists. Other moral reformers saw in the antislavery schism the dangers of tackling too many issues at once. By contrast, those who had cut their political teeth during the interracial moment in moral reform believed that any singular focus contradicted the movement's original commitment to eradicate licentiousness in all its forms. They considered all forms of oppression to be interconnected and mutually reinforcing. And while they shared an interest in reform physiology, they continued to maintain that social activism rather than personal discipline defined virtue.

The first signs of fallout appeared in the New York convention of 1838, which voted to regroup the following year as the American Female Moral Reform Society and to pursue a national campaign for the criminalization of seduction and sexual trafficking. Unlike the 1837 meeting, which drew African American reform women from a number of cities because it coincided with the First Convention of American Antislavery Women, the national moral reform convention of 1838 included very few black delegates. Two delegates from the Zion Female Moral Reform Society attended, as did an interracial group of Boston abolitionists, including Lydia Fuller. But Sarah Mapps Douglass, Hetty Burr, and other Philadelphians were too busy preparing to host the second women's antislavery convention to travel to New York.[34]

At this meeting, Secretary Margaret Dye declared that the national strategy must include southern white women. Although northern white women overwhelmingly dominated female moral reform, Dye insisted that a *"union of sentiment and effort"* united *"many thousands of virtuous females from Maine to Alabama."* Lydia Fuller and Mary Ann Johnson both expressed concerns: *Which* virtuous females? What had happened to the recognition of white women's complicity in the licentiousness of slavery? Where was the "bone of our bone and flesh of our flesh" bond between moral reformers and their enslaved sisters? The new physiological interests of the movement's white majority must not silence the "great question" of slavery. Johnson suggested a resolution that proved too controversial to record, and that was quickly tabled. Fuller urged the meeting to hold slavery at the center of sex reform, to recognize female slaves "as *women*" whose "dearest interests like our own are staked on the issue." With support from a coterie of abolitionists, Fuller's resolution passed—but only "after considerable discussion."[35]

Dye offered a weak olive branch. She refused to come out of the Methodist Episcopal Church because slaveholders preached in its southern branches. But she exhorted ministers to enforce the seventh commandment among all members. This concession, and the conversation that produced it, revealed the limits of the licentiousness of slavery as an abolitionist motto. At its best, this counterdiscourse could force a rethinking of the Jezebel stereotype, but sexual exploitation was only one aspect of slavery. Even if Methodist preachers managed to stop slaveholders from raping enslaved women, those women would remain enslaved. Dye's actions—and the support she received for them—suggested that white moral reformers prioritized sexual continence over the abolition of slavery.[36]

The next year, the new American Female Moral Reform Society fractured over this issue. Margaret Dye pushed again for outreach to white southern women, this time by reworking the licentiousness of slavery. Her version empathized with slaveholders' wives far more than with enslaved women:

> Resolved, That the universal prevalence of licentiousness among the enslaved females of our country, and the consequent contamination of those who, by their relation to the master and the slave, are compelled to witness those abominations without reproof, should render the abolition of slavery an object of earnest desire and fervent prayer to every lover of female purity.

Whereas other antislavery resolutions urged action—Mary Ann Johnson called for "our most vigorous efforts"—Dye substituted "desire" and "prayer." She vainly hoped to persuade southern women to pray along with northern moral reformers for slavery's quiet end. And she presumed that they could still be convinced to do so, since they shared a similar interest in "female purity." Beyond this naïveté, the real affront lay in Dye's use of licentiousness. Her resolution revoked enslaved women's claims on virtue and conflated female purity with white womanhood all over again. The real victims, she suggested, were slaveholders' wives, removed from the guilt of slavery yet "compelled to witness" its sexual "abominations." Worse, Dye construed licentiousness neither as a sin against God, nor a crime against liberty, but a "contamination" embodied by enslaved women. To reduce slaveholding men from perpetrators to passive vectors in the contamination of white "female purity" worked entirely against the logic of female moral reform to date. But it, too, passed. If any black delegates or their white allies spoke against the resolution, Dye did not record their remarks.[37]

The opposing positions staked by Fuller and Dye in 1838 and 1839—and the fact that either stance could carry a majority vote—indicated deep fault lines beneath the surface of the female moral reform movement. Disappointed, black women turned toward new projects. The Zion Female Moral Reform Society stopped sending delegates to national conventions in 1839. In addition to ongoing vigilance work, Zion leaders threw their energies into developing the national infrastructure of their own church. They particularly strove to facilitate meetings with African American women from border states such as Maryland and Missouri, where antislavery agitation was illegal and therefore best conducted within closed church conferences.[38]

Nancy Prince, embittered by the bickering among white reformers, set out for Jamaica, where she planned to institute moral reform within an autonomous black school. Writing a decade later, she recalled attending meetings of Boston abolitionists "and other philanthropists of the day." Prince had aligned herself with them "with much pleasure until a contention broke out among themselves." She judged squabbling to be a privilege shared by those who did not personally labor under "the weight of prejudice." Concluding that "much remains to be done," she confronted the sexual exploitation of black women and children, which continued after the abolition of slavery in the British West Indies. Prince blamed the island's sexual traffic on the ongoing schemes of capitalists (unlike white abolitionist travelers, who assumed that slavery had "demoralized" people of color).[39] She saw crowds of people who had "come to Jamaica under the impression that they are to have their passage free," only to be bound until they could pay the debt. She planned to use her school as a shelter for "these infant daughters of crime," and saw herself obligated to "guard their morals by salutary restraint and unremitting care." Once built, the school would be sustained by staff and students.[40]

In Philadelphia, Hetty Burr and Hetty Reckless successfully established a Moral Reform Retreat at the corner of Seventh and Lombard Streets in 1845. There, "colored females" could apply for aid "under the care of coloured persons" (almost all of whom were women). The retreat housed "between one and two hundred women" within its first two years. Residents stayed an average of six weeks in the retreat, a period of recovery, education, and skill building.[41] Believing that, "as in all cases, prevention is better than cure," the organizers solicited teachers to help by "drying up the sources from which destitution and wretchedness usually spring." Burr and Reckless described the women they sheltered as "victims of vice," but unlike white proponents of "rescue," they considered moral reform a type of mutual aid. Notices for the retreat downplayed distinctions between the residents and the larger community. The managers appealed to those "who are in possession of the comforts and conveniences of life" to support their work as a kind of resource redistribution. The Moral Reform Retreat provided much-needed employment for community leaders as well as their clients. While Reckless and Burr secured funding for the organization from elite black families and white Quaker philanthropists, both managers lived and worked among the laboring poor. Neither owned her home.[42]

This version of moral reform presaged uplift in African American women's organizing. By managing the retreat, both matrons did assert their own sexual respectability. But their primary goal was community empowerment, not to persuade whites of their moral worth. The physical space of the retreat served multiple functions. As cofounders of the Female Vigilant Committee, Burr and Reckless likely used the retreat as a shelter for fugitives from slavery as needed. White funders, on the other hand, expected, even demanded, austerities and exposés. They donated money to black institutions because they aimed to "shew the falsity of the charges so often brought against the coloured people of being more degraded and vicious in their moral character than the white."[43] Thus, Quaker philanthropists "regretted" that Burr and Reckless did not "enter more into detail as to the effects of the discipline of the institution upon its inmates." Practical, as well as ideological, reasons shaped their vague reports.[44]

The departure of African American women from the American Female Moral Reform Society left white women to argue about the movement's goals and priorities. Some white Garrisonian abolitionists such as Mary Ann Johnson also left moral reform around 1840. However, others who had participated in the interracial moment in moral reform, such as Sarah Towne Smith (now Martyn) and Paulina Wright Davis, stayed on. They pushed the American Female Moral Reform Society to "'exert their *whole* influence for the *overthrow of slavery*" on the grounds that "the horrible licentiousness that is 'part and parcel' of the system of American Slavery" made its abolition intrinsic to moral reform.[45] They also maintained that physiology intersected with moral reform. Through it, they promoted the sexual accountability of women such as themselves. Balancing activism with sexual self-control (not innate purity), this cohort still hoped to trouble conventions of white femininity. Paulina Wright Davis declared that "I am a rational creature, bound to think and act for myself" and extended this argument into the sexual realm.[46]

By 1844, however, Davis lingered as one of a few outliers in what was becoming a single-issue movement. A regional meeting of female moral reformers broke down when members of the Clinton, New York, society resolved that abolition and moral reform were one and the same. They argued that "all other efforts" to end licentiousness "except those put forth for the abolition of this great evil are 'comparatively futile.'" This perspective called forth "differences of opinion . . . that for a time seemed to indicate disastrous results" before being voted down.[47] Afterward, members of the Clinton society called upon the *Advocate* to publish their dissenting view. Editor Sarah Ingraham refused, writing that even if slavery were abolished, as long as "other existing causes of licentiousness to remain unchecked, the victims of vice would doubtless continue to increase." While the American Female Moral Reform Society regarded "all the great moral causes of the day as 'sisters of charity,'" she continued, "more will be accomplished by preserving their distinctive character, than could be done by their becoming merged in one."[48] After reading this exchange, Paulina Wright Davis wrote a letter of protest to be read in her absence at the next semiannual meeting in Albany. She demanded the national society "take decided action against slavery, as connected with impurity." Sarah Towne Smith Martyn spoke in support of Davis's letter, but its publication in the *Advocate* "was negatived by a large majority." When Ingraham reported this discussion to the national readership, she interjected that they "did not unite with an Antislavery Society, a Temperance Society, a Missionary Society, or a Society advocating any party, sect, or ism, *as such*—but simply a Society whose sole object is the promotion of moral purity."[49] The meeting voted to "sympathize" with enslaved women and to "raise our voices to heaven" for the abolition of slavery, but simultaneously affirmed that moral reform would henceforward be a single-issue movement.

Soon after this declaration, Davis and Martyn withdrew from the moral reform movement. Davis relocated to Philadelphia, where she joined the biracial Female Anti-slavery Society and commenced a physiological lecture career modeled on that of Mary Gove. Leaving moral reform was more difficult for Martyn, who had edited the *Advocate* in its early years, argued with Sarah Ingraham over the possibility that women such as themselves might as easily be licentious as pure, and declared enslaved women "flesh of our flesh." She had struggled to maintain these positions as an officer of the American Female Moral Reform Society ever since turning the *Advocate* over to Ingraham. Even as the majority continued to silence dissent within the ranks, Martyn held firm. Finally, in 1845, Ingraham found a way to be rid of her. A financial scandal broke around the treasurer's handling of the society's funds. Martyn defended the treasure's innocence and suggested that Ingraham had trumped up the allegations out of personal animosity. Ingraham retaliated by charging Martyn with violating the society's constitution, which forbade gossip "unless the interest of society require the exposure." After a nasty, complicated, and highly public dispute, the majority sided with Ingraham, and Sarah Towne Smith Martyn was stripped of her membership. In the aftermath, Ingraham revealed that the underlying contention had been over whether moral reform should be a single-issue or an intersectional movement. She declared her victory over those who "desired to blend this with other reforms."[50]

The movement contracted in personnel as well as focus as a result of the single-issue platform of the 1840s. Although Dye had begun this campaign as an attempt to court southern women, they never joined the female moral reform movement in significant numbers. Instead, the movement fractured and winnowed into a small corps of urban rescue operations. The schisms of 1839 and 1845 left the female moral reform movement in the hands of leaders who straightforwardly idealized female sexual purity, which they defined as virginity before marriage and monogamy afterward. Moreover, those leaders asserted the responsibility of women who lived by these standards to "rescue" those who did not.

THE RETURN TO RESCUE

Between 1834 and 1845, moral reformers exposed wrongdoing and trusted that an educated public would choose paths of virtue. After 1845, however, they lost faith in the prospect that informed people would—or even *could*—make righteous choices. Rather than *reform* morality, they now *guarded* chastity. The movement's press registered this shift. In a revealing turn of phrase, the *Friend of Virtue* eventually became the *Home Guardian*, while the *Advocate of Moral Reform* grew into the *Advocate and Family Guardian*.

Following in the footsteps of the gentlemen philanthropists who had created the nation's first Magdalen Asylums and prisons, female moral reformers now insisted that they, middle-class white women, could best "raise the fallen." Purged of black and white abolitionists, moral guardians no longer debated their own complicity in structures of power. At the same time, a surge in Irish immigration seemed to them to demand a return to rescue. The immigrants arrived destitute, only to be excluded from most employments; their mere presence made extreme poverty more visible than ever to urban reformers. The *Advocate* assessed the need for houses of refuge as "daily more apparent" and sought to place "matrons of the right kind" in charge of the inmates' "moral discipline" until they could be placed in domestic service. After securing antiseduction legislation in New York and a few other states, the guardians invested more heavily in such institutions than in all other moral reform efforts. Having mastered self-discipline, female moral reformers began to discipline others.[51]

This context transformed antimasturbation discourse. Female moral reformers had originally engaged the solitary vice in the context of intimate gatherings of equals who chose to study physiology and contemplate their sexual subjectivity. By the mid-1840s, however, self-appointed guardians acted as mothers, matrons, and missionaries to prevent those in their charge from succumbing to the solitary vice.

Because guardians were less interested than their predecessors in exploring adult women's subjectivity, they conflated masturbation with youth. Those with children felt a special duty to fight the "hydra sin" within their households. Motherhood had always figured into discussions of the solitary vice, but during the 1840s reformers named it as the primary reason for women to discuss it at all. We have seen that both Sylvester Graham and Mary Gove invoked motherhood in strategic rather than literal ways. By contrast, moral guardians justified speaking about sexual physiology, not to apply to themselves, but to better parent their children. In 1843, Rochester reformers agreed that "in the discharge of parental duty . . . knowledge of physical laws and obedience to the same, are indispensable to success." Three years later, a son thanked his mother for teaching him not to indulge in the solitary vice. "It is through your instrumentality," he wrote, "your plain and faithful instruction, that I have been saved from the snares of the destroyer.'" After women applied antimasturbation discourse to themselves, motherhood became an incredibly powerful mechanism for instilling bodily discipline in children. In the process, guardians erased the connections to sexual citizenship that their erstwhile rivals, the women's rights advocates, had drawn. They exchanged egalitarian sexual politics for maternalism. Uses of the phrase *solitary vice* declined, gradually replaced by terms such as *self-pollution* and *self-abuse*. By taking vice and virtue out of the equation, these phrases fit an infantilized discourse on masturbation. Maternalism, in turn, implicitly resurrected passionlessness.[52]

The racial politics of the guardians' return to purity became clear in the rush to build new houses of refuge and industry. In 1847, white moral reformers organized Philadelphia's Rosine Association, a philanthropic society that ran an asylum "for the *reformation, employment,* and *instruction* of females, whose habits and situation, have precluded them from the sympathies and respect of the virtuous part of the community."[53] Although black Philadelphians urgently needed social services—their demands far outstripped the resources of the Moral Reform Retreat—Rosine officers preferred to create a moral reform refuge that mirrored their own white households. Hundreds of African Americans had petitioned for years "to admit colored children to the House of Refuge."[54] White abolitionists such as Lucretia Mott withdrew their membership from the Rosine Association in protest when the majority voted to exclude African Americans from its newly built House of Industry.

The Rosine Association restricted its services to young white women whom its managers imagined as prodigal daughters—"young, friendless, and destitute females"—in need of motherly sexual advice. Believing white girls naturally pure, guardians blamed their prostitution on "deficient education, the want of proper remuneration for services, and the neglect of suitable maternal and sympathizing care." As white philanthropic women stepped into the role of surrogate mothers, they imparted the virtues of sexual restraint through physiology lessons. Teachers at Rosine's day school taught students the "laws of life and health," including the dangers of masturbation—a gateway to promiscuity learned from "evil companions." Such education was coupled with training in marketable skills like mantua making and therefore found readier acceptance among poor white women than institutional domesticity. While only fifteen women boarded in the Rosine house during the first year, its day school thrived.[55]

Beyond the houses of refuge, guardians did not confine their attentions to white women. They also institutionalized their authority in part by lobbying for positions in prisons, on the grounds that, as women, they could better reform female inmates. In an effort to prevent diverse inmates from returning to lives of crime, matrons took responsibility for warning them against the gateway sin of masturbation. The matron of Philadelphia's Moyamensing prison, for example, distributed Mary Gove's *Solitary Vice* among female prisoners in 1846.[56]

Moral guardians also spread antimasturbation discourse through missionary operations. The American Board of Commissioners of Foreign Missions fund-raised so heavily among moral reform women that by the mid-1840s, they had "adopted" several missionary institutions. For example, the missionary J. S. Green built multiple relationships with influential moral reform women in order to maintain his boarding school for Hawaiian girls in Wailuku. Similarly, Andalucia Condee cultivated the patronage of the Utica Female Moral Reform Society for her girls' school at Lahaina. Moral reformers approached these seminaries in maternalist terms: they could be called "moral reform schools" only because guardians assumed that Hawaiian mothers failed in the "training of children, watching over their morals, instilling sentiments of virtue, and guarding against vice in any of its forms."[57]

The Maternal Association in Hopkinton, Massachusetts, illustrates the maternalism involved in efforts to make the conversation about solitary vice both "general" and *global*. After hearing a "Physiological Lecture to Ladies" by Rebecca Eaton, secretary of the New England Female Moral Reform Society, members concluded that "the solitary vice we have reason to think is practiced to an alarming extent among children." It was this conviction that inspired them to send copies of the *Friend of Virtue* with a particular missionary, Mrs. Thurston, to her school in Hawaii; they also voted to raise funds for her daughter's teacher training at Mount Holyoke. Missionaries acknowledged receiving the papers and reported using them in sex education. Moral reformers supported physiological education for women in order to prevent masturbation among women and girls from Hopkinton to Hawaii.[58]

Reformers also created physiological primers for the indigenous youth of both sexes who attended missionary schools. In Honolulu, the medical missionary G. P. Judd translated excerpts from Sylvester Graham and others into a *Sandwich Islands Anatomy* textbook. His translation inspired Andalucia Condee to call for an especially woman-friendly "volume to be prepared in the native language on physiology and another on hygiene." Baptist missionary Stella Kneeland Burnett responded by translating William Alcott's *The House I Live In* into Burmese. Other texts made their way to Ceylon, Bulgaria, and Turkey.[59]

Despite these efforts, solitary vice discourse made fewer inroads abroad than it did in American institutions. In 1836, the missionary press published a questionnaire authored by none other than Sylvester Graham, who directed missionaries to interview the people they encountered, observe their habits, and even measure their body parts. If they would kindly report their findings about Native sexual habits (and fifty-three other biometric indexes), he would publish these data for the benefit of the global Christian community. Over the next three years, information filtered back concerning diet, exercise, dress, lodging, and vague impressions about "licentiousness." But neither Graham's private notebooks nor his published digest of the reports recorded anything about indigenous attitudes toward masturbation. The women and girls whom missionary teachers encountered answered the question about solitary vice with thunderous silence. Instead, Hawaiians repeatedly redirected missionaries' attention toward a bitter local truth about sex: it was syphilis, brought by Christians themselves, that decimated the population.[60] The obsession with masturbation that saturated American society during the middle of the nineteenth century—a period when white women, African Americans, and immigrants strove to demonstrate their fitness for citizenship—found its limits in missionary schools abroad. Colonized women were less interested in practicing virtue and civic worth than in disproving foreigners' fitness to rule. The sexual discourse that meant most to them was therefore not one of solitary vice, with its notes of self-discipline, but one of sexual exploitation, which exposed the hypocrisy and lawlessness of their so-called saviors.

CONCLUSION

The Ladies' Physiological Society helped several white women—starting with Mary Gove—to begin careers as professional lecturers on anatomy and physiology. By offering single-sex lectures to small moral reform societies throughout the New England hinterlands, these female educators spread the word about solitary vice without inciting riots. Audiences replicated the intimate culture of the Ladies' Physiological Society in their own female moral reform societies. Some members experienced a form of consciousness-raising that would have been familiar to feminists of the 1970s. Some, like Paulina Wright Davis, demanded "equal rights"—both within reform organizations and in American politics and society.[61] Others, having claimed and taken responsibility for their own sexual virtue, buried the process by which they had disciplined their passions beneath claims of innate purity. As the female moral reform movement grew, rural members carried the physiological argument against solitary vice into every corner of the Northeast and Midwest. By 1840, the female moral reform movement had decentered Sylvester Graham and made the case against solitary vice its own.

At the same time, conflicts within the movement drove away the very members—African Americans and white abolitionists—who had initiated the conversation about the nature of female desire and its relation to structures of power such as slavery and patriarchy. After the moral guardians redefined the movement as one centered on the protection of purity, they flexed their moral authority by disciplining others. The return to rescue transformed the politics of masturbation, with complex outcomes. On the one hand, matrons' use of antimasturbation discourse in reform and missionary institutions entrenched a sense of its special relevance to white women. Some institutions depended on a contrast between white matrons' own putative purity against the presumed licentiousness of diverse inmates, wards, or converts; others targeted white women as students of antimasturbation physiology in an effort to protect their purity. On the other hand, in order to defend (white) women's purity from men's predations, moral guardians defined male sexuality as essentially problematic and in need of motherly discipline. By reasserting passionlessness, they helped old associations between masculinity and "onanism" to return just when they succeeded in saturating the culture with warnings against masturbation.

The new emphasis on guardianship changed the movement's appeal to rural women. Many rural associations devolved into maternal associations and sewing circles whose handicrafts funded urban houses of refuge. Others, "languishing for want of work," simply stopped meeting during the 1840s. The return to rescue diminished the importance of self-culture and encouraged women in the countryside to focus on parenting pure children. This shift accelerated, rather than depressed, the spread of antimasturbation discourse in the hinterlands. Many white women who, a decade earlier, would have attended meetings to consider their own sexual passions turned their attentions toward the habits of other family members. The proscription multiplied exponentially as those children grew into parents who inculcated their own children with similar lessons.[62]

In separate institutions, African American women continued to define license in terms of white and male power. For example, Philadelphia's Moral Reform Retreat sheltered fugitives not merely from prostitution but also from slavery and exploitation. By applying an intersectional analysis, facilitating activism, and maintaining a mutual-aid orientation to moral reform, black moral reform diverged profoundly from white guardianship efforts during the 1840s.

As we shall see, African American reformers, moral guardians, and advocates of women's rights all brought the solitary vice into new institutions of their own making. Particularly in the realms of medicine and education, each of these groups would carry antimasturbation discourse to new groups and infuse it with new meanings. But the most pervasive popularizer of all would be the marketplace.

CHAPTER FOUR

A Philosophy of Amative Indulgence

Lectures on anatomy and physiology proliferated during the 1840s, shedding older associations with ultraism and reaching far greater numbers of Americans than ever before. As radicals departed from the moral reform ranks, female physiology lecturers were increasingly perceived as sensible matrons nobly imparting "the laws of life and health" to guard the nation's purity. Mary Gove, though not mobbed, initially faced harsh social disapproval for lecturing on sexual physiology: penny papers compared her to the infamous abortionist Madame Restell, and her Quaker meeting disowned her. Yet within a few years, the *Boston Medical and Surgical Journal* praised Gove as "the herald of truth" and declared it "nothing objectionable or indelicate for one woman to tell another those important facts."[1]

This change in perception took place alongside the transformation of the female moral reform movement. The turn away from social transformation and toward rescue and guardianship helped bring popular physiology into mainstream culture. Moral guardians' pursuit of purity cast married, middle-class white women as elevating sexual discourse rather than being sullied by it. In this context, "lectures to ladies on anatomy and physiology" appeared to threaten few social hierarchies. When white women gathered "alone" (that is, in the absence of men), they gave the appearance of containing sexuality in its appropriate, private realm. This fictive privacy shielded their meetings, whether held in domestic parlors or crowded lecture halls, from the appearance of challenging male dominance in public culture. Female lecturers transmitted antimasturbation discourse to growing numbers of women during the early 1840s without facing opprobrium. It had been years since a man had troubled the spheres by entering the imagined sanctum of the physiology lecture to women.

It would take a man on the make with extraordinary publicity skills to sensationalize the solitary vice all over again. That man, a British immigrant named Frederick Hollick, arrived on the scene in early 1844. Although now largely forgotten, Hollick achieved celebrity status during the mid-nineteenth century as a purveyor of sexual knowledge. His graphic lectures elicited outrage, obscenity charges, and equally fervent support. Like any showman, he knew how to generate conflict and profit from the resulting publicity. At the height of Hollick's notoriety, he claimed to have lectured to "upwards of thirty-nine thousands of persons," and he went on to reach many thousands more through books that sold hundreds of editions, traveled west, and were translated into Spanish. His most popular sex manual went through at least five hundred printings of between two thousand and ten thousand copies.[2] Hollick accomplished this widespread appeal by encouraging multiple audiences to interpret his physiology lectures in competing ways. On the one hand, he depicted female bodies as voracious and orgasmic, but ultimately dependent on men for their pleasure. This representation fit comfortably within the framework of libertine republicanism. On the other hand, by promoting contraception and marriage reform, Hollick appealed to many white women who read in his praise for female pleasure an alternative to moral reformers' fears of sexual danger.[3] By merging reform physiology with libertine republicanism, he avoided riots while popularizing the notion that the solitary vice caused illness, insanity, and death.

Hollick's career represented drastic changes in antimasturbation discourse. First, the market, rather than evangelical reform, became the main method by which people learned about the vice. Entertainments that spectacularized the body, such as anatomy museums, live model shows, and topless dancing, boomed during midcentury. Huge numbers of consumers also sought practical solutions to sexual problems by purchasing lecture tickets, home health manuals, and proprietary medicines.[4] Hollick brilliantly combined these two markets in his popular physiology lectures. Second, he participated in a growing print culture that celebrated pleasure for its own sake and revived *Onania*'s claim that limiting "healthy" intercourse drove people to masturbation and all of its dangers. Hollick called his pro-pleasure ethos "the philosophy of amative indulgence." Third, large numbers of white women consumed physiology lectures and books in search of instructions for female pleasure within heterosexual intercourse. Rejecting the old moral reform goal of "crucifying" sexual desire, thousands bought Hollick's *Marriage Guide* because it offered contraceptive advice, described the location and function of the clitoris, and advised readers how to achieve

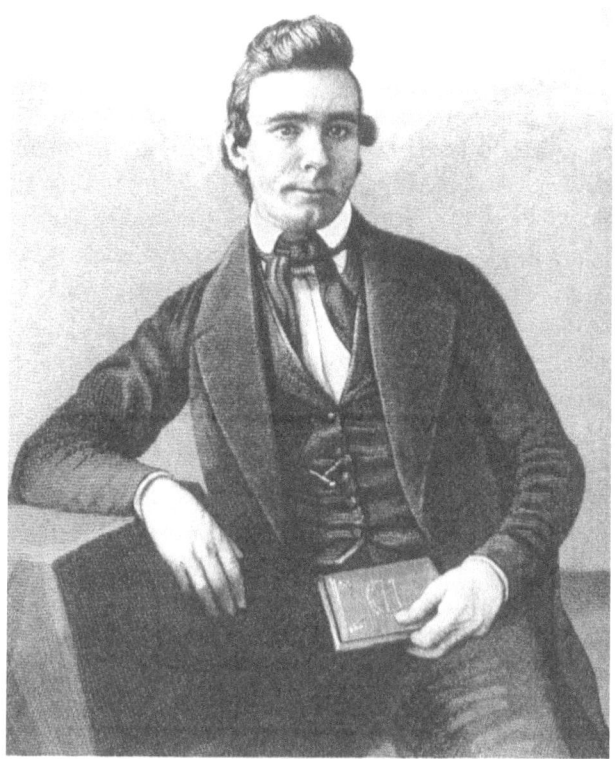

FIGURE 6. Portrait of Frederick Hollick.
(*Source:* Charles Arthur Hollick Papers, Institute of Arts and Sciences, Staten Island.)

mutual orgasms through penetrative sex. Such guides addressed middle-class women as both desirous bodies and virtuous citizens. They also diminished the importance of female masturbation. Moral reformers had cast it as the ultimate transgression of God's laws of life and health, a blight on women's capacity for self-government. Midcentury writers continued to insist that women harmed themselves by masturbating without knowing the dangers, but they invoked the vice primarily as a way of underlining women's need for *healthy* (marital) pleasure. While moralists associated the vice more with children than adults, entrepreneurs increasingly targeted young men, who provided a ready market for proprietary cures. Many unmarried, wage-earning young men also consumed advice that affirmed the healthfulness of their desire for women and promised to heal the lingering effects of "the imprudence and solitude of youth."[5]

Each of these broad cultural themes became apparent when Hollick was prosecuted for obscene libel in Philadelphia during the spring and summer of 1846. Once again, the conflict turned on challenges to the sexual double standard. The city's leading men considered it one thing for a man to describe ravenously orgasmic women in print for male readers, but quite another for him to lecture to women on the ecstasies of intercourse. Because Pennsylvania's obscenity law did not allow for prosecution of sexual speech, a grand jury had to decide whether his book *The Origin of Life* (a published compilation of the lectures) constituted a libel on the community. Many of the city's female reformers vigorously defended Hollick, just as they had Graham. While defending their own propriety, they also asserted their capacity to act as informed sexual citizens. They reframed the debate over *The Origin of Life* as one over women's right to assemble peaceably for the purpose of scientific education. At the same time, Hollick's defenders embraced the philosophy of amative indulgence, which named moderation, not chastity, as the basis of the laws of life and health. White advocates of women's rights—such as Lydia Maria Child, Mary Grew, and Paulina Wright Davis—resumed the pursuit of active sexual virtue during the late 1840s. In their view, virtue now lay in the ability to moderately indulge, rather than radically restrain, sexual impulses. They construed the solitary vice as inherently *im*moderate: secret and requiring no partner, it led naturally to addiction. Now, however, they disowned the solitary vice without denying pleasure itself. In doing so, advocates of women's rights contributed to "the invention of heterosexuality."[6] They embraced secular sex education as part of their more general shift away from moral suasion and toward legal reform, professionalization, and scientific rationalism.[7]

Popular physiology lectures simultaneously naturalized heterosexual desire in women and whitened the normative expressions of that desire. Anatomical texts represented black female bodies as inherently immoderate. White women who consumed these texts—even the reformers most attracted to active virtue and leery of prescriptive purity—defended their own interest in sexual physiology as a sign of "*true* delicacy and a really *pure* taste."[8] They did so instrumentally, for they sought to redefine normative femininity by replacing the emphasis on natural chastity with a new model of sexual citizenship. In the absence of cross-racial solidarity, however, the new feminist physiology reified black women's sexual abjection.

THE PEOPLE'S DOCTOR

Frederick Hollick first formulated the distinctive sexual politics that would become the philosophy of amative indulgence in Birmingham, England.

While working as a silversmith's apprentice during his teens, he attended free-thought lectures at the Mechanics Institute and embraced Robert Owen's utopian socialism. Eventually, he moved to the other side of the podium, becoming a secular "missionary" who argued against state religion.[9] Like other Owenites, Hollick insisted that neither church nor state should govern sexual conduct. Only the sacred individual—male or female, married or unmarried—could properly do so. He followed Richard Carlisle in considering pleasure a positive good and agreed with Fanny Wright that conventional marriage particularly disadvantaged women. Altogether, Hollick argued that each individual should pursue "the fullest liberty of thought and action compatible with the possession of like liberty by every other person." Sexual liberty required universal physiological education, including contraceptive information for every postpubescent person who wanted it. Critics in both England and the United States denounced Owenites as free lovers because of these arguments. However, Frederick Hollick did not oppose marriage per se. He married Eleanor Eliza Bailey before arriving in America in 1842. The couple originally moved to the United States because they planned to join the Owenite community at New Harmony. However, they learned upon arriving in New York that the utopian experiment had ended.[10]

Unknown and without resources, Hollick "cast about for a move" and decided to embark upon a thriving American career: that of a commercial lecturer. Inspired by Robert Dale Owen's *Moral Physiology*, he first tried lecturing about sex to New York's workingmen. He accused "medical Old Fogies" of monopolizing knowledge about anatomy and physiology. Although he identified as "a medical red republican," Hollick needed to sell lecture tickets to the masses in order to make a living. Ultimately, this proved financially unsustainable, for too few workingmen could or would pay for lectures that began with sex and ended with an appeal for socialism.[11] By contrast, advertisements for physiology lectures did attract evangelical women. In 1844, Hollick remade himself once more—this time as a Connecticut-born physician who had been trained at the University of Edinburgh. The self titled "Dr. Hollick" began to lecture "to ladies only."[12]

The cultural association between abolition, moral reform, and physiological lectures to ladies drew supporters of these causes to Hollick's earliest American lectures. The prominent abolitionist Lydia Maria Child (1802–80) noticed his "several courses of lectures on Anatomy, adapted to popular comprehension" in her widely read series *Letters from New York*. Child encouraged women to learn about sexual physiology in particular, for it was "most intimately connected with their deepest and purest emotions, and the holiest experience of their lives." To those who objected to the subject, she addressed the now-familiar barb, "How much *in*delicacy there is in thy delicacy."[13] By invoking false delicacy, Child signaled to other reformers the presence of a new lecturer who would address sex, including the solitary vice, in appropriate ways. Hollick's reputation as a trustworthy lecturer to ladies on physiology traveled with him from New York to Philadelphia. There he developed a full course, delivered separately to men and women but containing the same material, called "Lectures on the Origin of Life." Women would make up his most loyal supporters for the remainder of his career.[14]

However, Frederick Hollick was no Sylvester Graham. Rather than elaborating a prescriptive physiology of restraint, he advocated pleasure for its own sake—for women as well as men. Like other freethinkers, Hollick argued that "chastity," not indulgence, was unnatural and therefore unhealthy. Frequent sexual pleasure constituted a physiological necessity for all postpubescent human beings. Furthermore, sexual pleasure ennobled humanity: "The higher any being is placed in the scale of creation, the more multiplied are its means of enjoyment, and the more intense those enjoyments become." Sex itself was "a wholesome stimulus to the nervous system, at ordinary times, and a means of expending surplus energy when the vital functions are too active." Indeed, too *little* stimulation could throw the body out of balance. Hollick thus turned Grahamite regimen on its head. Intervening in cases of deficient—not excessive—desire, he promoted the medicinal use of aphrodisiac stimulants such as "coffee, tea, aromatics, and spices." He even sold *cannabis indica* (marijuana) through the mail as a remedy for those who needed additional excitement.[15]

Hollick's first book, *The Origin of Life*, preserved much of the content of his original lectures. Five years later, he responded to accelerating demand by bringing out *The Marriage Guide*, an expanded version with intensified focus on women's sexual satisfaction. These texts carried his sexual advice far beyond New York and Philadelphia. As with Graham's "Lecture to Mothers," the titles referred to reproduction and marriage in order to indicate and legitimize the discussion of sex within. However, they did not accurately describe the full range of subject matter. Both texts offered contraceptive information, and both explicitly addressed unmarried readers. Young men could find in Hollick's books arguments favoring prophylaxis, advertisements for mail-order condoms, and home remedies for gonorrhea and syphilis. But he also explicitly sanctioned women's contraceptive strategies with or without the approval of male partners. "No one person's decision should in any way affect another person," he argued; "in a word, I think it is everyone's own affair."[16]

Marriage needed to be reformed, Hollick maintained, and female pleasure was the key. His contraceptive advice, though flawed, was intended to enable women to enjoy sex.[17] Men must respect women's decisions regarding fertility and their sexual sovereignty. The best way to achieve this, however, was not by convincing listeners of the physiological necessity of periodic abstinence so that married women could authoritatively say *no* to sex. Instead, by carefully instructing men and women in the physiology of sexual response, Hollick hoped to improve marital sex so that women would want to say *yes* more often. Self-mastery and autonomy could—and should—coexist with pleasure. Hollick dispelled any assumption of passionlessness, insisting that "in both sexes, when the union is really desired," heterosexual intercourse led to "the highest and most absorbing excitement that animated beings can experience." Healthy women experienced orgasms. In fact, Hollick insisted that they felt them "much more intensely" than did men and that "several orgasms may follow each other in quick succession" without causing injury or depletion. Women who went *without* orgasm suffered "severe nervous afflictions." Arguing that it was the duty of their male partners to prevent this from happening, Hollick instructed men on clitoral stimulation, lubrication, and, above all, timing.[18]

Yet while representing the clitoris as "the principal seat of pleasurable sensation," Hollick also argued that the most rapturous experience of all—which should be intentionally pursued—was simultaneous orgasm in penile-vaginal intercourse. More than half a century before Freud, Hollick distinguished between vaginal and clitoral orgasms. "I believe," he wrote, "that sexual excitement is never known in its full intensity excepting when it is experienced in the neck of the womb, it being always weak and partial when confined to the clitoris and nymphae." This distinction was one of "considerable medical and moral importance"—after all, clitoral orgasm could be accomplished with or without a penis, with or without a partner.[19]

By instructing readers to pursue pleasure for its own sake, Hollick's physiology significantly differed from that of evangelical lecturers. Focusing on libidinous women, penetrative orgasm, and a live-and-let-live philosophy, his erotic priorities matched those of libertine republicans. Yet Hollick echoed Grahamites and moral reformers by describing desire as universal and validating women's equal sexual rights. Moreover, like these earlier reformers, he deemed the solitary vice "*the master evil* of the present day," because it depleted the nervous system. By relying on fantasy for satisfaction, the masturbator—who could be male or female—overtaxed the brain. By contrast, heterosexual intercourse reinvigorated both bodies by transferring nervous electricity from one partner to the other.[20]

Because Hollick perpetuated masturbation phobia, some scholars have interpreted his books as "primers for prudery."[21] But Hollick never lost his enthusiasm for pleasure itself; he set masturbation as the only "unnatural" limit to otherwise "wholesome" pleasure. What it threatened was specifically "the union of the two sexes." Men who overindulged would lose their "powers" (ability to achieve and maintain erection); women who could experience orgasms without submitting to marriage or risking pregnancy might lose their passions for men. His advice was presciently and aggressively heteronormative. In one telling example, he derided the vice in "fagging men of business" who showed "no love or reverence for the other sex." This use of the word *fagging* recalls Michel Foucault's argument that the masturbator preceded the construction of the homosexual as a (male) "type." Combining English slang for exhaustion with a critique of the sexual habits of wealthy businessmen, Hollick's language presaged the hetero/homosexual dichotomy of the late nineteenth century. Men were only half of the heterosexual equation, yet popular physiology made them responsible for more than simply refraining from masturbation. They now had to prevent it in women by skillfully stimulating them in partnered sex. This, too, was a drastic departure from earlier moral reform arguments, which foregrounded women's rational self-control. Nevertheless, women filled Hollick's lecture halls, eager to learn how they might experience legitimate pleasure while controlling their fertility. Later marriage manuals similarly urged husbands to strive for their wives' sexual satisfaction, enjoined women to channel their desires into coitus, and held out mutual orgasm as the ultimate sexual goal of every couple.[22]

THE TRIALS OF FREDERICK HOLLICK

If Hollick expected that his efforts to prevent masturbatory deviance and strengthen marriage would legitimize the argument for female pleasure, he was in for a rude awakening. By the spring of 1846, some Philadelphians strove to drive him out of the city never to return. Hollick blamed his "persecution" on "medical monopoly," a sinister conspiracy on the part of "regular" physicians to keep the masses sick and dependent. In reality, medical doctors had only recently begun to create professional organizations with the intent of lobbying for future license laws. They commanded no monopoly on knowledge about the body. On the contrary, unlicensed healers proliferated throughout the antebellum period, giving rise to alternative educational institutions. Many Americans doubted physicians' abilities, purchased home health guides to inform themselves of their options, and patronized practitioners of multiple healing systems at the same time. Hollick deftly positioned himself as a spokesman for this disparate popular health movement in an effort to galvanize support for his own case. There is no evidence to support his claim that doctors instigated the conflict.[23]

Instead, newspaper editors led the offensive against Hollick's "corrupting influence."[24] Two Philadelphia newspapers in particular—one a major commercial daily, the *North American* (edited by George Rex Graham, 1813–94), the other a failing penny paper, the *Daily Chronicle* (edited by Charles Alexander, 1796–1871)—attacked both the lecturer and his audiences. The *North American* had originally puffed Hollick's Philadelphia lectures but condemned them after George Graham noticed an advertisement to young people "of both sexes." The broadside promised that the lecture would introduce listeners to male and female genital anatomy so that courting couples might assess the "*adaptation*" of each other's genitals "*before* the [marriage] contract was formally completed." By instructing them in signs of trouble, Hollick hoped to prevent unfulfilling unions and teach young people how to avoid diseased partners. The editors, outraged by the thought of girls and boys listening to such descriptions, recruited a few other "gentlemen" to confront Hollick at a February 1846 lecture.[25]

There, Graham and Alexander uncovered a simple bait-and-switch operation. Verbally, Hollick merely described basic anatomy and suggested that, before marriage, parties should be certain of their intellectual compatibility. Those who wished to learn the lurid details mentioned in the racy advertisement would have to buy his book (available for purchase at the ticket booth). It was *The Origin of Life* that delivered the anatomical "signs" of sexual problems: "unnatural growth of nymphae," "cohesion of the external lips," "closure of the vagina," "stunted" penises and testicles, sterility indicated by "the tone of the organs," "doubtful or double sex," testicular "anomalies," "mutilated" genitals, and a whole range of sores and discharges. Technically, those who attended the plain-vanilla lecture could access this information—by buying the book sold within. In this way, Hollick foiled any plan to disrupt his lecture on the grounds of indecency. Graham, Alexander, and their comrades shouted at him from the balcony, then went home and set about exposing him in the press. Their investigative reporting, such as it was, brought Hollick's lectures to the attention of then district attorney William Darrah Kelley.[26]

On the surface, Graham, Alexander, and Kelley targeted Hollick in hopes of establishing clear standards of obscenity. Wave after wave of erotic prints, images, and services flooded a largely unregulated market in 1846. Common law, inherited from England during the colonial period, defined obscenity in local terms and assumed that communities shared a common store of sexual values. This legal orientation seemed ill equipped to manage the recent explosion of sexual discourse in the urban United States. Competing sexual ideologies had proliferated in the wake of religious disestablishment, reform movements, utopianism, and mass immigration; these "conversations" became cacophonous as itinerant lecturers and print culture amplified them.[27]

When, on March 17, 1846, a grand jury indicted Hollick for obscene libel, lawyers began to debate the moral effect of praising heterosexual pleasure for its own sake. The bill of indictment specifically listed as obscene the words *penis* and *vagina*, particularly when used together, as they were in one ardent section of *Origin*'s marital advice. Prosecutor Kelley deemed this juxtaposition a libel on the community, particularly when uttered before ladies. But defense attorney J. G. Clarkson responded that, as a science writer, Hollick had used the names of the genitals appropriately. And by informing readers that these organs *belonged* together—by showing the wholesomeness of heterosexual pleasure in contrast to the lethal solitary vice—the book *uplifted* the moral tone of the community. Given "the vast amount of wretchedness and insanity a certain practice had produced in the community," Clarkson maintained that even "if all the rest of the work were as vile as is represented," the "one chapter" on masturbation "would redeem the whole." Kelley rejoined that Hollick had disingenuously offered such "scientific" information to mask more prurient motives.[28]

The debate over whether exuberant heterosexual expression breached or reinforced community morals turned on the issue of women's exposure to and consumption of the philosophy of amative indulgence. The district attorney had to prove that Hollick had published and sold a book that offended community standards of morality within the state of Pennsylvania. The judge, Anson V. Parsons, would determine whether *The Origin of Life* could be considered an affront to Pennsylvanians' moral sensibilities; Kelley merely had to supply evidence of its local publication. As the prosecution and defense set about interviewing potential witnesses, the judge ordered Hollick to stop his lecture series until its obscenity or propriety could be determined. Yet the content of the lectures, however graphic, had no legal bearing on the case. Instead, Parsons aimed to protect women from hearing—and vouching for—obscenities disguised as physiology lessons.[29]

Editors such as George Graham and Charles Alexander also concentrated on Hollick's lectures to women, vowing "to put away an evil thing from the skirts of the community." Describing their publicity battle against Hollick as a campaign to protect "female delicacy," they rarely mentioned the printed text at issue in the obscenity trial. The *North American* wondered what kind of women would "recommend language and sights which to repeat or describe in company would be an outrage so infamous as to drive them from decent society." With regard to the lecture to ladies, editors doubted that the lectures had been as *"beautiful, plain, decorous,* and highly instructive" as the women claimed. They suspected the women of concealing "some ulterior object" and specifically pointed to an advertisement in which Hollick promised to explain certain "operations" that would result in "Foetal Expulsion."[30] In response, the women who had attended the lectures went public in their own behalf.

SEXUAL CITIZENS AND CONSUMERS

When newspapers called into question the moral standing of Hollick's audiences, reformers once again led the defense of a man who dared to address women on sexual subjects. In 1833, Sylvester Graham had blamed the backlash against his lectures on freethinkers, only to find himself at the center of a larger gendered battle between libertines and female moral reformers. Similarly, Hollick began by framing his 1846 trials as a contest between reactionary physicians and "the people" writ large. But it soon became clear that both detractors and supporters concerned themselves primarily with the question of women's right to hear "public" lectures—that is, those delivered by men—on sexual topics.

In order to support his image as a public benefactor, Hollick falsely represented his audience members as totally ignorant about their own bodies. One stock tale held that some were so shocked at the sight of the anatomical manikin he used as illustration that they fainted dead away.[31] However, many attendees had attended prior physiological lectures in the context of their ongoing activism. Hollick's audiences, like Graham's, participated in multiple reform movements. The story line of an embattled male lecturer who wanted to share lifesaving physiological knowledge with adult women was familiar to them. Many had already viewed manikins and other anatomical illustrations in the context of female moral reform and ladies' physiological societies; some had even dissected small mammals.[32]

Mary Grew, a well-known white abolitionist and moral reformer, first heard Hollick in 1844. By that time, she had held offices in the national conventions of antislavery women, served as corresponding secretary of the

Philadelphia Female Anti-slavery Society, helped organize the annual fundraising fair, and been denied a seat at the World Anti-slavery Convention in London in 1840 because she was a woman. She had witnessed opponents' efforts to quash abolitionist women's activism by appealing to feminine decorum; she had also gained ample experience using publicity for her own political ends. Two years before Hollick ever faced obscenity charges, she collected signatures from audience members attesting to the propriety and scientific importance of all that they had heard. By 1844, publishing resolutions had become a generic advertising strategy. Grew expected Hollick to pay for the publication of women's endorsements, so she drafted the resolutions carefully, lacing the resolutions of support with arguments for women's rights. She explained that women bought tickets to popular lectures because they could not access scientific knowledge "in any other way." Purchasing a ticket to Hollick's lectures entitled them to information that was "too generally regarded as belonging exclusively to the lecture room of a medical university." Surely women were entitled to learn the most recent explanations of conception, pregnancy, and contraception—"some of the dearest interests of our sex." Until women were admitted into medical colleges, they would continue to consume anatomy and physiology in any available form.[33]

Grew represented a larger group of savvy activists, not the fainting ingenues of self-promotional lore. Several of her fellow attendees—Margaret Jones, Olive Bacon, Elizabeth Bunting, Anna Brown, Esther Burr, Hannah Ellis, Huldah Justice, Mary Morris, Susan Shaw, Rebecca Stackhouse, and Eliza Webb—participated in the antislavery, antiwar, and prison-reform movements. Even Angelina Grimké Weld asked local moral reformers to "procure us a sight of Dr. Hollick's Manikin" when she visited Philadelphia in May of 1846. Some Hollick defenders belonged to the Rosine Association. Others, frustrated by the turn toward moral guardianship, went on to join the woman's rights movement.[34]

These reformers used the opportunity afforded by sexual scandal to articulate their citizenship and sexual subjectivity. Immediately after learning of the indictment, Mary Grew organized three hundred women to sign a new batch of resolutions. "Let men monopolize the sunshine," Grew exclaimed, "let them proudly claim and tax the very air we breathe; but do not let them lay their grasping hands on the means of intellectual culture [and] dole out to us that which they may judge to be our portion!" A month later, over one hundred more women assured "those self-appointed conservators of the public morals, who have sought to repress these Lectures by slandering their *fellow citizens*, and by other equally unworthy means, that we are not intimidated by the frowns or the slanders." *Slander*, a word they thought important enough to use twice in the same sentence, was a crime against an equal, a political agent. One historian has called suit for slander "the principal legal weapon of political rivals" in the early Republic. While Hollick had his day in court, Grew and over three hundred cosigners defended themselves against "the slanders" in the same way they had been attacked—as a group and in the press. By publishing their names, they recorded their individual identities as citizens.[35]

From the perspective of these reformers, the obscenity charges against Hollick amounted to nothing more than false delicacy. They pointed out a familiar and telling contradiction in the hostile newspaper coverage. On the one hand, Hollick's opponents claimed to protect "the skirts" of Philadelphia from a charlatan who exploited female innocence. On the other, they characterized the lectures as ministering to women's "private and loathsome curiosity." This contradiction, which rested on the virgin/whore dichotomy, aimed to silence and contain women audience members rather than the lecturer himself. Whether claiming to protect feminine innocence or to police female bawdiness, both sets of men assumed the prerogative of controlling women's access to public space and free speech—in short, their participation in civil society.[36]

While Hollick defenders differed from Grahamites by embracing a propleasure sexual ideology, both groups of women invoked citizenship rights to demand intimate knowledge. Both of the lecturers with whom they aligned linked the solitary vice to the self-government of republican citizens. For his part, Hollick adopted the language of false delicacy from his female supporters. Ignorance was not only "incapable of preventing vice," he argued, "it produces it, both directly and indirectly!"[37] Antimasturbation physiology promised freedom from vice. This defense was now well established, but Hollick framed it in secular terms. Where the older moral reform concept of true delicacy referred to the universal struggle to bring the flesh into subjection, the new discourse focused on women's education as a precondition for making virtuous choices.

Because false delicacy had become conventional, however, hostile editors were prepared to respond. Hollick, they alleged, hid behind "the truism, 'To the pure all things are pure." Charles Alexander summarized: "The argument amounts to this, that the greater the familiarity of the people with the secret vices to which a portion of our race are prone, and their consequences, the more they will shun them." But he doubted Hollick's sincerity. Despite his "soft words" to the ladies, his book seemed actually to teach youth of both sexes "the intricacies of vicious indulgences." The chapter on solitary vice could also be interpreted as instructions for self-stimulation. He might have referred to the following passage:

> The genital organs become . . . highly sensitive. This produces slight irritation and uneasiness, to relieve which the hand is directed to them; the friction of which produces a new and pleasant sensation before unknown. When once this has been experienced, the desire to create it again becomes irresistible, and with each new indulgence the habit strengthens and becomes more confirmed.

"Beware, the Trojan Horse!" replied Alexander.[38]

This skepticism derived in part from the drastic rise in proprietary healers claiming to treat the "solitary and destructive habits of youth"—a branch of the long-standing trade in venereal cures and abortifacients. A similar market had flourished in London as early as the 1720s, but this trend, like masturbation phobia itself, failed to make serious inroads in North America until the middle of the nineteenth century. Only after female moral reformers made the solitary vice a widespread concern did large numbers of consumers begin paying healers to reverse the damage they had apparently caused through the act.[39]

Hollick seemed to contribute to this growing industry. When the trial began, he made money not only by lecturing but also by selling sexual advice and commodities. The *Daily Chronicle* accused him of sexual quackery, taking particular note of his "private consultation room for the ladies" in the museum where he lectured. Readers of the penny press knew that women could, in fact, purchase sex therapy from a number of practitioners in Philadelphia. A Dr. Hunter, for example, invited "either sex" to his "Private Rooms" on Seventh Street, where he would cure "those who have injured themselves by solitary vice" as well as sufferers of "secret disease." At another office on Seventh Street, John Fondey sold electromagnetic instruments for men and women who experienced "diseases of excess or onanism." Another, Arnold R. Kinkelin, operated a Philadelphia Medical House with his wife, Augustina, including "separate rooms for private consultation" for women and men. Having long treated sufferers of syphilis and gonorrhea, by 1846 the Kinkelins also healed "persons who, by indulging in a secret habit, have entailed on themselves constitutional debility" among their patients. "Let no false delicacy prevent you," warned the Kinkelins in the very same language used by moral reformers, "but apply immediately and save yourselves from the dreadful and awful consequences of this terrible malady."[40]

Charles Alexander was right to suspect that Hollick participated in this marketplace of sexual therapeutics. Initially he saw patients in the museum where he lectured or in the Sanderson Hotel, where he lodged; later the consultations proved lucrative enough to rent a long-term office on Sansom Street. If regimen and medication failed, the ex-masturbator could purchase electrotherapy or "the shampoo" (genital massage). If even the shampoo failed, the client could apply for therapy with a special suction device that Hollick called "the congester," which promised to restore "the sexual powers" to even the most damaged organs. Neither Hollick nor his critics commented on the irony of massaging the genital area in order to restore sexual function lost through masturbation. Nor did contemporaries suspect him of selling a homosexual service when he advertised that "many a man has been saved by these means."[41]

The idea that Hollick might be selling his services to women proved so upsetting that it distracted editors from these interesting implications. Hollick repeatedly urged women to seek out treatment for sexual problems—which, left untreated, could cause insanity. And, at least by the time his second book appeared, Hollick openly advertised the congester to women as well as men. Altering its shape with "a modification," Hollick found the device "of great service in certain torpid states of the female organs." The shampoo also helped female ex-masturbators to recover normal sexual function. George Graham portrayed such consultations as trysts arranged by a seducer to attract women who were "easily led astray by [his] cunning pretensions." But Charles Alexander speculated that only "the abandoned class of females" would use these services. This implicated *all* women who attended the lectures, for there "ladies of good reputation" sat "cheek by jowl beside those who, in search of similar knowledge, may pervert it to wicked and criminal purposes." These critics recognized clitoral stimulation as sexual, even when framed as therapy. They did not, as Rachel Maines has suggested, consider such therapeutics asexual simply because they lacked penile-vaginal penetration.[42]

The women of Hollick's audiences may also have recognized the shampoo and congester as sexual services, but these were trivial matters in light of their larger goals. They therefore sidelined further debate about the nature of these therapies in favor of directly defending their civil rights to free speech and peaceable assembly. As Philadelphia women transformed the lectures into organizing meetings, they consistently elected as officers the most politically experienced of their peers rather than the most respectable. Mary Grew and her sister Susan presided over or recorded the proceedings of meetings in 1844, 1845, and 1846.[43] Neither of the Grew sisters played the role of the dignified matron. Neither married, each expressed her own keen interest in sex, and both subscribed to the model of active virtue rather than passive purity. That their fellow audience members chose them as leaders also challenges the image of white, middle-class women maintaining an appearance of sexual modesty in order to camouflage their best chance at sexual release. Instead, the Grew sisters and their peers had begun to formulate a new politics of positive sexual rights for women and to redefine what counted as *true delicacy* and *pure taste*. Fusing the philosophy of amative indulgence with their pursuit of civil rights, Philadelphia women campaigned openly for their right to discuss sex and pursue pleasure.

The physiology lecture itself offered some women erotic stimulation as well as sociability and politicization. For example, Mary Grew listened to Hollick's rhapsodies about clitoral stimulation and multiple orgasms while seated next to Margaret Jones Burleigh. The two women had been active together in antislavery and moral reform since 1836 and would go on to live together in a "closer union than that of most marriages." They never hid this intimacy from family members, friends, or the activist community. Nor did they mask it as mere friendship or companionship. Far from construing themselves as essentially pure, and therefore too chaste to experience or act upon sexual desire, both Grew and Burleigh publicly endorsed free sexual expression for women during their defense of Hollick. Historians have extensively debated the extent to which such romantic friendships may have been overtly sexual. When Margaret Burleigh died in 1892, Mary Grew grieved in a letter to a friend that her loss was greater than that of most widows, for "love is spiritual, only passion is sexual." Some interpret this statement as an endorsement of white feminine passionlessness. But it might also be read as Mary's attempt to describe the depth of her loss after fifty years of intimacy. To say that such a relationship *surpassed* sexual passion is not to say that it *never included* it.[44] In any case, we know that Mary and Margaret listened together to physiological accounts of female sexual response, read about mechanical instruments that could induce orgasm, became public sexual activists in 1846, and never subordinated their romantic relationship to heterosexual marriage. However they may have behaved physically when alone, it is clear that they did not conform to prescriptions of passive white femininity. Thus, Hollick's paeans to female pleasure, though clearly meant to incite desire for sex with men, allowed for multiple readings.

When female audience members voted for Grew to represent their interests, they chose a capable publicist, not an exemplar of white feminine purity. Yet few other reformers flouted marriage. In the long term, most of

Hollick's defenders embraced heterosexual pleasure and, as we shall see, helped to popularize it as part and parcel of ideal white femininity. They used sexual knowledge, not innocence, as an entry into public debate. However, citizenship carried duties as well as rights in the early Republic. Women continued to assume responsibility for stopping the solitary vice, the outer limit of permissible pleasure. Since "the dissemination of knowledge" would "diminish the awful amount of vice and crime which abounds in our land," they proclaimed it "the duty they owe to the public, to Dr. Hollick, and to themselves" to lead in this dissemination. Defining their sexual rights *and* responsibilities, most of Hollick's female defenders embraced desire, pleasure, agency—and conformity.[45]

THE FRIENDS OF DR. HOLLICK

While women's rights advocates battled conservative editors, the obscenity case against Hollick stalled on a technicality. None of William Darrah Kelley's witnesses could "prove that the book had ever been, legally speaking, 'published' by Dr. Hollick in this city." Witnesses had purchased copies of the book at his lectures "from the person who sold the tickets, but he was only the agent of the Doctor for the sale of the tickets, and not for the sale of the books."[46] Lacking evidence, the district attorney asked to enter a nolle prosequi, but the defense demanded a verdict. Hollick had lost income by suspending his lectures, raised bail, and endured public censure—he wanted the court to declare *The Origin of Life* not obscene. Without proof that he had published the book in Pennsylvania, the jury was forced to find him not guilty.

Immediately, the commonwealth charged Hollick with a different count of obscene libel. This time Kelley accused him of publishing a specific passage, which differed from the original charge of publishing the whole book. The passage "inculcated the doctrine that sexual intercourse was proper, moral and essential to health immediately on attaining puberty, and ought to be encouraged." With no time to prepare, Kelley called himself as a witness. He testified that he had seen a note in Hollick's handwriting attached to a copy of the book. Didn't this prove his publication? The strategy failed. The *Daily Chronicle* blamed Kelley's "manifest incompetency" for bungling the case, while sporting-press editors laughed at the irony of an obscenity prosecutor who "mounted the witness stand himself, to give his testimony 'against the doctor's opinions on sexual intercourse'!" Hollick, for his part, delighted in advertising the "VERDICT OF NOT GUILTY," and returned to the full range of "his professional duties."[47]

The lecturer did not exactly leave free and clear, however. Judge Parsons still intended to read the book and give his opinion of its content. For the prosecution, this hearing would reopen the question that Kelley wished to resolve: what constituted obscene content? For Hollick, it would occasion a chance to argue the merits of popular physiology in court—and benefit from free publicity in the trial reports. After reading the book, Parsons pronounced that Hollick violated the spirit of the law and held him to two thousand dollars' bail, pending a new trial.[48]

Undaunted, Hollick spotted an opportunity to go back to business—now "to give all an opportunity of judging for themselves . . . the character of Dr. Hollick's lectures." Between the indictment and the subsequent hearings, he delivered several courses of "Lectures on the Physiology of Organic Life" (a title intentionally easy to confuse with the suppressed "Lectures on the Physiology of the Origin of Life"). "THE LAST LECTURE BEFORE THE TRIAL!" advertisements screamed, "single admission, or LADY AND GENTLEMAN, 25 cents." The classes had been separated by gender in March; in April, Hollick lectured to men and women together. This tactic gave the appearance of observing Judge Parsons's order to suspend the original lectures. Perhaps the new lectures contained no sexual content. If, on the other hand, Hollick did describe reproduction, the new gender arrangement suggested that he had said nothing to women that he could not say before mixed audiences. Patriarchs could take comfort knowing that women were now chaperoned, while female reformers could celebrate women's equal access to the identical information men received. Hollick could not resist playing on the irony that "promiscuous" lectures were deemed more respectable than those to single-sex audiences. Admitting couples at bargain prices, he invited them to experience heterosocial titillation in the physiological lecture hall. Audiences grew as a result of all of these strategies.[49]

As the trials dragged on, Hollick also attracted new support from a group of male audience members. In May, the "Friends of Dr. Hollick" invited him to lecture on "the equal rights of all men to the possession of scientific knowledge; and the moral, social, and religious benefits which result from its universal dissemination." Within a month, they had appointed a finance committee for the purpose of raising bail. Then, learning that some unscrupulous opponents had allegedly been mailing lascivious notes to female audience members over the lecturer's signature, they raised a reward for information about their identities. Finally, the Friends of Dr. Hollick explicitly supported the statements of female audience members. They pronounced "the information imparted by Dr. Hollick in his Lectures to us, our wives and daughters, as eminently beneficial in their moral and physical tendency," and asserted that "females have a right in common with us to obtain a knowledge of their own structure."[50]

Representing themselves as benevolent husbands and fathers, the Friends claimed to speak for female audience members. But Philadelphia women had already been advocating for themselves for two years before these Friends first convened, and they had consistently maintained that male protection was not what they sought. Moreover, very few "wives and daughters" of the men's society actually attended the lectures. In reality, the social distance between the women who defended Hollick and his male "friends" was far greater than it had been between the Grahamite women of 1837 and the male American Physiological Society.

Hollick's male and female advocates were in fact deeply divided—especially over slavery. About a third of the women had signed antislavery petitions or membership rolls, but only 2 percent of male supporters were abolitionists. Moreover, a significant subgroup opposed abolition: vocal leaders among the men's society ran for public office as proslavery Democrats; other members belonged to the American Colonization Society. None of the female defenders publicly supported these stances. Whereas the abolitionist Mary Grew repeatedly headed women's petitions, the Friends of Dr. Hollick elected a proslavery Democrat, Col. Thomas B. Florence, to preside over their group. Wealthier members could be found, but Florence's populist appeal—he also served as alderman, postmaster, comptroller of public schools, and organizer of the Philadelphia Fire Engine and Hose Company Parade—better served Hollick's man-of-the people image. In short, Florence fit the profile of one of the anti-Graham "street brawlers" of 1834.[51] Perhaps the Friends—despite oddly vowing to defend Hollick "by all legal and honorable means"—actually organized in order to instigate a riot if his books were suppressed. The Whig *Daily Chronicle* hinted that Florence ("the rubicund faced, full-fed, alderman-sized individual") attempted as much; soon after Hollick's first inconclusive trial, he "mounted the stage and endeavored, in the midst of hisses and laughter, to make a speech in favor of universal information in general, and the Doctor's science in particular." The fear that an audience made up of like-minded men could quickly become a mob may also have contributed to Judge Parsons's order to suspend the lectures until Hollick's case was settled.[52]

Whether they knew it or not, Philadelphia's abolitionist women were rubbing elbows with the enemy. That the political gap within Hollick's audiences breaks down most clearly by gender suggests that men and women embraced his sexual advice for different reasons. A substantial number of female moral reformers participated in the defense. Determined to demolish the sexual double standard, they were willing to support even a sexual enthusiast such as Hollick because he supported women's sexual autonomy and maintained that similar physiological principles governed female and male sexuality. Men, on the other hand, likely saw the philosophy of amative indulgence as an expression of libertine republicanism. Hollick's explicit themes of freedom and penetrative pleasure mattered more to libertines than the rest of the text.

The obligatory chapter in *The Origin of Life* on solitary vice would have reminded some libertines of other erotic books that playfully warned against onanism while fetishizing masturbating women. For example, Leopold Deslandes's *Treatise on the Diseases Produced by Onanism*, originally published in Paris in 1835, arrived in the United States in 1845.[53] Deslandes suggested illicit sex as a "less dangerous" means than masturbation by which a young man should "gratify his feelings." Other libertines knew of William Greenfield's *The Secret Habits of the Female Sex*. Ostensibly addressed to the "young solitudinarian," it clearly targeted sporting men with its self-cures for syphilis and condom advertisements. Moral reformers warned one another not to fall for this "most miserable catch-penny," published under the pseudonym *Jean Dubois*. Over time, *Secret Habits* made its way into multiple obscenity prosecutions.[54] At least one of the Friends of Dr. Hollick, T. B. Peterson, certainly knew of Deslandes and Dubois. Peterson published and sold such racy books as *Wildness of Woman, History of a Flirt, The Beautiful French Girl, The Divorced*, and *The Insnared: A Story of Woman's Heart*. His better-known productions included the salaciously anti-Catholic *Awful Disclosures of Maria Monk* in 1836 and a novelization of the murder of Helen Jewett in 1878 ("full of illustrations"). No moral reformer, Peterson defended Hollick because he opposed the censorship of pornography. After the trials, he went on to publish some of Hollick's later works (*Neuropathy*, 1847, and *Outlines of Anatomy and Physiology*, 1861). Moral reformers had feminized physiology during the 1830s; now libertine republicans looked for popular scientific justifications of *their* worldview. Their warnings against masturbation dovetailed with those of physiological reformers, and the discourse on solitary vice reached growing numbers of consumers across the political spectrum.[55]

RIGHTS, DUTIES, DESTINIES

With leaders such as Lydia Maria Child and Mary Grew endorsing Hollick since 1844, Philadelphia's abolitionist women reasonably assumed that he fit into the chain of ultraism that linked reform physiology to abolitionism.

Sylvester Graham's universalist notion of sexual restraint had inspired interracial audiences of abolitionists. But Hollick, unbeknownst to many of his supporters, had declared war on abolitionists in 1843. In a little-known pamphlet entitled *An Inquiry into the Rights, Duties, and Destinies of the Different Varieties of the Human Race*, he argued, first, that black slaves fared better than white wage laborers and, second, that abolitionists advocated interracial marriage in order to "destroy all distinction" between the races. Moreover, the pamphlet asserted the superiority of the white race and attacked "amalgamation" on physiological grounds. Interracial sex, he argued, produced children destined by "physical deformity and mental imbecility" for sterility and early death. Such "offspring" were already "fast dwindling away, and there is no doubt but they will soon become extinct." Because "all the inferior forms, the subordinate varieties of the human race" were "destined to a limited period of existence," Hollick argued that a "natural repugnance" to interracial sex pulsed through white bodies. Drawing on a hodgepodge of extant proslavery theories, the pamphlet offered nothing original to American racial thought. Instead, Hollick assumed the prejudices and resentments of his intended audience of white workingmen and pandered directly to them.[56]

The pamphlet had a limited run. In 1849, a sporting editor scoffed that Hollick had written it in search of fame and fortune before he knew that middle-class northern women would become his meal ticket.[57] He wrote the pamphlet in desperation, shortly after the failure at New Harmony, and brought it on a southern trip. Representing himself as slaveholders' "intended champion," he "told them of his brilliant exploits in England, and what he would do for them by speech and pen." This lifelong ability to tell people what they wanted to hear may have financed his subsequent career in sexual physiology.[58]

Whatever his actual opinion of abolitionists, Hollick never repudiated the antislavery women who came forward to defend his lectures. On the contrary, he cultivated this following while also publicizing the support he received from proslavery men. Did Child, Grew, or other antislavery women know about *Rights, Duties, and Destinies*? If so, they never mentioned it publicly. It is quite possible that the pamphlet went unnoticed by abolitionists: it reached a very small readership, contained little to distinguish it from other proslavery tracts, and was published by the Democratic *New York Sun*. However, Hollick's lectures to ladies did capitalize on the emergence of racial science. And rather than protesting the racism that infused his sexual physiology lectures, white abolitionists and women's rights advocates bought lecture tickets, challenged the obscenity charges, and circulated his books widely. The old Grahamite universalism had faded from their memory, especially after the female moral reform movement stopped addressing the intersections of race and sex.

In order to convince white women that their passion could be virtuous, Hollick encouraged them to believe that they possessed an inherent tendency toward moderation. In fact, he appropriated the word *moderation* from Grahamites to describe the kind of disciplined conformity that, according to him, made certain kinds of *indulgence* healthy. Abstaining from the solitary vice, which he described as an "addiction," was one way to exercise this virtue. Another way lay in cultivating pleasure within loving ("amative") heterosexual relationships, which tended naturally toward moderation. A supremely flexible concept, moderation became a prescriptive norm to which many people could happily subscribe.[59]

At the same time, Hollick suggested that black women were physiologically given to excess. Reviving colonial natural histories that represented African bodies as "curiosities," Hollick wrote that, unlike "normal" (white) women, black women's genitals were covered by an "apron" of flesh. Here he drew upon the science writing of travelers such as Georges Cuvier and Henri de Balinville, who used the word *apron* to describe what they considered to be "enlarged" labia minora and clitorises. Incredibly, he even claimed to have personally inspected Sara Baartman, the South African woman described by Europeans as "the Hottentot Venus," while she was displayed in England. He did not, in fact, see Baartman—she died before he was born. But to sustain the illusion, he copied Cuvier's autopsy notes as if he himself had dissected her body. "In these females," wrote Hollick-as-Cuvier, "the whole of the external organs, differ much from the those of white females; the Mons Veneris being less prominent, the external lips smaller, and the passage itself much larger, while the mouth of the opening is more underneath, or farther back so that, when stooping forward, it is nearly in the same position as in some animals." This association of black women with bestial sexuality illuminates the dehumanizing underside of the liberating self-knowledge that Hollick promised to his audiences of white "ladies." He also reified the Jezebel stereotype by suggesting that black women generally had "enlarged" clitorises and "elongated" labia minora. This explained what he assumed readers considered a stable fact: black women lived in a constant state of desire. He added that the disorder known as "nymphomania" resulted from enlarged *nymphae*, the contemporary term for labia minora. Hollick revived an old racial ideology for the benefit of white female consumers of popular physiology manuals.[60]

What is especially striking is that Hollick pathologized black women's anatomy at the same time that he naturalized white women's sexual passions. What should we make of white abolitionist women's enthusiastic support for Hollick? What does it mean that female moral reformers, so concerned with eliminating the sexual double standard when it came to white men, endorsed a racialized version of the double standard among women? Once again, it is possible that they supported him while unaware of his racist imagery. Hollick may not have remarked on Sara Baartman and nymphomania in his lectures to ladies (these sections did not appear in 1845 editions of *The Origin of Life*, the title at issue in the obscenity defense; they appeared in *The Marriage Guide*, a sex advice manual first published four years later). Even so, we cannot assume that those who defended him against obscenity charges did not also buy and endorse the later works. One 1846 Hollick defender, Susan A. Nudd, went on to buy and inscribe an 1851 copy of *The Marriage Guide*. She was one of thousands who purchased that book. Moreover, while some white abolitionist women fought "prejudice against color" as "the very spirit of slavery," others clearly shared in problematic attitudes toward black female sexuality. Recall Margaret Dye's contention that slavery should be abolished because the "licentiousness among the enslaved females" sullied white women's homes, or the semipornographic images of sexual violence that white abolitionists circulated after the licentiousness of slavery argument lost its critical edge.[61] Many well-meaning white women accepted and perpetuated the racialization of sexual physiology. Without them, it never would have achieved such popularity.

Hollick's second trial dragged on for the next year, being suspended no fewer than four times before he was finally acquitted in March of 1847. After he closed his office and left Philadelphia in 1848, national demand continued to increase for his lectures on "the maternal and paternal systems." His works exploded with popularity beyond the reform community and among middle-class women. As late as 1861, the very voice of respectable femininity, *Godey's Lady's Book*, recommended his *Anatomy and Physiology*, published by T. B. Peterson, as "a most useful work."[62] The idea that solitary vice offset legitimate pleasure reached these women, as well as sporting men, through the expanding market in sexual information.

CONCLUSION

Hollick's writings, trials, and defense illustrate how the sexual messages of popular physiology changed as they entered the mainstream. He initially attracted the attention of female reformers who associated physiology lectures—especially those that warned against the solitary vice—with the chain of ultraism. Over time, however, a broad swath of the American public found his secular, propleasure remarks on sex more palatable than Sylvester Graham's admonitions to chastity. His insistence that women naturally desired heterosexual intercourse appealed strongly to libertine republicans, and the emphasis on male sexual potency made the new secular physiology both more masculine in tone and more popular in reach than evangelical physiology had ever been. Midcentury physicians responded to patients' growing concerns. Despite suspecting *Origin* of being "a nine-penny skeleton of a pamphlet written with a view to excite diseased minds," the *Boston Medical and Surgical Journal* still preferred Hollick's physiology over "the unblushing impudence, officiousness, and offensive" lectures of Sylvester Graham. As we shall see, reform women actively contributed to the medicalization of masturbation through midcentury asylum reform and educational campaigns. Although male physicians built upon women's crusade against *solitary vice*, they increasingly pathologized masturbation through the masculine idiom of *onanism*.[63]

By emphasizing heterosexual mutuality and moderation over solitary chastity, Hollick explicitly invited women into a pleasure-affirming discourse on sexuality. The notion that an individual's freedoms and privileges in the Republic could be measured by his entitlement to pleasure had formerly been the central ethos of libertine republicanism. By 1846, some reform women applied this idea to themselves. They equated sexual demands—to participate in sexually explicit discussions, to experience heterosexual pleasure, and to control their fertility—with political rights. In doing so, they did more than politicize sex; they also presented themselves as sexual citizens—subjects whose sexual virtue proved their civic abilities. The new popular physiology valorized female sexual agency; at the same time, it specifically conditioned women's sexual citizenship on heteronormativity and whiteness. The notion that African American women *embodied* excess implied that white women, like white men, might never reach that limit. The new moderation could include amative indulgence only if lovers were white. White women who consumed the new popular physiology thus purchased sexual subjectivity through black women's abjection.

Yet white women were not alone in redefining sexual physiology. The black abolitionist Sarah Mapps Douglass lectured for decades to African American women and girls on anatomy, physiology, and hygiene. An early participant in the interracial moment in moral reform, Douglass clearly understood the ideological differences between moral guardians and proponents of women's rights. As a critic of the discourse of white feminine purity and an advocate of universal virtue, she leaned toward the women's rights cohort. However, Douglass never signed a pro-Hollick petition. Instead, as chapter 5 argues, she carefully crafted an affirming counterdiscourse on black female sexuality. In an ironic appropriation, she titled these sex education lectures "The Origin of Life."

CHAPTER FIVE

Flesh and Bones

In a Philadelphia schoolroom in 1859, seven students—African American girls, ages fourteen to seventeen—stood in a neat row at the head of a classroom, reciting a passage from an anatomy textbook in unison. Their teacher, Sarah Mapps Douglass, listened, now and then correcting a student's pronunciation. Suddenly, the door creaked open and four white women entered the classroom, their gray dresses quietly conspicuous against walls glowing with watercolor paintings, a botanical alphabet, and maps of Africa. A few students saw Mrs. Douglass inhale, stand, and walk crisply over to greet them; their chorus slowly abated. The teacher turned her back to the strangers for an instant, gestured encouragement, and the recital resumed. In another part of the room, a young poet returned to her contemplation of the human skeleton while two students catalogued the bones, shells, and fossils of the science cabinet.

These impressions are drawn from a source both deeply problematic and unusually revealing: the journal of a southern white woman, Anna Maria Davison (b. 1783), then in Philadelphia on a summer tour.[1] Pleading her health, she enjoyed exploring a northern city each year—a temporary escape from the "dependence" that anchored her to her slaveholding son's Louisiana plantation. On one of these trips, Davison met Rebecca White, a philanthropist from a wealthy family who attended the same Quaker meeting as Sarah Mapps Douglass and contributed financially to her work at the Institute for Colored Youth. White had targeted Davison as a special project for moral suasion and introduced her to the astonishing reach of women's reform culture in the antebellum North. Every year the aging widow toured its institutions with subversive glee before returning to her slaveholding family. She attended Quaker meetings, listened to Lucretia Mott's antislavery lectures, visited the House of Industry for "Fallen Females," and witnessed the creation of the Female Medical College of Pennsylvania in 1850. Now she interrupted Sarah Douglass's class for a surprise visit (in Davison's words: "that I might judge for myself if they [free black students] were capable of receiving instruction—of being elevated—and fitted to take care of themselves").[2]

Sarah Mapps Douglass had once welcomed visits of this kind. In her youth, she had proudly invited whites to view "the hearts" of her "wronged people." She had begun teaching the daughters of the wealthiest black families privately in 1827 and delighted at first in showcasing their intellectual accomplishments. During the visionary 1830s, antislavery activism had changed her goals: no longer interested in proving African American mental and moral worth to whites, she had come to believe that education could uproot exploitive institutions. After the interracial moment in moral reform ended, she turned toward autonomy and immersed herself in all-black spaces. When black abolitionists demanded that "the Public Schools of this city, for our youth" should be "furnished with well-qualified and well-paid colored teachers," she saw a new path. Teaching in one small, private institution, Douglass could not solve this larger problem. However, with the financial support of white philanthropists, she could provide students who passed rigorous qualifying exams with a tuition-free liberal education. They, in turn, would become teachers and start their own black schools throughout the nation. In order to finance the long-term goal of self-sufficiency, Douglass courted white funders to sponsor her educational vision at the Quaker-owned Institute for Colored Youth.[3]

When philanthropists gave unannounced promotional tours to women such as Davison, they revealed a class deeply engaged in learning the sciences of the body. Teaching physiology was both necessary and risky in a social context that maligned all black women with demeaning bodily stereotypes such as promiscuity, corpulence, and gaudy fashion.[4] Those risks intensified during the early 1850s, when Douglass began teaching sexual physiology to adult women and her students at the Institute for Colored Youth.

This chapter examines Douglass's classroom as a case study from the first wave of sex education in the United States, which developed out of the female moral reform movement's physiological crusade against solitary vice. As one of the leading thinkers of the interracial moment in moral reform, Douglass had helped to construct the distinction between innate purity and sexual virtue that motivated many white women to contemplate their own sexual subjectivity. As a result, white reformers focused incessantly on eliminating the solitary vice. By the 1850s, two camps had emerged: those who promoted purity by preventing children from acquiring precocious sexual desires, and those who asserted the sexual rights of virtuous women. The latter group argued that female bodies required both solitary restraint and amative indulgence. The sex education they developed should be recognized as a primary institution in constructing female heterosexuality. Their efforts to cultivate sexual citizenship in schoolchildren dovetailed with the movement for women's rights, especially those who supported medical training for women. As the first female physicians institutionalized the study of anatomy, physiology, and hygiene, they contributed to the medicalization of masturbation and gathered widespread support for the sexual education of youth.

Douglass, despite having become more interested in black autonomy than interracial dialogue, continued to discuss the politics of sex with some white physiological reformers. In her classes and public lectures, however, she foregrounded the specific needs of black women. As the elocution lesson observed by Davison illustrates, she prepared African American girls to "stand and speak"—to talk back to the sciences of the body that permeated popular culture.[5] She also provided useful information for sexual protection, health, and enjoyment.

The solitary vice engendered an elastic discourse on sexual health that spurned false delicacy and introduced new possibilities for female pleasure and civil rights. Douglass deployed its terms in order to safely deliver a unique version of sex education that addressed the specific conditions faced by African American women. For this, she met praise rather than censure or riots. The *Weekly Anglo-African*, for example, warned every female reader that "any feeling that leads her to shrink from the study of this great work is not of God's implanting, and should be repudiated by her."[6] By the 1850s, lectures on sexual physiology were presumed to include lifesaving warnings against masturbation. The necessity and propriety of women's physiological education had been forged through the two decades of crusades against solitary vice. Subtle references to "the laws of life and health" now enveloped Douglass and her students in protective armor. Yet within the walls of her classroom, she prescribed neither perfect restraint nor amative indulgence. Instead, she prepared young black women to navigate real sexual dangers while gently affirming the delicacy of their bodies. By normalizing black female heterosexuality, she affirmed racial equality—and also prescribed sexual conformity. Her classroom bespeaks a wider counterdiscourse of embodiment that free black women forged across class lines during the years leading up to the Civil War.

"THE DIFFUSION OF KNOWLEDGE"

How did Sarah Mapps Douglass, an elite African American woman, become a sex educator in antebellum Philadelphia? At first glance, she appears highly exceptional. Raised in a prosperous, activist household, Douglass had enjoyed educational opportunities unavailable to most antebellum African Americans. She had attended a school cofounded by her mother, Grace Bustill Douglass, and the wealthy black abolitionist James Forten. There she had learned to see her privilege as a debt to her peers, and teaching was "chosen for" her as a means of repayment. Visitors such as Davison recorded detailed observations of the Institute for Colored Youth in part because they found Douglass remarkably cultivated. Many also considered her classroom singularly focused on science. While other girls' schools had emphasized botany for two or more decades, "No other school at present has a mineral cabinet and philosophical apparatus." Martin Delany endorsed the Institute for Colored Youth as "foremost" among Philadelphia's "several good select schools . . . for colored youth," in large part because of this emphasis.[7]

However, Douglass preferred to diminish her uniqueness. She resisted being singled out as "one who is more intellectual than the mass" and challenged stereotypes of an "ignorant and unrefined" black majority. She especially resisted those who held her up as a standard by which to judge other women of color harshly. Anna Maria Davison, for example, construed the teacher's "striking" intelligence, "accuracy" of language, and demeanor "of a Lady" as attributes that "would grace the circles of any white society." Particularly galling was the assumption that she must have inherited her intellect, along with her light complexion, from white ancestors. Like other black abolitionists, Douglass protested that "to be intelligent [was] to have one's Negro blood ignored." Davison tested her on this point by inquiring about "any difference of intellect in the very black scholars from the lighter, or mixed, ones." Whatever her internal response, Douglass replied with studied calm that "she did not think there was any difference, the black ones being equally capable of receiving instruction."[8]

In reality, Douglass came to the study of physiology through long years of collaboration with African American and white women. First in the all-black Female Literary Association and later in the Philadelphia Female Anti-slavery Society, she participated in cross-class and interracial discussions about the body. Well before the rise of Grahamite reform physiology, Douglass's African American peers impressed upon her the potential connections between moral reform, community health, and black women's empowerment. Over time, Douglass also formed a few cautious friendships with white women who fused physiological reform with agitation for women's rights. They introduced Douglass to the campaign to include physiology in the public school curriculum and showed her how to become a public lecturer to ladies on anatomy and physiology. As we have seen, Douglass also challenged white feminists to rethink the racial logic of licentiousness, purity, and virtue. Before, during, and after the interracial moment in moral reform, she remained an independent thinker on sexual physiology.

Douglass began discussing health, moral reform, and the politics of education with other black women as early as 1831 in the Female Literary Association, one of several peer-education groups comprised of African American women from diverse backgrounds.[9] Associated with the cultivation of a free black elite in the antebellum North, literary associations also included working-class women. Members shared multiple forms of knowledge, from basic literacy to poetry, science, and political debate. As secretary, Douglass represented the group's "capacity of receiving a liberal, a classical education" while encouraging less privileged members to express themselves verbally. Topics of conversation included discriminatory state legislation, medical resources for black Philadelphians, white women's complicity in slavery, and black moral reform efforts.[10] Several members—including Grace Douglass, Margaret and Sarah Forten, Hetty Burr, Elizabeth Butler, Amy Cassey, Rebecca Hitchins, Margaret Bowers, Sarah Dorsey, and Mary Woods—went on to cofound the Philadelphia Female Anti-slavery Society in December 1833.[11] Having mustered their own educational resources, this cross-class group began to envision a political role for themselves in abolishing slavery.

The Female Literary Association also connected Douglass to a national black women's community of discourse on moral reform, science, and the body. For example, she learned about the formation of Boston's Afric-American Female Intelligence Society through Lavinia Hilton, one of the African Americans involved in the moral reform movement. The Boston society's first president, Elizabeth Jackson Riley, was employed as a nurse, and members valued her expertise in matters of health and the body. Riley and Hilton agreed that "the diffusion of knowledge" would achieve "the suppression of vice and immorality."[12] In New York, the Ladies' Phoenix Society also formed "for the purpose of acquiring literary and scientific knowledge" in a moral reform vein.[13] Members Louisa Plete and Abby Matthews hoped that by sponsoring "lectures on the sciences," the Phoenix Society would inspire other African Americans "to form moral societies" in their neighborhoods and churches. President Henrietta D. Ray, like Elizabeth

Riley, lacked "an extended systematic education." Nevertheless, her "persevering industry in making investigations" made her one of "the brightest stars in the female literary society." (Her daughter, Henrietta Cordelia Ray, went on to publish, among several poems, one that bore the evocative title of "Self Mastery.")[14] By participating in an emergent national black women's peer-education network, Douglass learned to engage intellectual subjects in terms of their moral and political applications.

In 1835, Douglass joined the biracial Philadelphia Female Anti-slavery Society, where she worked closely with Hetty Reckless, a working-class black abolitionist concerned with aiding fugitives from slavery. Reckless further sensitized Douglass to the experiences of black women beyond the elite circle into which she was born. For Reckless, moral reform meant theorizing the connections between slavery and prostitution, two institutions that thrived on black women's material vulnerability and sexual commodification. From this perspective, the role of education in moral reform became literal and not just rhetorical. By providing literacy and marketable skills to poor African American women, Douglass hoped to furnish them with economic alternatives to prostitution and domestic service. Thus, when Hetty Reckless and Hetty Burr cofounded the Moral Reform Retreat in 1847, Douglass invested her educational talents and resources in Philadelphia's only shelter for African American women. By that time, she had intentionally transformed her own school from one that catered to students "selected from our best families," into a cross-class project, ultimately aiming to train future teachers.[15]

Keeping an independent black school was difficult: Douglass struggled so much with financial hardship, overwork, and occasionally intractable students that friends considered it "almost the certain sacrifice of life for her to continue."[16] But as teaching professionalized, feminized, and expanded during the 1840s, Douglass strove to make the growing field of employment accessible to a range of young black women by preparing them to fill new schools. As the Philadelphia Female Anti-slavery Society joined a widespread push to increase the number of schools "for colored children," Douglass argued that the society's funds should be directed to schools in which black students could advance beyond primary education under the guidance of black teachers. In 1838, she convinced the society to fund her classroom and for the first time made her school available without tuition to all qualified black applicants. In doing so, she joined a larger pool of African American women educators in Philadelphia, most of whom taught in "infant schools" designed primarily to care for children while both parents worked.[17] Douglass distinguished herself by offering advanced education to economically diverse African American girls. Yet nothing in her experience had prepared her for white abolitionists to critique her pedagogy, as some members of the antislavery society began to do. After two years, she chose to separate her school from the society's oversight. Her decision to assert the autonomy of her own school in 1840 resonated with the conflicts dividing the national antislavery and moral reform movements that year.[18]

However, independence came at the cost of financial stability. After years of fretting over low enrollments, Douglass approached Edward Needles of the Pennsylvania Abolition Society to apply for a more secure position as principal of the girls' department of the society's Institute for Colored Youth. Upon beginning that position in 1852, Douglass could count on an annual salary of two hundred dollars for instructing twenty-five aspiring teachers at a time.[19]

Douglass emphasized the sciences at the Institute for Colored Youth partly to ensure that her students received the same education that middle-class white women had begun to receive at female seminaries such as Mount Holyoke. There, Mary Lyon made chemistry, botany, and physiology central to women's education because she believed that science provided a template for a moral society and hoped future teachers would disseminate that model throughout the nation. Douglass shared Lyon's hope that her students would transmit the moral lessons of physiology to new generations of students. At Mount Holyoke, male experts lectured on chemistry or anatomy, after which female faculty led students in "recitations" of that material. By contrast, Douglass wrote her own lectures, thereby controlling the content of the physiology curriculum. The institute, later renamed the Cheney University of Pennsylvania, grew into one of the earliest African American normal schools.[20]

Through the Philadelphia Female Anti-slavery Society, Douglass met white reform women who also politicized physiology. For example, Paulina Wright Davis joined the society in 1845, on the verge of a new career as a lecturer to ladies on anatomy and physiology. Bereaved by the death of her first husband and "entirely isolated" after the split in the female moral reform movement, she regrouped in Philadelphia before setting out on a tour of the mid-Atlantic states. Wright used the science lecture as a space of organizing for women's rights, challenging physiological justifications for female subordination while her old moral reform associate Mary Ann Johnson dissected an anatomical manikin. Douglass shared this politicized understanding of female bodies. Years later, after Paulina Wright Davis remarried and left Philadelphia, Douglass continued to support her newspaper, the *Una*. In it, Davis refuted physiological explanations of women's scarce employment options. "Delicacy and propriety have little to do with the occupations of women," she editorialized; "the one thing required is, that they should be subordinate." After all, those who considered white women too physically delicate for labor beyond the household never made the same claims about enslaved women. Douglass maintained a cordial acquaintance with Davis and called the attention of other white reform women to *Una* articles such as these. She was also struck by the visual power of the manikin and purchased one to illustrate her own lectures as soon as she could afford it. Personally, however, she kept an amicable distance.[21]

Douglass's earliest and closest interracial friendship was with Sarah Grimké, who had begun to visit her family as early as 1835 and later encouraged her to expose racism within Philadelphia's Society of Friends. Grimké moved to rural New Jersey with Angelina and Theodore Weld in 1838 and withdrew from activism just as schisms began to divide abolitionists and moral reformers. White activists critiqued the sisters for retiring to domesticity, but Sarah Grimké's distance from the painful debates that ended the interracial moment in moral reform may have saved her friendship with Sarah Douglass.[22] Over their decades-long correspondence, sex and the body remained recurring themes. Grimké had converted to the Graham system during the early 1830s, and for years afterward she dispensed unsolicited advice about diet, exercise, and water cure. Douglass once playfully rejoined that her own grandfather had baked brown bread long before Sylvester Graham had the idea. At other times, however, she frankly confided in Grimké about her own "trials" while "passing thro' a fearful conflict with the world, the flesh & the devil." During long visits, they sometimes discussed "things that perhaps it is best neither of us should commit to paper."[23] For the majority of their friendship, both women remained celibate. But in 1855, at age forty-nine, Sarah Mapps Douglass agreed to marry the Reverend William Douglass. She expressed anxiety to Grimké, who advised her not to "shrink from sexual intercourse" and assured her, "I have always calculated on being with you when you are married." After the wedding, Douglass regularly alluded to the "painful results" of what proved to be an unhappy marriage. Long after the end of the interracial moment in moral reform, the Douglass-Grimké friendship proved unusually intimate and enduring.[24]

Closeness evolved into mutual instruction as Douglass undertook the study of physiology in her own right. During the 1830s, she had attended popular scientific lectures but remained ever conscious of being one of a very few African Americans present.[25] Over the subsequent decade, therefore, she turned toward black institution building. Along with Amelia Bogle, another black abolitionist teacher, she cofounded the Gilbert Lyceum, a coeducational literary society. At first, Douglass merely hosted the lyceum's courses on "Physiology, Anatomy, Chemistry & Natural Philosophy" at her school. In order to include those who could not afford to pay, she requested a grant of five hundred dollars from Rebecca and Catherine White to fund a series of "mothers' meetings."[26] By 1853, 217 adult women had enrolled in the night school where Douglass delivered lectures on these subjects. Still, only after her marriage to a minister had lent her "unimpeachable respectability" did Douglass take the bold step of advertising her first physiology lectures to the public.[27] White abolitionists sometimes purchased tickets to her lectures at antislavery fairs. One "gay young lady, a Hixite Friend," had "attended my first lecture," she recalled. On another occasion, a wealthy white woman named Edith Elkington attended with her daughter and husband. While white audience members contributed to the support of the lyceum and school, their presence discouraged African American women from speaking frankly and may also have deterred some from attending at all. To remedy this situation, Douglass began to lecture in her home to black women only.[28]

Throughout this period, Douglass occasionally entered white-dominated spaces in search of various sources of scientific information to discuss within Philadelphia's black public sphere. While pursuing black autonomy, she remained informed of shifting discourses on the body in white institutions. This enabled her to update her old friend, Sarah Grimké, as she participated in a significant transformation of the 1850s. Reform physiology, formerly rooted in moral suasion, gained an institutional foothold as it merged with an organized movement for women's rights. After years of agitating for access to public space and claiming a unique need for sexual information, women now claimed the right to practice medicine. In 1849, Elizabeth Blackwell became the first woman to earn a medical degree in the United States. When Geneva Medical College admitted her as a rare exception to its usual policy of excluding women, female healers elsewhere began to challenge barriers to formal medical training. Harriot Keziah Hunt, for example, had practiced without a degree in Boston since 1835. After learning about Blackwell's experience, she applied to Harvard Medical College. When Harvard rejected Hunt, she publicized the injustice at the first national woman's rights convention in 1850.[29]

Blackwell and Hunt inspired a new generation of women, who no longer felt satisfied by the moral guidance and regimen advice offered by popular physiology lecturers. Medical feminists demanded the kind of education that would prepare them for professional employment. The reform physiology movement of the prior generation had raised their expectations: public lectures to ladies had become so commonplace that many considered physiology a distinctly feminine science. Activists insisted that medical practice would benefit from women's special understanding of the body. To this end, reformers created medical colleges for women in Boston in 1848 and Philadelphia in 1850. The New England Female Medical College appealed to gender difference by arguing that women, not men, should deliver babies and treat women's reproductive ailments. The Female Medical College of Pennsylvania, founded by Quakers, tended to endorse women's equality and worked harder to provide educational parity with male medical students at other institutions. When the college awarded Harriot Hunt an honorary medical degree it 1853, it declared support for a known leader of the woman's rights movement (a step the female college in Hunt's own city of Boston did not take). Despite these differences, both schools continued to focus especially on women's physiological education. Male medical colleges did not emphasize physiology until after the Civil War.[30] Reform physiology had given rise to a movement for women's medical education.

Female medical reformers inherited a physiological tradition that deemed sexual behavior a critical factor in determining health or disease. Moral reformers had taught physiology to other women as a set of warnings against licentiousness and the solitary vice. In more recent years, popular physiologists such as Frederick Hollick had counseled women to seek pleasure in heterosexual intercourse and suggested that total chastity could be as damaging to the nervous system as masturbation. The medical women of the 1850s updated these ideas in light of the women's rights movement and their own need for professional employment. Their distinct politics of sexuality shaped the physiology curriculum within women's colleges and beyond. Amid the turn toward medical institutions, popular lectures to ladies continued to disseminate sexual instruction coded as physiology. Female physicians gave public lectures because they needed to supplement the meager income earned by treating patients who, by and large, remained skeptical of "lady doctors." Both Harriot Hunt and Elizabeth Blackwell supported themselves by lecturing on "the laws of life" early in their careers. Their lectures to ladies denounced licentiousness, warned against masturbation, and promoted healthy sources of pleasure.[31] Similarly, the Female Medical College of Pennsylvania raised funds by selling tickets to courses on anatomy, physiology, and hygiene. Graduates such as Hannah Longshore and Ann Preston became members of the faculty and lectured to "LADIES ONLY," finding this work "quite profitable pecuniarily."[32]

Although Sarah Mapps Douglass did not intend to become a physician, she enrolled in Ann Preston's courses and introduced Sarah Grimké to

Hannah Longshore.[33] Both Preston and Longshore were active in the antislavery movement and the Society of Friends, and Douglass delighted in their lectures.[34] However, she probably took classes at the Female Medical College of Pennsylvania despite, and not because of, white abolitionist women's involvement. Several white members of the Philadelphia Female Anti-slavery Society joined Douglass in attending Preston's first anatomy, physiology, and hygiene course in 1851. Most of this cohort, which included Mary Grew, had defended Frederick Hollick against obscenity charges; more than half also belonged to the all-white Rosine Association.[35] Douglass had argued with some of these same women within abolitionist and moral reform meetings. She knew that, despite belonging to an integrated antislavery society, color prejudice continued to shape their attitudes toward sexuality in significant and damaging ways. At the same time, as one of only a very few black women who could attend any college, Douglass persevered at the medical school. Amid her overarching pursuit of black autonomy after the end of the interracial moment in moral reform, she learned physiology with the goal of teaching African American women to think and speak for themselves about their bodies.

THE FLESH

Whether Douglass liked it or not, the Female Medical College exposed her to white women's sexual politics, including enduring disagreements over the nature of female desire. Some medical reformers suggested a need to protect feminine purity, while others portrayed women and men as equally desirous and encouraged listeners to cultivate their own virtue. Proponents of both positions were affiliated with the Female Medical College of Pennsylvania and with reformers within Douglass's friendship network. Few white women analyzed the racial implications of these concepts, but purity increasingly referred to a unique spiritual dimension of white femininity while virtue represented a standard of bodily discipline that theoretically anyone could achieve. As one of the original theorists of this distinction, Douglass remained alert to its meanings for African American women. She selected and elaborated on physiological explanations of sex and reproduction for their specific benefit.

In order to understand Douglass's unique sexual thought, it is necessary to first reconstruct the ideological context in which she formulated her lectures. On the one hand, midcentury medical feminists continued the moral trajectory of reform physiology. They stressed obedience to a set of divine "laws of life" and declared the solitary vice a violation of the body's "proper government."[36] On the other hand, the advent of an organized woman's rights movement changed the terms of sexual citizenship. Grahamite discourse on solitary vice had included women in the ideology of republican virtue but only rarely made reference to the specific civil rights they lacked. As moral suasion gave way to practical activism, women's rights advocates challenged the principle of coverture that subsumed a woman's legal identity under that of her husband. Coverture had special sexual implications: it granted a husband authority over his wife's body and negated any legal recognition of marital rape. Wives were simply expected to submit to their husbands' sexual demands. While feminists worked to change these laws, they also used physiology lecturers to change social attitudes. Paulina Wright Davis, for example, argued that coverture and "the bread question" (female economic dependence) entrapped women in "false marriages." Coercive marital sex caused dangerous pregnancies and disordered reproductive systems. Moreover, yielding to husbands rather than responding to one's own desire caused overstimulation and nervous diseases. Davis attributed widespread invalidism among women to legal and economic oppression rather than the frailty of the female body.[37] Reformers who cast women's physical suffering as a violation of their rights replaced Grahamite rhetoric of self-government with calls for bodily sovereignty. Instead of stressing the individual's duty to control internal urges, they prioritized her liberty from external forces—including a husband's sexual coercion.

Advocates of women's bodily sovereignty ranged across the reform spectrum. Some radicals, branded free lovers by their opponents, called for the abolition of legal marriage. Mary Gove Nichols, who had helped formulate the older notion of women's sexual citizenship, turned from moral reform to radical individualism. Along with her second husband, Thomas Low Nichols, she believed that no woman could achieve liberty or health within the confines of "indissoluble marriage." The Nicholses promoted a radical form of voluntary motherhood: they considered every woman a "passional queen" who should be free to choose whether, when, and with whom to engage in reproductive intercourse.[38] Gove had profoundly influenced many medical feminists: Paulina Wright Davis, Harriot Hunt, and Ann Preston all began to study physiology after hearing her lecture to ladies. But when she began to argue that voluntary spiritual unions should replace marriage, most woman's rights advocates turned their backs on her. Harriot Hunt admired Gove's early career but considered her "present convictions" unfortunate; Sarah Grimké judged her "preeminently repulsive."[39] They feared that free love would leave women completely vulnerable to exploitation and agitated to strengthen wives' legal rights instead. Liberal reformers worked hard to distinguish themselves from sex radicals in order to make marriage reform respectable and broadly relevant.

When it came to physiology, however, radicals and liberals actually shared significant ideas about sexual health. Reformers of all stripes agreed that women and children suffered the consequences of involuntary motherhood. Mary Gove Nichols described the ravages of "amative abuse"—frequent pregnancies, miscarriages, uterine tumors, and nervous disorders—as slow and systematic "murder." Harriot Hunt, despite disagreeing with Gove about marriage, also traced the "secret springs" of women's invalidism back to "the vice of their husbands."[40]

Moreover, diverse reformers produced physiological arguments that naturalized heterosexual pleasure for women. Thomas Low Nichols celebrated the female ability to have "six or seven orgasms in rapid succession, each seeming to be more violent and ecstatic than the last," as long as they occurred within intercourse between loving partners. Sex radicals argued that women's "ardor" and "great capacity for enjoyment" had been repressed by the "enslaved and unhealthy condition" of marriage.[41] Elizabeth Blackwell rejected free love but agreed that women naturally felt desire and pleasure. The presumption of "superior force of sexual attraction or passion in the male," she wrote, was "a common but mischievous fallacy." Both Blackwell and Nichols argued that sex "in a union without love, or where all the enjoyment is on one side" caused disease in women, while mutually pleasurable intercourse soothed the nervous system. "There is nothing necessarily evil in physical pleasure," Blackwell told women, for "righteous use brings renewed and increasing satisfaction to the two made one in harmonious union."[42]

Liberals and radicals alike also deemed masturbation "a sin or crime against nature," a foil for healthy heterosexual intercourse. Mary Gove Nichols never changed her mind about this; Thomas Low Nichols deemed even sodomy "less hurtful than the far more common practice of solitary vice."[43] Unlike the masturbatory "paroxysm," mutual orgasms did not deplete the nervous system, for "when two persons, loving each other, and adapted to each other, come together in the sexual embrace, nature has provided that a portion of the nervous expenditure of each goes to strengthen the other." Sex radicals and medical feminists agreed that one of the most dangerous aspects of masturbation was that it destroyed the "natural" desire of one sex for the other. In women, Nichols argued, it "transferred" sexual sensation from the vagina to the clitoris. Blackwell told students that "erectile tissue, mostly internal" was "the direct seat of special sexual spasm." By irritating the clitoris, "self-abuse" lessened women's physical craving for penile-vaginal intercourse. "Love between the sexes," Blackwell summarized, "is the highest and mightiest form of human sexual passion."[44]

The contrast between "self-abuse" and "love between the sexes" reverberated throughout women's physiological discourse during the 1850s. Within the Female Medical College of Pennsylvania, Sarah Mapps Douglass might have heard Anna Longshore Potts lecture that women should experience a "healthy ... nervous thrill" during "the normal act of coition," the opposite of the "unnatural mania" that accompanied masturbation.[45] Even Catherine Beecher—known for opposing both free love and the liberal woman's rights movement—conceded that "pleasure is a healthy stimulus to the brain & nerves." Beecher credited Elizabeth Blackwell for introducing her to physiology and argued that social pleasures were superior to solitary ones and that all should be pursued in moderation ("secret vices," of course, must be avoided at all costs). Across the political spectrum, women's physiological discourse returned again and again to parsing healthy pleasure from unnatural abuses.[46]

As arguments for women's pleasure within heterosexual intercourse overlapped, liberal women's rights advocates distinguished their own position by emphasizing spiritual ecstasy in loving marriages. They admitted women's physical desire but increasingly subordinated it to the "love principle," a concept popularized in 1844 by the phrenologist Orson Squire Fowler.[47] Fowler had defined "amativeness" as the mental faculty responsible for sexual desire and the love principle as its spiritual component. The love principle made sex pleasurable and reproduction sacred, for the sexual act only had the potential to reproduce *bodies*. It was the love principle, Fowler explained, that transmitted the *soul* from parents to children. The love that parents felt toward each other at the moment of conception infused children with positive character traits, whereas the absence of love wrought psychic and physiological disaster upon offspring. Thus, "love alone can sanctify this indulgence." People who sought mere physical sensation were "BAD CITIZENS." By "perverting" the *"normal or natural"* use of the amative faculty, they damaged their organs and eventually lost the ability to feel even bodily pleasure.[48]

Yet precisely because love sanctified sex, Fowler considered "mutual pleasure" within a loving marriage to be important in its own right. In this way, he helped to lay the groundwork for heterosexuality, which later sexologists would define as the desire for intercourse with the opposite sex regardless of the potential for reproduction.[49] Fowler presciently employed the word *sexuality*—a term few other antebellum writers used—to refer to "the mental and physical characteristics and differences of the sexes."

Those differences included eroticism: a man was a man partly because he desired a woman, and vice versa. Because the sexes embodied opposite and complementary spirits, they thrived only in connection. "The fundamental basis of love," Fowler argued, "is laid in the adaptation, especially mental, of the sexes to each other." The love principle superseded the physical need to procreate. Although spouses should *only* indulge when they were both moved to become parents, sexual reciprocity also constituted the backbone of an intimate relationship ("the tie that binds" and "bane of contention"). In heterosexual intercourse, "the man . . . gives off his masculine fluid or mentality, which his loving consort imbibes, and incorporates with her own, and vice versa as to woman."[50]

The problem with the solitary vice, from this perspective, was that it diminished "the manliness of the male, and the feminineness of the female." Women innately possessed a greater measure of the love principle than of amativeness. They needed their "physical and mental sexuality" to be cultivated by their spouses. A sexually selfish husband could permanently damage normal female desire, whereas an attentive husband made his wife "prize his sex." More than parentage, sexual pleasure involved a magnetic "attraction," the mutual exchange of spiritual and sexual affinities. Increasingly, it also struck reformers as a right of woman—one too long monopolized by men.[51]

Amativeness proved flexible enough to inspire libertarians such as Frederick Hollick, radicals such as Mary Gove Nichols, and liberal feminists such as Sarah Grimké. The latter group, especially, invoked the love principle to sanctify women's pleasure and safeguard their sexual rights within legal marriage. It was this group who composed the bulk of the physiology lectures that Sarah Mapps Douglass attended. Both in the Female Medical College of Pennsylvania and in her correspondence with Sarah Grimké, Douglass encountered the love principle as a legitimate source of female sexual pleasure. However, the medical reformers and woman's rights advocates in her discursive community did not agree among themselves about the implications of amativeness. The idea of the love principle enabled some feminists, such as Harriot Hunt, to turn once again toward the goal of protecting white feminine purity.

Hunt agreed with Fowler that women possessed a greater measure of spiritual than carnal love; she added that they could therefore elevate society's moral tone in the political realm. Unlike most liberal feminists, she remained active in the female moral reform movement well into the 1850s. Fusing political rights with the rhetoric of moral guardianship, she argued that "society needs women with good legal knowledge, as administrators, as guardians for children, and as a protecting feminine element for women." Hunt also typified the increasing whiteness of purity discourse. As an abolitionist, she protested the licentiousness of slavery—but she did so by condemning slaveholding men's adultery, the desecration of their vows to their wives. Writing in 1855, Hunt echoed Margaret Dye's 1838 contention that the main victims of licentiousness were white women of the slaveholding class.[52] But now, few fellow reformers noticed or condemned this perspective. Hunt invoked the love principle to purify white women's political aspirations. Yet even as she championed woman suffrage and other political rights, her sexual ideology emphasized external control over individual virtue. Once empowered, moral guardians would mobilize the state against licentiousness and thereby protect other women against sexual exploitation. This ideology would come to characterize the feminist wing of the postwar Social Purity movement, which agitated for laws against prostitution and sexual trafficking (tellingly called "white slavery").[53] With regard to both slavery and woman's rights, Hunt deemed purity the moral property of white women.

Other antebellum feminists, such as Paulina Wright Davis, invoked the love principle to endorse an egalitarian model of sexual citizenship. The *Una* reprinted sections of *Love and Parentage*, editorializing that sexual virtue could only occur alongside bodily sovereignty. The sexual commodification of *all* women—enacted in brothels, slavery, and marriage laws—neutralized their virtue, which could only be exercised by sovereign individuals. The "correction of these abuses," she concluded, "is the starting point of all other reforms." In an ideal relationship—a union formed by two self-governing individuals—true love naturally encouraged sexual moderation. Rather than an essential trait of whole races or sexes, virtue followed the love principle. In doing so, it also structured heterosexuality. Davis explained to her listeners that it "was intended in the divine order" that women should enjoy sex with men, for "the blending of the two [sexes] constitutes the progress, and will result in the perfection of humanity." The love principle made a virtue of heterosexual pleasure.[54]

The purity/virtue split also characterized midcentury women's physiological societies. The Ladies' Physiological Institute of Boston and Vicinity, for example, promoted sexual purity. A special committee chose women to nominate for membership, vetted their "character," and reported their findings before calling a vote on each name. Having confirmed members' purity, the institute's board of officers protected it by censoring racy books and lectures. They invited Orson Fowler to discuss woman's "love-nature" in 1852, but drew the line at Frederick Hollick's philosophy of amative indulgence. When Hollick donated copies of his newest book, *The Marriage Guide*, to the institute, an officer moved to restrict access to the book "to such persons as their judgment approved." With only one dissenting voice, the board agreed and further voted not to list Hollick's books in the institute's catalog.[55]

By contrast, the Providence Physiological Society, which formed in 1850 under Paulina Wright Davis's leadership, considered virtue an attribute gained through learning and open discussion. Although this society was also comprised entirely of women, its name did not define them primarily as "ladies" and its bylaws included all who sought physiological education. Davis explained the "necessity of woman's nature to love," adding that "this love is not debasing but purifying."[56] She cited both Fowler and Hollick, inviting members to consider the implications of their physiology for women's rights. Hollick had written in the *Marriage Guide* that refraining from sex for nine months of pregnancy was unhealthy. Though Davis broadly supported the philosophy of amative indulgence, she feared this passage could be interpreted to suggest that pregnant wives owed their husbands regular sexual intercourse. She maintained "that it was a matter which woman must take into her own hands, and give the law upon the subject."[57]

The disagreement between the two groups should not be overstated. Both included liberal advocates of women's rights and endorsed the love principle. But only the Providence society treated the solitary vice as a matter of concern for adult women.[58] The Boston Institute, comprised of women whose purity had become a qualification for membership, departed from the older tradition of self-scrutiny. Ideological tensions between reformers who attempted to build white women's moral authority (purity) and those who sought political rights based on egalitarian principle (virtue) persisted. These issues, rooted in competing sexual ideologies and racial assumptions, would profoundly divide the postwar women's rights movement.

Douglass participated in a community of discourse that included both views of amativeness. Sarah Grimké, though presumably celibate, considered heterosexual pleasure sacred and Americans "impure that we do not so regard it." She wrote in 1855 that "if the intercourse of the sexes is at once placed on the high & holy ground it ought to occupy . . . marriage, generation, birth will be full of purity & interest, full of solemn wonder & tender recognition." On the eve of Douglass's marriage, Grimké called sexual intercourse "as much the natural expression of affection as the warm embrace & ardent kiss" and advised Douglass to focus on the love principle, for "the more intimate your union with Mr. D. the less you will turn from it."[59] Grimké also brought these ideas to Harriot Hunt, whom she had befriended during the late 1840s. At first, she argued against Hunt's assumption of essential feminine purity. For example, when Hunt lectured on sex and reproduction, Grimké urged her to include men. Mixed audiences would be a "noble testimony to the oneness of man & woman."[60] But over time, she came to admire Hunt's medical knowledge and feminist activism so much that she stopped critiquing her sexual ideology. Grimké also introduced Douglass to Hunt in hopes that their shared interest in physiology would engender dialogue, if not friendship.[61] But Douglass continued to prefer Ann Preston, whose sexual physiology turned on virtue rather than purity. She attended her lectures for "the pure intellectual enjoyment they give me," and praised Preston for "bringing great truths clearly before her pupils"—that is, for emphasizing universal physiological laws and suggesting all could cultivate virtue by obeying them.[62] As one of the architects of the purity/virtue distinction during the 1830s, Douglass remained acutely aware of its racial implications.

By advocating sexual virtue rather than feminine purity, Douglass also necessarily promoted the idea that all women must rise above the solitary vice. African American women came into focus as self-governing individuals in her physiology lectures. Members of her public audiences thanked her for this, resolving that "women owe it to themselves, as well as posterity" to obey the laws of life.[63]

THE INVENTION OF SEX EDUCATION

By teaching the same physiological laws that adult women learned in public lectures and female colleges to young people in her classroom, Douglass participated in the nation's first wave of sex education in schools. This movement used the newly widespread fear of masturbation to advocate for laws mandating physiology as part of the public school curriculum. Having accepted that adult women needed to learn physiology partly in order to avoid the consequences of solitary vice, reformers of the 1850s extended this argument to children. After more than a decade of imploring mothers to teach their own children not to masturbate, reform women concluded that state intervention would be necessary because the false delicacy of parents kept the rising generation ignorant and in danger.

Women's medical colleges especially supported measures requiring teachers to pass a qualifying examination in physiology before they entered the classroom. Their own graduates would gain professional opportunities when normal schools and teachers' institutes hired them to lecture on physiology to aspiring female teachers. Administrators also hoped that in exchange for this public service, states would allocate public monies for the medical colleges to maintain operations and attract new students. Women's rights advocates such as Ann Preston supported this reform because they sought to cultivate virtue in youth of both sexes while also meeting a practical need. Those such as Harriot Hunt who subscribed to the purity model agreed that masturbation endangered the nation's health. Calling it the "especial temptation of the child," they deemed women the proper authorities to prevent it.[64] Although their motives differed, both sets of activists helped to revive the association of masturbation with young people by campaigning for physiological education as a means to prevent the solitary vice.

In order to achieve mandatory physiological education, reform women had to convince male politicians and voters that investing in female medical colleges and teacher training would serve the public good. They did so by stressing the old association between the solitary vice and mental illness. In doing so, evangelical women who warned that the solitary vice harmed the nervous system unknowingly contributed to what would become a secular and medicalized view of "masturbatory insanity."[65] Until the 1850s, most antebellum physicians remained skeptical of the notion that the solitary vice caused insanity, but moral reformers had promoted this etiology as early as 1833. They focused particularly on the neurological issue after 1836, when their interests began to intersect with those of a self-promoting asylum superintendent named Samuel B. Woodward. That year, Woodward named masturbation as the second leading cause of insanity among patients of the Worcester Lunatic Asylum. He also issued a tract called *Hints for the Young*, which described masturbators of both sexes "reduced to idiocy" by a habit that proper education would have prevented. These claims were directed at taxpayers, who financed his controversial "moral treatment" of patients in the public asylum. Moral treatment involved expensive architectural changes to asylum buildings and paying staff to distract patients from their baser appetites with edifying literature, uplifting lectures, and sewing circles. Female moral reformers reprinted Woodward's arguments again and again in the *Advocate* and the *Friend*. They also distributed *Hints to the Young* in every village from Maine to Ohio and canvassed their neighbors to take Woodward's statistics to heart. Partly as a result of this publicity, states built numerous public asylums on the moral treatment model over the next two decades.[66]

During the same period, however, reform women began to lobby state officials such as Horace Mann, creator of the common school system and Massachusetts secretary of education, to redirect funds from asylum building to professional training for women. Moral guardians cited Woodward's statistics to argue that women, who increasingly predominated among teachers, could prevent what appeared to be a cresting wave of mental illness. Medical feminists, for their part, hoped to convince male politicians and voters that public investments in physiological education would save taxpayers money by *reducing* the need for state asylums such as the one at Worcester—institutions that "abound through the prevalence of secret vice."[67] No longer willing to be relegated to the popular lecture circuit, they appealed to the state to formalize a new cadre of female experts on the science of sex.

Horace Mann introduced this logic to the attention of taxpayers and jurists, arguing that "a general diffusion of physiological knowledge will save millions annually to the State"—primarily by reducing "the size of those deplorable necessities of an imperfect civilization, Hospitals for the Insane." Until his last year on the school board, Mann insisted that the solitary vice—about which too many educators were silent—gave "direct birth to insanity."[68] In 1850, Massachusetts's General Court passed a law requiring qualifying exams in physiology for all teachers, and American sex education was born.

As the asylum reform movement grew up alongside the feminization of physiology, women's medical colleges sought to place their students as physicians, matrons, and educators in state institutions. Samuel Gregory—founder of the New England Female Medical College and author of two pamphlets denouncing solitary vice—hoped alumnae would staff "insane and general hospitals, alms-houses, and prisons, in asylums for the deaf, dumb, & blind; and in reformatory schools for girls" throughout the land.[69] Relatively few women secured such positions at first, but those who did institutionalized female moral reform discourse on the solitary vice. Douglass could witness as the matron of Philadelphia's Moyamensing Prison proselytized female inmates with copies of Woodward's *Hints to the Young* and Mary Gove's *Solitary Vice*.[70] She may also have known Mary Stinson, the first woman to practice medicine in an asylum, for they both attended the Female Medical College of Pennsylvania. In 1869, Stinson joined the very epicenter of masturbatory insanity: Worcester State Lunatic Hospital.[71] The scarcity of such opportunities, however, continued to push many medical women to earn their living as lecturers on physiology.

The movement for women's medical education both contributed to and profited from the antebellum feminization of teaching. Between 1837 and 1848, more than twenty-five hundred women gained employment in the Massachusetts schools, outnumbering men by two to one at the end of this period. Envisioning "a nobler professional class," Horace Mann initially encouraged teachers to consider "apprenticeship with a physician," so that "by acquiring a knowledge of human physiology" they could "preserve and insure the healthfulness of the young." Samuel Gregory agreed that "a matron-physician should be attached to every seminary for the education of girls . . . to draw out revelations (before it should be too late) on which future health, or life itself, might depend." Upon passage of the physiology law, the New England Female Medical College pledged an annual quota of graduates to teach physiology in normal schools and teachers' institutes. Others went further, arguing that "our female teachers ought to attend at least one term in a medical college, to qualify them to preserve their own health and that of their pupils." Sarah Mapps Douglass did exactly that.[72]

Teacher training could endorse a vision of feminine purity or of virtuous heterosexual pleasure, as long as it prevented the "insanity, idiocy, and various other physical infirmities" associated with solitary vice.[73] Students at the New England Female Medical College could read Frederick Hollick's *Origin of Life* and *Diseases of Women*, while the Ladies' Physiological Institute considered its own lectures best suited to "the first classes in the Public Schools."[74] Local school committees that checked compliance with Massachusetts's physiology law expected teachers who had learned physiology under "physicians of their own sex" to find an appropriate way to instruct children on the dangers of solitary vice. In 1858, school visitors in the town of Boxford chastised teachers who failed to teach physiology, reminding them that the law required them to impart, among other virtues, "chastity." The Plymouth committee considered teachers more likely than parents to recognize the symptoms of masturbation. In Sturbridge, townspeople held that even the youngest children could understand "the great laws of human existence, the violation of which produces disease, suffering and death."[75]

The Massachusetts campaign inspired other states to follow suit in subsequent decades and had a long-term impact on sex education. When Pennsylvania passed its own law in 1881, the Institute for Colored Youth had already produced generations of black teachers equipped to teach physiology. Educators continued to pathologize masturbation, whether to promote abstinence or "wholesome" married intercourse, well into the twentieth century.[76]

Douglass participated in this trend for her own reasons: she worked in a private school and in a state that did not yet require even public teachers to teach physiology. Nor did the Institute for Colored Youth require it of her. Charles Reason, the principal of the male department, did not teach physiology to boys. Though intent on giving girls exactly the same classi-

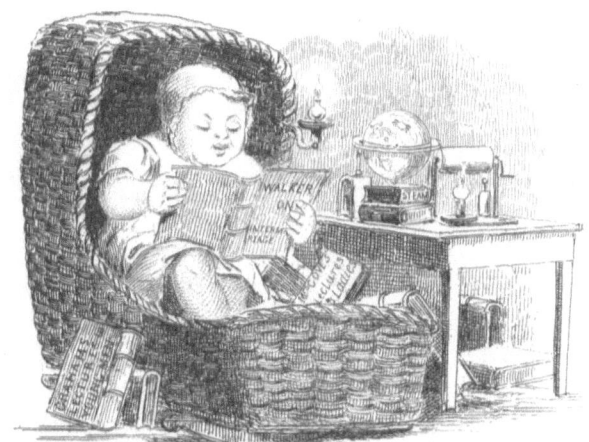

FIGURE 7. In this parody of "Juvenile Studies in the Nineteenth Century," humorist David Claypoole Johnston mocks the campaign for physiology in the public schools by depicting a very young child learning about the solitary vice from books such as Sylvester Graham's *Lecture to Young Men* and Mary Gove's *Lectures to Ladies*. (*Source:* D. C. Johnston, *Scraps*, 1840. Courtesy of the American Antiquarian Society.)

cal education that boys received, Douglass added physiology to the girls' curriculum.[77]

Antimasturbation physiology legitimized sex education for girls in her school, just as it had done for women in public lecture halls. Douglass invoked this discourse when she argued that students "wholly ignorant of the laws" of health could not exercise "proper government" over their own bodies. "Then light, more light," she urged, "that they may read, mark, learn and inwardly digest!"[78] By teaching the "laws of bodily and *mental* well-being," she contributed to the association between solitary vice and mental illness.[79] But she also depended on that association to mask the rest of her sexual content.

So what exactly did students learn about sex in their physiology lessons at the Institute for Colored Youth? In the absence of student notes or lecture transcripts, Douglass's teaching materials shed some light. When Anna Maria Davison observed Douglass's classroom, she recalled seeing *Cutter's Anatomy*. The Institute for Colored Youth's library contained nine hundred volumes; the fact that Davison saw this one in use during an unannounced visit suggests that students used it frequently. Its author, Calvin Cutter, an abolitionist doctor, supported mandatory physiology as sex education. He and his wife, Eunice P. Cutter (herself a teacher), wrote physiology textbooks to be "placed in the hands" of normal school students. Douglass catalogued his *Anatomy and Physiology* as part of the institute's library. She may also have lectured from his *Female Guide*, which warned against "a solitary, but fatal vice." Cutter prescribed home recipes for "suppressed menstruation," including known abortifacients such as aloe and pennyroyal. He also publicly endorsed Savage's Bilious Deobstruent Pills (possibly a commercial emmenagogue) and lost his membership in the New Hampshire Medical Society as a result. *The Female Guide* further advised women to wash with a mixture of zinc, laudanum, and water if they suffered from leukorrhea—a common complaint that sometimes masked gonorrhea. Some editions of *Anatomy and Physiology* contained the same recipes without identifying them with women or the reproductive system.[80] Alternative physiology primers certainly existed, from the didactic (e.g., William Alcott, *The House I Live In*, 1834) to the soporific (e.g., William Carpenter's *Elements of Physiology*, 1846).[81] Douglass chose *this* textbook because it offered valuable information for her physiology classes without advertising its sexual content.

By teaching Cutter's book, Douglass also aligned herself with liberal reformers who rejected purity in favor of virtue. Davison seems not to have registered the sexual politics of the selection, but other reform women considered Cutter a controversial advisor even for adults. In 1851, the Ladies Physiological Institute of Boston debated his propriety. Cutter fared better than Frederick Hollick had in a similar discussion—members narrowly voted to hear him lecture—but both men raised hackles by prescribing fertility-control methods in their printed works. As reform women increasingly accepted that parentage and the love principle sanctified sex, these men suggested the possibility of love and pleasure without reproduction. While purity advocates considered this a perversion of amativeness, proponents of voluntary motherhood subtly welcomed information that might help women control their own fertility. To be sure, white reformers publicly stressed women's negative rights as the key to voluntary motherhood; some also condemned abortion as a brutal consequence of seduction. But many more understood that in the absence of negative rights, practical tools were necessary to manage the effects of unwanted sexual contact. Thousands of them bought books, such as Cutter's or Hollick's, that taught them how to prevent unwanted pregnancies and infections.

Douglass gave students access to Cutter's text as a protective strategy for African American women of all economic classes. At least some of her students performed paid domestic labor to help support their families, while others undoubtedly lived with mothers, sisters, and aunts employed as cooks, maids, and laundresses. (We know this because she reported using domestic examples when describing the physiological consequences of overwork and struggling to use accessible language in her lectures; she probably also accounted for work schedules when excusing tardiness and absence.)[82] As we have seen, African American women who worked in white homes experienced sexual harassment and assault. Nor were they alone in their sexual vulnerability: middle-class black women also faced the possibility of being accosted for sex by white men who presumed that they were promiscuous. In this context, Cutter's recipes could meet a deep and urgent need.

Davison might have picked up this complex of meanings had she not been so fixated on the skin color of the student reading the volume ("remarkably black") that she could not see its sexual implications. Douglass closed the conversation by loftily declaring it "a pleasure to her to teach Physiology" since "a knowledge of the construction of the human frame taught morality."[83] Antimasturbation discourse both authorized a frank sex education and concealed its explicitness in strategic ways.

Yet Douglass also conveyed a joyous approach to the body, not merely a defensive one. When Davison entered the classroom in 1859, she vividly recorded an active and colorful pedagogy in motion. The teacher had "hung various paintings of her own" on the walls: "the circulation of the Blood from the Heart . . . the Muscles, and the different parts of the human system." She also used her own botanical art, a series of floral watercolors, as teaching tools, which may have functioned as erotic allegory. Dorri Beam argues that flowers—which are, after all, plants' reproductive systems, replete with soft creases and folds—naturally allude to female genitals. Douglass strategically depicted brightly colored, "exotic" flowers (such as fuchsia and hibiscus) as emblems of modesty.[84] She painted the fuchsia for one of her wealthiest students, Mary Anne Dickerson, and inscribed her friend Amy Matilda Cassey's album with a direct simile between black women's bodies and delicate flowers:

> No marvel woman should love flowers
> They bear so much of fanciful similitude
> To her own history; like herself repaying
> With such sweet interest all the cherishing
> That calls their beauty or their sweetness forth
> And like her, too, dying beneath neglect.

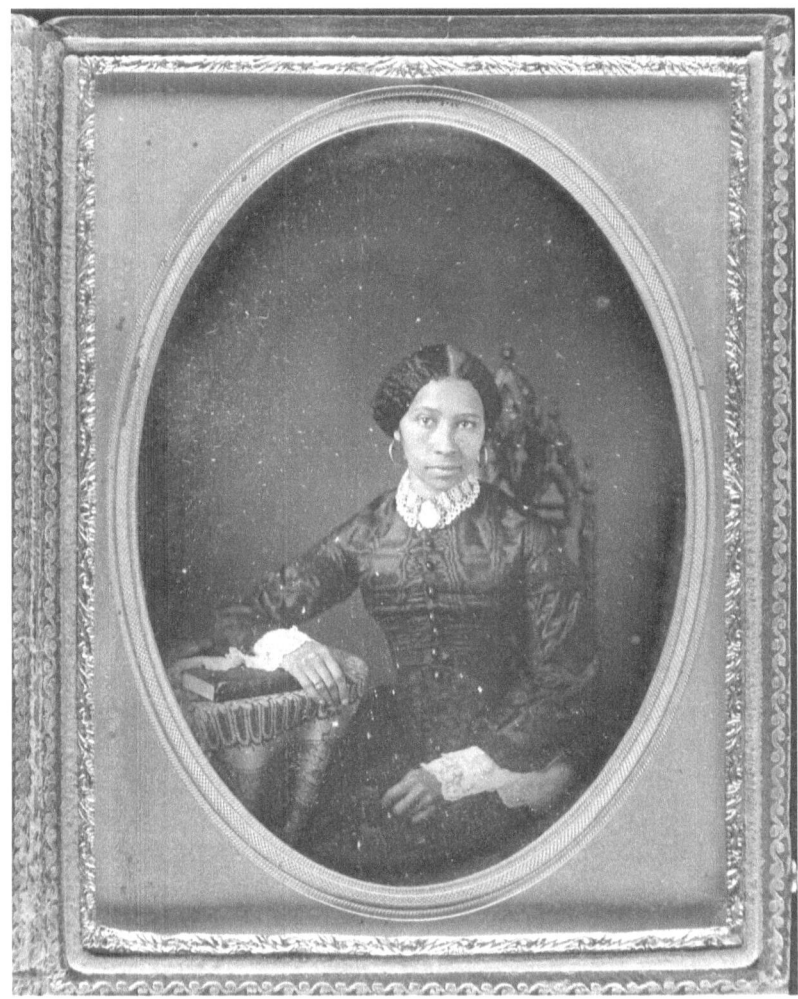

FIGURE 8. Portrait likely taken by Robert Douglass, brother of Sarah Mapps Douglass. The sitter has not been identified but may have been one of Sarah Mapps Douglass's wealthier students, Mary Anne or Martina Dickerson. (*Source:* From the Dickerson Family Collection, courtesy of the Library Company of Philadelphia.)

Douglass copied these lines from an elocution primer that she used in her classroom alongside Calvin Cutter's sex education textbooks. The aspiring teachers who attended the Institute for Colored Youth learned anatomy through elocution rather than passive listening precisely so they would be able to pass it to future generations. The fuchsia thus illustrated a lesson in which students and peers learned to speak for themselves about black and female bodies.[85]

As historians Erica Armstrong Dunbar and Erica Ball have noted, Douglass, like other black abolitionist women, presented refined sentimentalism as a counterdiscourse on black womanhood.[86] While the drawings certainly marked sex education as a respectable endeavor, they might also be interpreted as a contribution to the larger feminist discourse on the love principle. Bodies that experienced love ("cherishing") bloomed with beauty and sweetness; without it, they died "beneath neglect." Teaching black girls to regard their bodies as beautiful, she also raised their expectation for pleasure. Speaking to adult women, she *directly*—and not just allegorically—defined pleasure and love as intertwined and legitimate needs. She conveyed this message by advertising a special lecture on "the Origin of Life." After Frederick Hollick's trials, this phrase became a kind of sexual shorthand signifying conception, fertility control, and amative indulgence. Douglass may or may not have read the book from which it was lifted; she may or may not have known that the author represented black women as anatomically predisposed to nymphomania. Perhaps, like Paulina Wright Davis, she used the opportunity to critique the offending passages. If so, she reserved this exercise for adult lectures while shielding younger students. (The Institute for Colored Youth did not include *The Origin of Life* in its library; Cutter's *Anatomy and Physiology* could serve similar practical purposes from an abolitionist perspective.) In any case, the phrase subtly invoked heterosexual pleasure as a physiological need and a woman's right. Over many years of dialogue with white reform women about the nature of female sexuality, Douglass came down strongly on the virtue side of the debate. Yet in a culture that stereotyped black women as hypersexual, endorsing heterosexual pleasure for women was far riskier for her than for white lecturers. At the same time, teaching African American girls and women to define sexual health in terms of voluntary motherhood and the love principle was in many ways a radical act.

Douglass's sexual radicalism existed not in her explicitness but rather in guiding students toward practical information in a cautious *and* affirming atmosphere. Anna Maria Davison accidentally observed a moment in this process, and knew at some level that she had stumbled upon something remarkable. But its actual significance eluded her. She thought nothing of requesting a souvenir—one of Douglass's floral prints. The teacher demurred, telling Davison she needed "more time to select me something." The following day, she sent along a copy of her best student's physiology composition. Davison judged the student's essay "a *fair* specimen," crudely punning on the color of the author ("the only girl of unmixed blood in the school"). Douglass had bundled the essay within her own drawing. Signed with apparent ambivalence—"I cannot help loving you, because, I believe, you love the truth"—the drawing depicted a crocus, "abuse not" in the "language of flowers."[87]

Douglass communicated through flowers with deliberate, studied clarity. She depended on Davison, an elite white woman, to be literate in the language of flowers and therefore able to translate her message. She needed the crocus to speak for her, to command what she called "delicacy." In asking Davison to "abuse not," she reminded her that she had witnessed a delicate scene and instructed her not to "abuse" the students with unguarded or malicious words. She also used physiology, art, and poetry to portray black women's bodies as themselves delicate—neither hardened against pain nor immune to desire—exclaiming, "how marvelously has God fashioned these poor bodies!"

This affirmation came at the cost of normalization and discipline, for she also charged *students* to "abuse not"—to avoid the "self-abuse" of masturbation. In challenging the stereotype of black female voracity, she taught both self-mastery and self-love. Her blend of antimasturbation discourse, sexual frankness, and racial affirmation reached several generations of children. For Douglass, self-abuse also included a false delicacy that could prevent them from learning how to control their fertility, heal a sexually transmitted infection, and exercise informed virtue. She exhorted her students to treat their own bodies as theirs alone to "govern," "steward," and "tend."[88] For these efforts, Philadelphia's black community rewarded her with respect. When, in 1877, Rebecca Cole became the first African American woman to graduate with a medical degree from Female Medical College of Pennsylvania, she took over Douglass's duties as principal of the girls department of the Institute for Colored Youth—including the responsibility for teaching "physiology, preventive medicine, and hygiene."[89]

THE BONES

While white reformers hoped physiology education in schools would end what they perceived as an epidemic of masturbatory insanity, Douglass deployed this discourse on sex education to her own ends. Similarly, she taught anatomy in a way that would equip students to respond to anatomical racism. Douglass emphasized the bones as much as the flesh. In addition to Cutter's textbook, Davison watched as students handled "a Skull and Vertebra," quizzing one another on the names of each part. Their elocution lesson consisted of "the 'Skeleton,' a poem" ("well recited," Davison noted). Later, they circulated "several pieces of their own composition" on the bones.

This attention to skeletal anatomy occurred amid the rise of craniology, the study of skulls as indexes of racial traits. Samuel George Morton—physician of the Philadelphia Almshouse, and like Douglass, a Quaker—launched the American school of craniology with his 1839 book *Crania Americana*. The book, though replete with methodological errors visible to some contemporaries, met immediate acclaim. In addition to cementing what Dana Nelson has called "an imagined fraternity of white men," craniology served the interests of physicians then searching for professional credibility.[90] At the height of popular physiology, doctors resented competition from self-taught lecturers. They asserted their unique expertise on the body by improving the anatomical education of medical students while barring women and African American men from theaters of dissection.[91] Morton's work, based on comparative anatomy, promised to breathe new life into a science long thought to contain "nothing particularly novel." Setting out to "make these dry bones speak," he appealed to the self-interest of members of the Philadelphia Association for Medical Instruction. Donors contributed more than fifteen hundred skulls to his collection, most of which were taken in wars of conquest against American Indians. From these, he concluded that skull measurements indicated brain size, which in turn determined the character and intelligence of "the five races of man." The rapid acceptance of Morton's theory alarmed black abolitionists, who noted his particular "contempt for Negroes."[92]

Eighteenth-century scientists had also identified "distortions of the human head" with broad racial groups, but their environmental theory of race tempered biological explanations of racial hierarchy with a recognition of human unity. African American intellectuals had responded to the older discourse by stressing that historical and literary examples of black genius disproved claims of their inferiority. But Morton argued that evidence of racial superiority could be found, not in the cultural accomplishments of a group (evidence that allowed for speculation and debate), but in the deepest, hardest, and most enduring matter of bodies: the bones. Morton's craniology seemed to support a theory of separate, hierarchical races.[93]

Lecturers popularized the new science of immutable racial difference in part by merging it with sexual physiology. At approximately twenty times the cost of most popular physiology books, *Crania Americana* found a limited readership. However, the new ethnology reached wider audiences through the lecture circuit. Popular lecturers such as Josiah Nott and

Frederick Hollick told northern workers that the abolition of slavery would inevitably increase interracial sex, adding that the differences between the races were so profound that such "hybridity" would decimate the population. This interpretation stretched Morton's theory beyond its original claims. To support it, lecturers represented "mulattoes" as weak, sterile, and on the verge of "extinction." Colonizationists especially favored this doctrine, for it added a scientific justification for their campaign to remove free blacks to Africa. Morton, for his part, thanked the American Colonization Society and white missionaries to Liberia for their support.[94]

When Sarah Mapps Douglass foregrounded cranial and skeletal anatomy in her classroom, she prepared students to rebut the claims of craniology. Previously, black antiracist protest had generally used a strategy of "decorporealization." By emphasizing religious and historical arguments, in other words, African Americans had minimized the importance of bodily differences. But the popularization of racial anatomy changed the terms of the debate. It became necessary to engage the new sciences of the body in their most popular forums. For example, the popular science of phrenology seemed to dovetail with craniology. Morton was himself an avid phrenologist when he authored *Americana*, and the writings of popular phrenologists such as George Combe and Orson Fowler attracted the attention of northern readers and audiences to craniological arguments. Black abolitionists such as James McCune Smith responded by warning against the "pretentions" of phrenology. Smith had received his medical degree from the University of Glasgow in 1837, where he met George Combe. In the spring of 1839, Combe traveled to Philadelphia and specially invited Smith to his lecture series. For several weeks, Smith sat in the same building as Samuel George Morton, listening to Combe expound on the bodily signs of character traits. Afterward, Smith would watch as Morton testified to the scientific soundness of phrenology. And, when *Crania Americana* began to be reviewed, he would see that Combe returned the favor by heartily endorsing craniology. Disgusted, Smith created a lecture course of his own to "uproot" the claims of these men. With "the aid of skulls," he "demonstrated the fallacy of the attempt to designate the developments of the brain by external convexities upon the skull."[95]

Other black intellectuals joined Smith in expressing their growing concern over what the *Colored American* called the "influence upon an unthinking community" of scientific claims. William Whipper challenged "the learned phrenologists" to "cultivate a new science, and tell us what organs a man ought to have to render him a slave." African American lecturers intervened in these shifting discourses of the cranium so as to rework them in popular venues. "Fashion is not confined to dress but extends to philosophy as well," wrote Frederick Douglass in 1854, "and it is fashionable now, in our land, to exaggerate the differences between the Negro and the European." But there had very recently been a time "before the Notts, the Gliddens, the Agassiz, and Mortons," and it was still possible to change the intellectual tide once more. This possibility required widespread and early education.[96]

Sarah Mapps Douglass taught African American women to study the cranium so they could intervene in these debates. Although she embraced a qualified version of the phrenological love principle, she denied the premise that physical differences indicated moral and intellectual traits. Instead, she assigned readings that stressed the universal qualities of skeletons. Calvin Cutter's textbooks all began with a sketch of an idealized skeleton. His representation of the "bones of the head" was just as teleological as Morton's—but here one cranium, ingeniously sculpted by a single creator to protect the brain from injury, imparted health advice, instilled faith, and modeled discipline. A helpful skull met students' eyes, beaming mutual recognition: "Know thyself." A catechism quizzed them on cranial invariability: "What is the form of the skull? How does the base of the skull compare in thickness with the top and sides?" This universalism struck phrenologists and craniologists as antiquated, one of the anatomical errors that Cutter committed in his enthusiasm for reform. A reader of the *American Phrenological Journal* asked the editors whether Cutter was right to state that the part of the brain responsible for intellect was unknown. "No," replied the editors; intelligence could be measured in "the front part."[97]

Sarah Mapps Douglass's physiology surpassed an investment in respectability and uplift (or, in Davison's word, "elevation"). She taught black women and girls to care for themselves and to speak back to scientific racism. Once, she bragged, a woman in her audience rose, "took up the skull, and . . . explained several things connected with it, quite satisfactorily to me, and to the wonder of her companions." The woman's anatomical literacy constituted a tool to which she could refer in conversations about phrenology or craniology. By training her students to teach future generations how to respond to racial science, she politicized the sciences of the body.[98]

CONCLUSION

As racial science fused with sexual imagery and inundated popular culture during the 1840s and 1850s, African Americans moved away from decorporealization as a mode of resistance. This strategy included particular risks for black women, for white popular culture degraded their bodies on the one hand as unwomanly and on the other anatomized them as spectacles of hypersexual femininity. Nevertheless, Douglass chose not to disavow the body. She jarringly combined the signs of racial science and sentimental femininity—skulls and flowers—to unsettle these discourses. Through poetry, art, research, and elocution, students practiced their own responses to racial science.

Well into the 1850s, diverse women continued to deploy physiology as a tool in their struggles against white and male supremacy. White feminists, such as Paulina Wright Davis, Ann Preston, and Harriot Hunt, transformed physiology lectures into direct discussions of sexual autonomy and legal rights. Reform women also institutionalized solitary vice discourse in women's medical colleges, normal schools, hospitals, and prisons. They argued that sexuality should be considered a proper subject of scientific study; however, unlike later sexologists, they denied that an elite intellectual class should be designated experts in the field. By seeking the widest possible dissemination of their version of sexual science, they medicalized masturbation in the eyes of most Americans. Pitting solitary deviance against a naturalized and empowering view of female heterosexual pleasure, the new sex education tied women's sexual autonomy to active heterosexuality and associated masturbation with children.

Sarah Mapps Douglass contributed to these developments as part of her larger deployment of physiology. She considered sex education a means for improving African American women's immediate material reality and a discursive tool for challenging social hierarchies. Far from proving the morality of African American women to whites, she demanded racial justice. In the process, she instilled in her students a self-respect premised in sexual sovereignty. Her physiology lessons promoted solitary discipline, but not absolute purity. Instead, Douglass encouraged black women and girls to see their bodies as normal—even beautiful—and deserving of the pleasure that came with virtuous love. Long before the rise of sexology, such affirmation powerfully incited heterosexuality.

Epilogue

Around the same time that Anna Maria Davison surprised Sarah Mapps Douglass in her classroom, Sarah Grimké's eighteen-year-old nephew, Theodore Grimké Weld, also tried to pay her a visit. Sarah had asked Sody (as he was known to friends and family) to check in on her old friend, from whom she had not heard in an unusually long time. Sarah Douglass was away when the young man called, but she passed a message along through mutual friends that her health was fine, and she remained absorbed in the duties of a wife, stepmother, teacher, and activist. What little time remained, she reserved for her continuing education in physiology. She simply could not find time to write.[1]

Sody, on the other hand, was not well. He had come to Philadelphia on the first of many trips in search of relief from a mysterious illness that affected him with weakness, reverie, melancholy, and occasional paralysis of the limbs. He also insisted that he could "read the thoughts of others, obtain & retain the contents of an unopened volume in a few minutes, see truth in the operations of nature without the laborious inductive sciences." His anguished family consulted numerous healers and subjected him to several experimental therapies—mesmerism, electricity, boxing, gymnastics and a low-starch diet—before committing him to the Westborough Asylum in 1895. The 1859 visit to Sarah Douglass coincided with a Philadelphia trip to seek treatment from Professor C. H. Bolles, "the electrical M.D.," who promised "almost miraculous cures" with the use of galvanic batteries at the Electrical Institute on Walnut Street.[2]

Other healers determined that Sody suffered from an involuntary loss of semen called spermatorrhea. In 1860, Sody visited Orson Fowler, who examined his urine under a microscope and discovered "considerable amounts of the seminal fluid" mingled with it. Although the adults in the household had done all they could to stop Sody and his brother Charley from masturbating in early childhood—Sarah Grimké had even sewed up trousers to discourage wandering hands—Theodore Dwight Weld considered his son's involuntary leakage a long-term consequence of the solitary vice. Whether or not Sody believed that masturbation had caused his illness, he appears to have resented such surveillance. Yet family members continued to meddle well into his adult years. Relieved that the condition had "a *physical* cause which can be entirely removed," they implored him to give up the habit. If his did so, "all consequences" would vanish. If he refused, "this draw upon the Seminal fluid will, if not stopped, lead ultimately to *insanity* or to *idiocy*." Sarah Grimké, once a champion of universal sexual physiology, now explained the physiology of masturbatory insanity in distinctly masculine terms: "The fluid instead of coursing in its proper channels was diffused through the system." Semen in the bloodstream "rendered the muscular system which should be firm & wiry soft & flaccid," but "the effect on the brain is different there it consolidates." Certain that the feminine love principle could set Sody straight, she engaged a spiritual medium named C. A. Coleman to "rouse into action a desire for the healthful love of woman." Mrs. Coleman proposed a magnetic therapy in which she would place one hand over the small of Sody's back and the other over her ovaries. In this way, "he may discharge the seminal fluid, without the contact of the sexual organs" and "get rid of the fullness of the brain."[3]

Sody's case reflected important changes in the sexual thought of the Weld-Grimké family and the culture at large. His mother and aunt had been among the first to insist that women were neither more nor less virtuous than men in order to call for female accountability, activism, and citizenship rights. In combination with reform physiology, the same argument had inspired moral reformers to make the solitary vice a national—rather than strictly masculine—concern. By midcentury, however, female moral guardians distanced themselves from the solitary vice and staked their authority on claims of intrinsic sexual purity. Meanwhile, women's rights advocates who sought professional opportunities institutionalized antimasturbation physiology in schools, further distancing adult women from the vice. With female moral guardians projecting the solitary vice onto others and women's rights advocates agitating for sexual citizenship in terms of healthy indulgence, antimasturbation discourse slowly reverted to its earlier concern with male genital hydraulics.

Although reform women had helped to medicalize masturbation, male physicians wrested control of its diagnoses. After the American publication of Claude-François Lallemand's treatise on spermatorrhea, the widespread

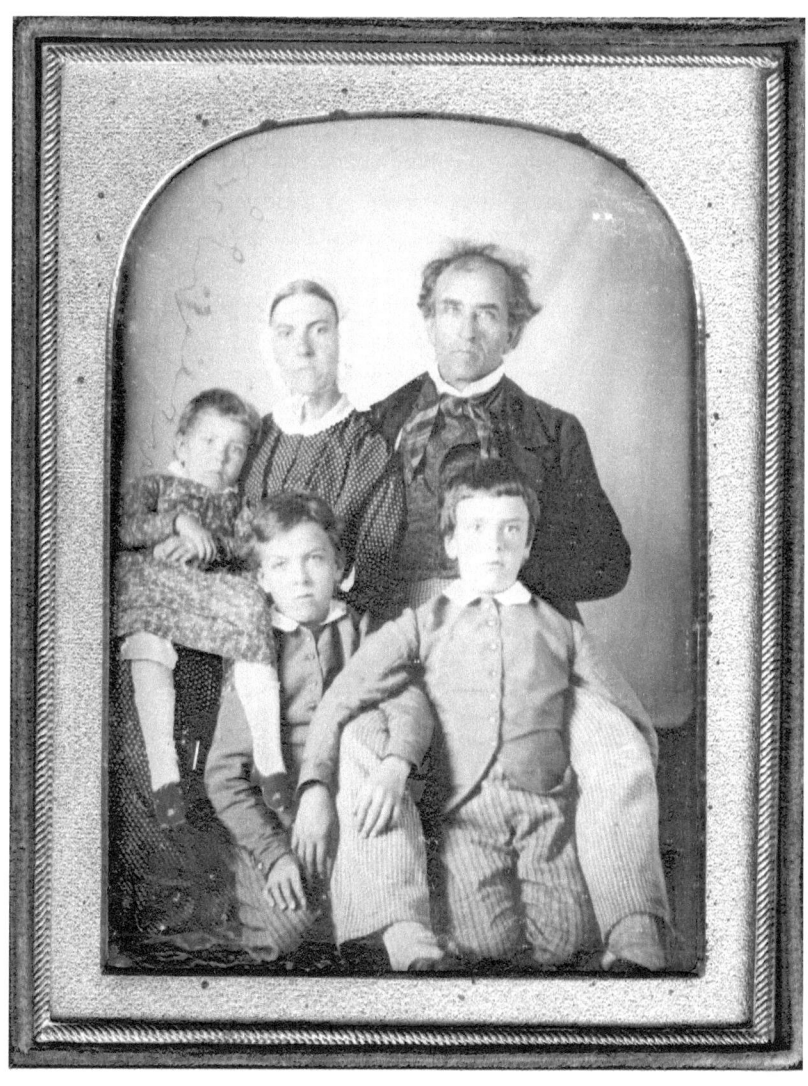

FIGURE 9. Portrait of the Weld family, late 1840s. Charles (Charley) Stuart Weld, *front right*; Theodore (Sody) Grimké Weld, *front left*; Sarah (Sissy) Grimké Weld, *rear left*; Angelina Grimké Weld, *rear center*; Theodore Dwight Weld, *rear right*. (Courtesy of the Clements Library.)

concern over youthful masturbation focused heavily on male youth.[4] Even those such as the Grimkés who had once rejected the notion of gendered morality now subscribed to Orson Fowler's theory of amativeness, which premised virtuous sexual pleasure on mutual desire between a masculine and a feminine spirit. Thus, while the Weld-Grimké family went to great lengths to stop the male children from masturbating, none expressed concern that Sody's *sister* needed the same sexual guidance. By 1860, the solitary vice had reverted to onanism: a problem of male youth who required amative contact with women. But unlike the eighteenth-century discourse, it now claimed the attention of most Americans. Female moral reformers, including Sarah Grimké and Sarah Mapps Douglass, had made it a national obsession.

Douglass's cool response to Sody's inquiries in 1859 also revealed deep and lingering conflicts between women about the goals of sexual reform. Despite the unusual intimacy and duration of their friendship, Sarah Douglass and Sarah Grimké had in fact begun to drift apart. Prior to this period, the two had always maintained a steady correspondence no matter how busy, even when they traveled. But this changed when Sarah Grimké began writing to friends that she had begun to consider women superior to men, rather than morally equal. Without women's "love nature," she insisted, masculine lust would brutify all of humanity. Decades earlier Grimké had famously challenged Catherine Beecher's domestic ideology; now she recommended Beecher's treatises on housewifery. By the end of her life, she had completely abandoned the notion of universal virtue. "After much reflection," Grimké declared, she had concluded "that woman in the matter of licentiousness is the greater sinner." In a complete reversal of her earlier stance, she wrote that "sexual passion in man is ten times stronger than in woman." Therefore, women, "being gifted with greater moral power than men, fall so much the lower when they do fall."[5] Thus, by the 1870s, many white liberal feminists who longed to demolish the sexual double standard found themselves trapped in its circular logic.

Sarah Grimké's revised beliefs about gender and desire hardened further when Sody exhibited signs of masturbatory insanity. After he was diagnosed with spermatorrhea, she wrote to Sarah Douglass about his delicate health and her own changing sexual philosophy. The first signs of a rift occurred when Grimké suggested that Douglass should read Eliza Farnham's *Woman and Her Era*. Aware that Douglass would not like "the author's theory of the superiority of woman," Grimké nevertheless maintained that Farnham's book should be read by all women, because it inspired "appreciation of our nature & destiny."[6] *Woman and Her Era* defined "purity" as one of the "actual qualities of Woman's nature" and "the everlasting barrier against which the tides of man's sensual nature surge." Farnham even argued that "the slave system" had "furnished" opportunities for white women to demonstrate their moral superiority—a line that must have made Douglass shudder. The racial politics of purity, though never articulated in Grimké's letters, remained clear.[7] Douglass remained silent for four years after this recommendation, leaving Grimké to "marvel greatly why my last letter remained so long unanswered."[8]

Then, in 1869, the Grimké sisters discovered the existence of three adult nephews—Archibald, Francis, and John Grimké—the children of their brother Henry and Nancy Weston, a woman he had held as a slave. Sarah Douglass reconnected with Sarah Grimké when two of the brothers came to Philadelphia to meet mentors within the aging black abolitionist community. Afterward Douglass regularly invited "Archie" and "Frank" to her home. But she would never again discuss sexual politics with their aunt. In the end, it was Frank Grimké who informed Douglass of Sarah Grimké's death in late 1873, just when the organized Social Purity movement burst onto the national scene. Douglass mourned the distance that had parted them, a symptom of the more general distrust that would divide postbellum black activists from white advocates of women's rights and sexual purity.[9]

By 1860, then, four major elements of American sexual culture had settled into place. First, masturbation had become firmly associated with mental illness in the minds of most people. Second, although evangelical reformers crusaded against the solitary vice during the 1830s because they considered it a danger to women such as themselves, the very process of spreading the word beyond the feminized reform circuit revived its older associations with masculine sexuality. Both medicalization and commercialization contributed to the new focus on spermatorrhea, yet neither would have occurred without the earlier women's crusade. Third, white feminists such as Sarah Grimké forgot the critical distinction that they and their African American comrades had once drawn between purity and virtue. Once bitterly alienated from one another, liberal feminists and moral guardians now agitated together for Social Purity and "white women's rights." Finally, purity reformers revived the very same racialized sexual discourse that the radicals among them had once denounced. By doing so, they snuffed out the few remaining embers of coalition between white and African American sex reformers and ushered in an era of profoundly segregated women's movements.

Social Purity advocates would not have the last word about female sexuality, even when it came to the solitary vice. A countervailing trend toward sexual liberalism began to reverse antimasturbation discourse in the early twentieth century. Amid cultural changes such as the advent of sexology, the birth control movement, and the sexual revolution, masturbation ceased to be defined as a cause of mental illness. Along with heterosexual pleasure—and eventually, in some circles, surpassing it—*self*-pleasure became an "erotic right of woman."

FROM MASTURBATORY INSANITY TO THE EROTIC RIGHTS OF WOMAN

Both the cultural phobia of masturbation and its destigmatization depended upon understandings of its relationship to mental illness. When Sylvester Graham offered his first course of "private lectures to married ladies" on sexual physiology in 1833, he argued that the solitary vice could afflict people regardless of gender because it overtaxed nerves and not because it wasted semen. The female moral reformers who championed Graham's lectures were the first group to seriously connect the solitary vice with mental illness in American culture; male physicians did not use the phrase *masturbatory insanity* until the 1860s. Male lecturers and crusaders such as Samuel Woodward and Frederick Hollick, who hoped to win the support of these vocal women for their own projects, learned to stress the gender neutrality of nervous disorders caused by overstimulation. Reform women took the threat of nervous collapse seriously because the twin threats of "insanity and idiocy" dramatized the lack of self-possession that came with compulsory dependence and mental thralldom. Politicized by the experience of anti-Graham riots, moral reformers set out to convince women everywhere that physiology concerned them. By disaggregating masturbation from masculinity, women could justify meeting in groups, articulating their subjectivity, organizing for political activism, taking pleasure in sexual speech, learning practical skills, and positing diverse feminist theories of sex.

During the 1840s, lecturers to ladies justified their public sexual speech on the grounds that by teaching the dangers of the solitary vice, they saved the sanity and the lives of all who listened. In the process, they made physiology into a cultural synonym for sex education. Within all-female spaces, white moral reformers testified to their own past errors and warned one another that the vice could make a rational woman into a "confirmed idiot."[10] Month after month, rural women attended intimate physiology meetings where they could—indeed, must—focus on their own sexuality.

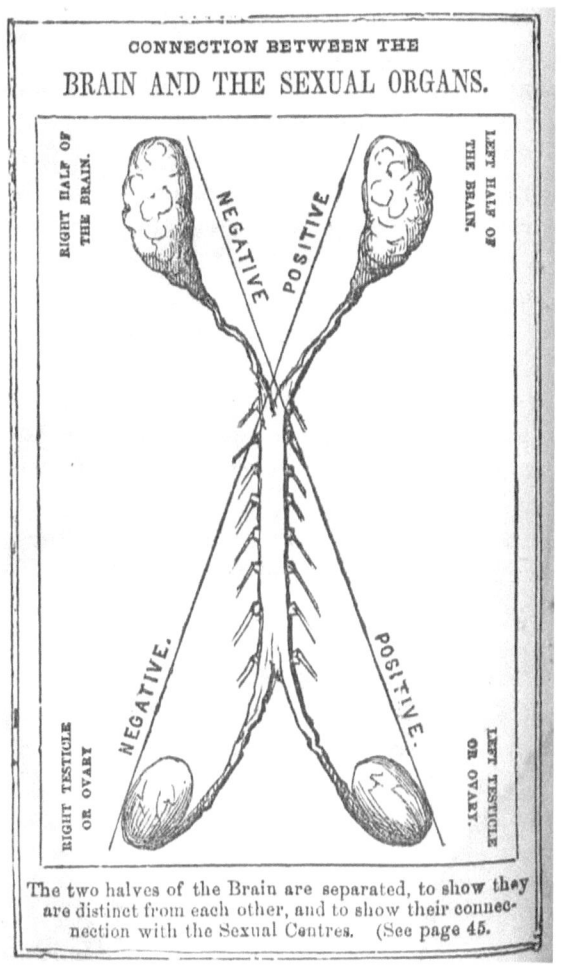

FIGURE 10. With regard to the nervous damage caused by solitary vice, the brain-ovary relationship mattered as much as the brain-testicle relationship. (*Source:* Frederick Hollick, *The Male Generative Organs in Health and Disease* [New York: T. W. Strong, 1853], 368. Collection of the author.)

With so much invested in self-mastery, lecturers such as Mary Gove Nichols, Paulina Wright Davis, Ann Preston, and Sarah Mapps Douglass vowed to "prevent insanity, idiocy, and various other physical infirmities" by institutionalizing antimasturbation discourse. Moving beyond public lectures and female physiological societies, they mentored students at female medical colleges and normal schools. Their students, women such as

Mary Stinson, brought the association between masturbation and mental illness into institutions across the North and West. The institutionalization of women's antimasturbation discourse continued after the Civil War and reached all corners of the nation by the 1880s.

However, even as the women who followed Mary Stinson into asylum administration built this network, the "moral treatment" of insanity began to crumble. Neurology and sexology eroded the discourse of masturbatory insanity. Critics disparaged Samuel B. Woodward's asylum statistics as unscientific and backward. Inappropriate or excessive masturbation was increasingly seen as a symptom of a preexisting mental illness, not the cause of insanity. Matrons and female physicians in women's institutions resisted this change at first, for their cultural influence had come to depend on the existence of sexual threats that they alone could prevent.[11]

Near the turn of the twentieth century, some asylum women began to doubt the reality of both masturbatory insanity and white feminine purity. Between 1890 and 1908, Clara Barrus, the physician in charge of women at the Middletown, New York, State Homeopathic Hospital wavered between the antebellum assumption that sexual self-government was the necessary predicate for sane living and the modern skepticism that masturbation could ever, in itself, sufficiently explain insanity. Barrus warned that correlation should not be confused with causation: if in rare cases masturbation could be shown to have caused mental illness, "it is the concomitant and the result of existing insanity in many more."[12] She especially feared that family members used the diagnosis of masturbatory insanity to subdue ambitious or unruly daughters by having them committed to an asylum. While conservatives argued that rigorous study endangered female minds and bodies, Barrus responded that those who truly valued young women's mental health should encourage them to "engage in some occupation, pursuit or study, with all the earnestness we look for in their brothers." Mental cultivation, not the preservation of innocence, benefited young women. When Barrus did occasionally treat female patients who masturbated in the common areas of the asylum, she refused to use "padded mitts, restraining of hands and feet, [and] the protections sheet." Barrus considered these spectacular weapons in the war against masturbation worse than useless. Such moral splints only increased young women's dependence on external authority when, in order to recover their faculties, they needed to exercise *mental* restraint. The most extreme example of external restraint was clitoridectomy. The British doctor Isaac Baker Brown famously recommended removal of the clitoris in cases of masturbatory insanity and nymphomania. Barrus found such surgeries "reprehensible" precisely because they forever negated the need for willpower. In effect, Barrus suggested that women could only be self-possessed with their hands free and clitorises intact. Masturbatory sanity required masturbatory capacity.[13]

Such ambivalent observations on the relationship between "insanity in young women," moral autonomy, and masturbation made an impact. The British sexologist Havelock Ellis quoted Barrus in his *Autoeroticism* (1899), a watershed publication in the history of masturbation.[14] Ellis held that psychological damage was not caused by masturbation but by what he saw as "ignorant and chaotic notions among the general population," which bred neurosis about harmless behaviors. In reality, he argued, "active, intelligent, and healthy women who otherwise lead a chaste life" could masturbate in moderation without harming themselves. Although adult women are often marginalized in the historiography of masturbation, they loomed large in *Autoeroticism*. Female patients and case studies suggested that masturbation may actually be "beneficial." One woman exclaimed, "I felt that I should go mad and I thought that it was better to touch myself than to be insane."[15]

Yet Ellis was no feminist icon. He promoted gender essentialism and eugenics, drew unapologetically on imperial anthropology, and, while sympathetic to male inverts, pathologized lesbians. He also hedged his claim of relatively harmless masturbation with warnings that "excess" led to neurasthenia (nervous exhaustion)—and, in women, created an aversion to "normal coitus." Women might very reasonably prefer masturbation over "normal coitus," he wrote, because they "experience greater difficulties than men in obtaining sexual satisfaction, and so are impelled by unsatisfying coitus to continue masturbation after marriage." Furthermore, when marital sex proved unsatisfying, the sexual double standard gave men extramarital opportunities for obtaining "sexual gratification with the opposite sex," while "women are . . . shut out from such gratification." Here Ellis unwittingly drew on the philosophy of amative indulgence that had circulated among American feminists since the 1840s. While promoting "the love rights of woman," he simultaneously freighted heterosexual pleasure with social responsibility.[16]

American feminists popularized Ellis's work—including, unfortunately, its most problematic aspects—because it authorized their "erotic rights."[17] As Linda Gordon has argued, Margaret Sanger and Emma Goldman disseminated the new sexology during their national lecture tours because they believed free sexual expression to be a fundamental component of social revolution. When they cited Ellis's *Studies in the Psychology of Sex*, they encouraged other women to explore the topic independently. Local organizations, from Socialist groups to birth control leagues, continued the discussion long after lecturers left town. Early twentieth-century feminists spread the new sexual discourse through the same method used by the female moral reformers who came before them—small groups promoting political discussion and the "scientific knowledge of sex-physiology."[18]

Some evidence of impact can be found in Katharine Bement Davis's 1929 survey of twenty-two hundred women's college alumnae. While several respondents still blamed the practice for "increased nervousness," fully half reported no bad effect. Only one associated masturbation with "dread of insanity." They masturbated because they felt a sense of erotic entitlement, including "desire for full satisfaction" and to avoid "long periods of sexual starvation." More ambivalent beneficiaries linked the act with "will power," as had moral reformers and asylum matrons before them. They were glad they had masturbated, because *quitting* gave them "a sense of power." But chief among the benefits, according to sixty-one respondents, was *improved* mental health. One woman volunteered, "I think it has kept me sane"; another felt "more normal because of it."[19]

The race and class biases of Davis's sample make it useless for tracking the spread of these ideas. But the very elitism of the survey is itself significant. Davis was a penologist with a history of tracking the sexual behaviors of incarcerated women. But she limited *this* questionnaire to wealthy white women with the expressed aim of capturing "norms of sex behavior" for the purposes of future sex education.[20] White writers such as Havelock Ellis and Katharine Bement Davis construed moderate female masturbation as normal, even aspirational.

During the same years, by contrast, leading black Progressives shunned any act that might threaten the mental or physical health of African Americans. Michelle Mitchell has argued that the intersecting crises of lynching, Jim Crow segregation, extreme poverty, epidemic diseases, and racist explanations of these problems impelled African Americans to turn "increasingly inward" and "focused upon changing individual and collective habits" in the struggle for survival. In this context, race leaders infused the concept of racial destiny with "a welter" of intraracial prescriptions for sexual health. During the same years that the white-dominated medical profession reassessed the presumed consequences of masturbation, African American experts connected masturbation to "sexual morbidity." William Hannibal Thomas and Dr. A. Wilberforce Williams correlated masturbation with syphilis and racial degeneration. In Williams's words, "chronic self-abusers" gave birth to "idiots, epileptics, imbeciles, and the hopelessly insane." African American club women and hygiene instructors at black colleges also condemned masturbation. By the early twentieth century a few radicals, including Archibald Grimké's daughter Angelina Weld Grimké, protested that racial violence damaged black women's sexual and reproductive health far more than did masturbation or promiscuity. Unlike white feminists, however, they did not construe masturbation as a rational enactment of women's "erotic rights." It would be a mistake to assume that African American women ignored masturbation during the Progressive era solely because they had more serious concerns. On the contrary, Mitchell shows that contested definitions of sexual health became all the more compelling when survival itself seemed at stake.[21] African American women turned away from white reform women such as Katharine Bement Davis, who, despite their changing stance toward masturbation, continued to conflate normal feminine sexuality with whiteness.

MASTURBATORY SANITY

By 1968, when a new generation of feminists began exploring erotic liberation as part of women's liberation, much of this history had been buried under neo-Freudian discourse and antifeminist backlash.[22] White feminists especially rejected Freud's characterization of clitoral orgasms as "infantile." What was infantile, they argued, was to wait passively to be awakened by a male partner. Armed with physiological studies that proved clitoral stimulation a healthy part of mature women's sexual expression, they quickly launched "a campaign to recognize masturbation as normal."[23]

Hoping to "liberate" masturbation from its associations with deviancy and insanity, some white feminists raised it to the level of a fetish. Amid multiple campaigns in the realms of reproduction, health, education, and law, they created a "women's culture" in which masturbation became the reigning symbol of female independence and self-love. Promasturbation writers conflated the sexual prescriptions of white femininity with women's oppression writ large. Betty Dodson, for example, implored her sisters to "step down from the pedestal to become a sexual equal" (without acknowledging that the "pedestal" of sexual purity and moral superiority had historically constituted *white* femininity).[24]

Dodson found the presumption of sexual innocence so unhealthy for most (white) women that she founded Bodysex Workshops, in which groups of women masturbated together to orgasm. Echoing Mary Gove Nichols, she argued that the sexual double standard depended on women's "deprivation of direct sexual knowledge—especially [regarding] masturbation." Now, however, it seemed that physiological ignorance kept women *from* masturbating. Without actually being taught how to do it, women remained depressed and dependent. Dodson set out to remedy this problem by distributing images of female genitalia, selling vibrators, and providing live demonstrations that sometimes became women-only orgies.[25] Yet even Dodson was no hedonist. Eating only raw vegetables, fruits, and seeds, she advocated a dietetic restraint that would have put Grahamites to shame.[26] Moral reform societies had struggled together against temptation. Now women's liberationists accepted the same premise, stated by Shulamith Firestone, that "self-regulation is the basis of freedom." In small groups, women rediscovered "disciplinary intimacy." They discovered together their "right to pleasure," and also urged one another to take "responsibility for obtaining it." As consciousness-raising sessions became self-help groups, masturbation gained therapeutic, as well as liberatory, potential. By the mid-1970s, masturbation was better than normal—it was a panacea. It had come to seem almost insane for a feminist *not* to masturbate. One member enthused, "Masturbation gave me the knowledge I could achieve orgasm. Now I know I'm normal."[27]

Once again, peer education gave rise to a new crop of feminist experts. Lonnie Barbach, a sex therapist who created "preorgasmic women's groups," argued that consciousness-raising was not enough. Members needed "peer pressure and group reinforcement" to overcome the stigma of masturbation that kept them dysfunctional. But they also needed "trained therapists" who could break down their "resistance." Some eroticized this discipline, reporting that they "visualized the whole group" at the moment of their first orgasm. But others lusted after affirmation. Karen Sandler, who became orgasmic in a women's group, was even tempted to "rent a billboard on Wilshire Blvd. with I CAME, I CAME, I CAME in big red letters." Sandler longed to tell because she longed for belonging—for normalcy—as proof of her feminist autonomy.[28]

Within seven years, a new psychiatric diagnosis, primary orgasmic disorder, would define Sandler's "preorgasmic" friends as mentally ill. Even masturbatory insanity itself had not made it this far: it was discredited before the American Psychiatric Association published the first *Diagnostic and Statistical Manual* in 1952. *DSM-III* relied on a criterion established by Masters and Johnson, one of the most quoted research teams in 1970s feminism. Its sole symptom, "anorgasmia," disproportionately pathologized women. Masters and Johnson defined as anorgasmic "women who have never had an orgasm." The diagnosis was revised in 1990 to include "persistent or recurrent delay in, or absence of, orgasm in a female following a normal sexual excitement phase, during sexual activity that the clinician judges to be adequate in focus, intensity and duration." The baseline activity by which therapists test for normal excitement is, of course, masturbation. This diagnosis continues to be used under the name "female orgasmic disorder."[29] The twentieth-century feminist pursuit of sexual autonomy has become codified as a psychological imperative.

What are the consequences of promoting a feminist sexual norm? The strange career of solitary vice suggests that one such historical process has impacted women's movements in unpredictable and problematic ways. This book has argued that, before the advent of sexology, evangelical women created a normative discourse on sexuality. Initially an assertion of female subjectivity and virtue, the solitary vice ballooned into a national obsession that did little to change the structural dimensions of women's sexual oppression. Diverse women engaged in sexual discourse as a means to political ends, yet they could only bring about finite changes in gender and racial hierarchies in this way. Despite profoundly challenging white male sexual entitlement within marriage, slavery, and urban culture, these changes could not in themselves topple patriarchy, abolish slavery, or empower otherwise disenfranchised people in civil society.

Changing sexual discourse itself also proved elusive. Profound power differentials and political differences undermined women's shared sexual protest. It therefore became if not easier at least more seductive for white women to focus on a sexual practice that seemed subject to no external control. The result was that sexual discourse, though always embedded in and signifying other power relations, took on an activist life of its own. Many women devoted time, resources, and intensity to their crusade against solitary vice quite out of proportion to its political impact because it seemed to promise them an achievable form of sexual selfhood. The ephemeral coalition between black abolitionists and white moral reformers collapsed, leaving behind only a *symbol* of female passion, virtue, and autonomy in the form of solitary vice discourse. As it traversed beyond the reform community, the discourse took on the racism of the dominant society. African American women who battled racist discourses found themselves bound by the sexual terms of normal, healthy femininity that their predecessors had inspired.

Twentieth-century feminists reversed the terms of their foremothers' discourse on masturbation but continued the same political cycle. At first, heralding women's sexual autonomy seemed to require recognizing masturbation as normal. Later, self-pleasure became a normative discourse of its own. White women invested most heavily in this reversal: while black feminists of the 1970s also claimed "the power of self-definition" over their sexuality, they had never been placed on a sexual pedestal. Defining self-help in terms of social transformation rather than individual rights, many feminists of color tackled issues of sexual violence, reproductive justice, poverty, and public health. Yet prioritizing these movements did not stop black feminists from revolutionizing sex on their own terms, including through the autoerotic writings of Audre Lorde and Alice Walker. The point, according to Hortense Spillers, was that feminism should not *stop* at sexual counterdiscourse: feminists must pursue "a global restoration and dispersal of power." In the pursuit of such a goal, sex would be "rendered one of several active predicates."[30]

Spillers wrote this caution in the midst of the sex wars between antipornography feminists and sex-positive feminists during the 1980s. Both groups consisted largely of white women who subscribed to two radically different views of sexual power. Antipornography feminists emphasized the dangers of sex and demanded protection from male violence and exploitation, while sex-positive feminists considered pleasure a form of power that women should also possess and insisted upon freedom from state oversight (and that of other feminists) in order to exercise it. This bifurcated model has been interpreted as a continuation of disagreements between late nineteenth-century purity reformers and advocates of free love.[31] Looking back still further, the roots of the sex wars may actually lie in the tension between passive purity and active virtue that black abolitionist women such as Sarah Mapps Douglass suggested to white women's rights activists such as Sarah Grimké. During the 1980s, the battle between pleasure and danger seemed to Spillers to silence all other discursive possibilities. In much the same way, female moral reformers who argued among themselves about sexual politics drowned out African American voices during the 1840s, ending the fragile interracial coalition of the 1830s.

Katha Pollitt has recently named sex-positive feminists the undisputed victors of the sex wars.[32] In the wider society, however, the battle raged on between those who wanted to protect young women's sexual innocence and those aiming to empower them to make their own sexual choices. In 1994, President Bill Clinton fired Surgeon General Joycelyn Elders, purportedly for recommending that masturbation should be discussed in public schools as a legitimate alternative to sexual intercourse. More than masturbation was at stake: Elders favored programs aimed at preventing HIV/AIDS and other sexually transmitted infections. When conservatives deemed her the "Condom Queen," she accused them of having "a love affair with the fetus." The lasting impact of the debacle was that the so-called last taboo of masturbation effectively distracted political debate from the AIDS-prevention policies that Elders had tried to launch.[33] Two years later, Clinton signed into law the Personal Responsibility and Work Opportunity Act. In addition to "ending welfare as we have known it," the new law slated fifty million dollars annually in federal funds for states whose school systems promoted abstinence before marriage. The sex education programs of prior decades had aimed to prevent teenage pregnancy, but abstinence-only education promoted purity and especially celebrated female virginity. Like the physiological education demanded by Massachusetts school committees, abstinence-only teaching materials described masturbation as a gateway to further sexual experimentation, which would in turn cause disease.[34]

On the other side of the issue, the sexual marketplace of the early twenty-first century took the place of feminist therapists in defining sexual pleasure as a female entitlement. Even nonfeminist women subscribed to an ideology that normalized masturbation and reconciled it with heterosexual pleasure. The hugely lucrative Passion Parties enterprise sold vibrators and other "sex toys" without necessarily promoting gender equality. Modeled on the iconic Tupperware party of mid-twentieth-century suburbia, Passion Parties revolved around the sale of sex toys to groups of women in private homes. Hosts "experienced the ultimate girls' night in" by inviting friends to learn about sex toys "designed to promote intimacy and communication between couples." These messages appeared to reassure a very different segment of the vibrator-buying population than those who searched for feminist autonomy in the Bodysex Workshops of the early 1970s. Yet Passion Parties Inc. shared Betty Dodson's view that women needed detailed instruction about their own sexual response.[35] Similarly, Kandi Burrus, a cast member of the reality show *The Real Housewives of Atlanta*, marketed a line of sex toys for women. Her "Bedroom Kandi" online catalog coded vibrators as "massagers" and instructed women to "tickle his pickle." Although these products had been designed for female masturbation, both Passion Parties and Bedroom Kandi normalized them by encouraging women to use them within a partnered, heterosexual context. At the same time, they brought a particular version of twentieth-century feminists' discourse on masturbation into the cultural mainstream: "The best things in life empower us to be free, free to explore, free to discover, free to live, free to be." Masturbation, a perfectly healthy and normal behavior, bewitchingly promised to make any woman powerful without challenging thorny social hierarchies.

ACKNOWLEDGMENTS

This project has been generously supported and substantially improved by many insightful readers over several years of research, writing, and revision. I owe my first and greatest debt to Patricia Cline Cohen, an unparalleled teacher, brilliant historian, and dazzling beacon of inspiration. She attentively read draft after draft of each chapter, always raising generative questions grounded in her deep knowledge of early American women's history and intended to help me clarify my own contribution. She continues to mentor me, as well as many other women in the historical profession, long after completing her official advisory duties. Eileen Boris, who also encountered my work in its earliest incarnations, has continued to productively engage with my changing ideas ever since. I remain extremely thankful to both of them, as well as to Leila Rupp, Ann Plane, John Majewski, and Michael Osborne, for early and sustained guidance.

A Central Fellowship from the University of California at Santa Barbara enabled me to begin the research process, and fellowships from the Social Science Research Council and the Library Company of Philadelphia saw me through the first full draft of the work. I wish to particularly thank Phil Lapsansky at the Library Company for his practical help researching the city's black abolitionists and for sharing his thoughts about one of the images used in chapter 5. During the same period, Anne Boylan invited me to give a talk at the University of Delaware, where collegial interlocutors offered new angles of vision on my findings. I am also grateful to the University of Texas Press for allowing me to reprint portions of a very early article about Frederick Hollick, published in the *Journal of the History of Sexuality*, in chapter 4.

More recently, Lori Ginzberg and Carol Faulkner read the entire manuscript twice, and together their constructive criticism profoundly reshaped and strengthened my analysis. Carol pointed out significant omissions, made specific research suggestions that proved extremely fruitful, and wrote helpful letters of support. Lori challenged me to sharpen and clarify my interpretation and showed great consideration by setting aside other tasks in order to attend to this project in a time-sensitive manner. Bruce Dorsey read a draft of *Riotous Flesh*, too, and prevented me from including an erroneous statement in the book. His comments about the stakes for rioters significantly shaped my revision of the first chapter. Nancy Isenberg gave cogent and useful feedback on an earlier version of chapter 1 as well. Carol Lasser discussed our different interpretations with the perfect blend of intellectual rigor and gracious collegiality. Sharon Block read and commented on rough drafts of new chapters, offering helpful interventions and kind encouragement.

In 2009, financial support from the National Endowment for the Humanities and the Massachusetts Historical Society enabled me to delve into key collections and substantially expand the argument. I was lucky enough to overlap there with Crystal Feimster, whose insights proved formative. Nina Dayton and Conrad Wright coordinated my participation in the Seminar in the History of Women and Gender at the Radcliffe Institute for Advanced Study in early 2010. Helen Lefkowitz Horowitz gave thorough and vital feedback on the paper I presented there, which was my first public exploration of the interracial moment in moral reform and the counterdiscourse on licentiousness. Barbara Krauthamer read a revised version of that paper in 2013, and her comments deeply influenced the way I present my conclusions in this book.

No part of this project would have been possible without the American Antiquarian Society's Hench Postdissertation Fellowship, which I held from 2009 to 2010. The book benefited from its wonderful scholarly community and its extraordinary collections of early American print culture. I wish to thank staff members Caroline Sloat, Paul Erickson, Jackie Penny, Elizabeth Pope, Laura Wasowicz, Vince Golden, and Ashley Cataldo for routinely going beyond the call of duty in their assistance. Mary Kelley, Steve Nissenbaum, Diane DiMauro, and Ezra Greenspan read a much longer and rougher version of *Riotous Flesh* and offered wise counsel about how to streamline its narrative and refine its argument. Emma Lapsansky-Werner and Manisha Sinha provided detailed, helpful notes on portions of the manuscript. An unforgettable cohort of long-term fellows, including Emily Pawley, Jessica Lepler, Lloyd Pratt, Mary Beth Sievens, and Michael Winship, made the work a pleasure. Emily and Lloyd very kindly gave feedback on chapters in process, and I continue to marvel at their brilliance. Emily also offered personal support during a family health crisis, as did Ezra and Rikki Greenspan. Jessica Lepler and Paul Erickson each drove me home from the archive on many wintry Worcester evenings; they also patiently accepted my feeble efforts at repayment in the form of oddly knitted items.

A newly minted PhD could not ask for a warmer welcome into the profession than that which the Department of History at Case Western Reserve University extended to me in 2010–11. Renée Sentilles, Jonathan Sadowsky, and Miriam Levin offered much-needed professional advice and generous intellectual engagement. Jim Edmundson showed me the research possibilities of the Dittrick Medical History Center, including an example of the anatomical manikin used by the physiology lecturers discussed in this book. I am also grateful to Wendy Fu, Marixa Lasso, John Flores, John Broich, Gillian Weiss, Stephen G. Hall, and Zebulon Milestky for their collegiality.

A 2012 Margaret Storrs Grierson Scholar-in-Residence Fellowship at the Sophia Smith Collection of Smith College funded research that vastly improved the epilogue and introduction. Maida Goodwin went out of her way to introduce me to sources that I would not otherwise have discovered. Elizabeth Pryor and Jerry Stordeur opened their home to me for an extended stay. Liz has an amazing gift for encouraging one's best thoughts while keeping one honest and accountable at the same time. I have admired her analytical clarity and eye for historical detail since graduate school. I am also thankful to Dawn Peterson for talking through my very new Smith findings over dinner in Northampton and for participating in a provocative session at the Organization of American Historians several months later.

In 2013–14, the William L. Clements Library granted me the Earhart Fellowship in early American history, which allowed me to add important new material to chapters 1, 5, and the epilogue. Cheney Schopieray made some of the newest, uncatalogued portions of the Weld-Grimké Family Papers available to me. These letters revealed a new side of Sarah Grimké, which influenced my conclusion. Clayton Lewis introduced me to key images. Diana Sykes and Jayne Ptolemy furnished secondary sources and other technical assistance that made it possible to stay productive while far away from home.

During the past four years, the University of Oregon has been the site of this book's most intense revision. Within days of my arrival on campus, Michelle McKinley invited me to participate in a seminar with Hendrik Hartog, where I received encouraging and helpful feedback on the first chapter. She has been an incisive interlocutor and unofficial mentor ever since. The Center for the Study of Women in Society and the Américas Research

Interest Group provided space, resources, and professional networks in which to try out many of the new ideas that have made their way into the book. Lizzie Reis, Carol Stabile, Jennifer Burns, Courtney Thorsson, and Lise Nelson have commented on portions of this book and extended various kinds of institutional support. The Department of History has collectively enriched the book. The Spencer Brush Faculty Fellowship enabled me to conduct research in the Oberlin College Archives in summer 2012 and supported my writing new sections based on those findings in 2013. Colleagues Ellen Herman and Matt Dennis somehow manage to find time to notice articles relevant to my work and forward them to me. Marsha Weisiger offers professional mentorship, holiday mirth, and feedback on work in progress. Jim Mohr drops by regularly to discuss nineteenth-century medicine and women's education. I am very thankful for the friendship of Melissa Stuckey, Lindsay Braun, and Julie Weise. Jeff Ostler's running advice has energized me during stressful moments. Former and current graduate students Carrie Adkins, Hillary Maxson, and Quinn Akina all share a knack for asking the right questions, and observing their progress has been inspiring. Shelley Grosjean helped the project in a practical way by watching my dog during various trips. I thank my lucky stars that I get to work within such a fabulous intellectual community.

I am also grateful to past and present staff members at the University of Chicago Press. Robert Devens shepherded this project through the first stages of approval for publication and met with me at more than one convention of the Society for Historians of the Early American Republic to keep me on track. Ed Gray, Timothy Mennel, and Mary Corrado also fielded my inquisitive emails and dispensed wisdom along the way. Nora Devlin helped me coordinate logistical publication details in a timely way. Susan Cohan's careful copyediting vastly improved the book.

Family and friends have sustained me through this process. Nadine and Frank Servedio, Kathleen and Brandon Halbert, Jennifer Black, Julie Avery, Eve Shapiro, Krista Smith, Mel Corn and Tanner Johnson, and Bev Hart have hosted and nourished me en route to archives and during the off-hours of history conventions. Marsha Lawson took me under her wing in 1993 and passed away in 2010. I thank her in memoriam for finding power in the queerest of thoughts.

Hex Hassinger deserves my untold gratitude for all the patience, joy, and pleasure she has given freely over the last ten years. Today and every day, she shows me "a love that baffles all expression." This book is dedicated to her.

NOTES

The following abbreviations are used to identify frequently cited publications and organizations:

AAS American Antiquarian Society
AHR *American Historical Review*
AMR *Advocate of Moral Reform*
APS American Physiological Society
BMSJ *Boston Medical and Surgical Journal*
BPL Boston Public Library
CL William L. Clements Library, University of Michigan
FOV *Friend of Virtue*
GFP Graham Family Papers
HSP Historical Society of Pennsylvania
LCP Library Company of Philadelphia
LPI Ladies Physiological Institute of Boston and Vicinity
LPS Ladies' Physiological Society
MHS Massachusetts Historical Society
PPS Providence Physiological Society
RIHS Rhode Island Historical Society
SL Schlesinger Library
SSC Sophia Smith Collection
WG MSS Weld-Grimké Family Papers

INTRODUCTION

1. Shere Hite, *The Hite Report: A Nationwide Study on Female Sexuality* (New York: Seven Stories Press, 1976), 62.

2. Dell Williams, quoted in *Passion and Power: The Technology of Orgasm*, directed by Wendy Slick and Emiko Omori (First Run Features, 2008), DVD; and Anne Koedt, "The

Myth of the Vaginal Orgasm," in *Notes from the Second Year*, ed. Anne Koedt and Shulamith Firestone (1968; repr., New York: New York Radical Feminists, April 1970).

3. Alfred C. Kinsey, Wardell B. Pomeroy, Clyde E. Martin, and Paul H. Gebhard, *Sexual Behavior in the Human Female* (1953; repr., Bloomington: Indiana University Press, 1998); William H. Masters and Virginia E. Johnson, *Human Sexual Response* (Boston: Little, Brown, 1966); Koedt, "Myth"; and Boston Women's Health Book Collective, *Our Bodies, Ourselves* (New York: Simon and Schuster, 1973), 46–48.

4. Boston Women's Health Book Collective, *Our Bodies, Ourselves*, 47–48; Joan W. Scott, "The Evidence of Experience," *Critical Inquiry* 17, no. 4 (Summer 1991): 773–97; Betty Dodson, *Liberating Masturbation: A Meditation on Self Love, Dedicated to the Women* (New York: published by the author, 1974); and Dodson, quoted in *Passion and Power*.

5. Patricia Hill Collins, *Black Feminist Thought: Knowledge, Consciousness, and the Politics of Empowerment* (New York: Routledge, 1991).

6. Toni Cade Bambara, *The Black Woman: An Anthology*, 2nd ed. (New York: Washington Square Press, 2010), 2, 4–6, 207; Combahee River Collective, "The Combahee River Statement," in *Home Girls: A Black Feminist Anthology* (New York: Kitchen Table, Women of Color Press, 1983); and Kimberly Springer, *Living for the Revolution: Black Feminist Organizations, 1968–1980* (Durham, NC: Duke University Press, 2005).

7. Audre Lorde, "Uses of the Erotic: The Erotic as Power," in *Sister/Outsider* (1978; repr., New York: Crossing Press, 1984), 55.

8. Alice Walker, *Possessing the Secret of Joy* (New York: Harcourt Brace, 1992), 216.

9. *Off Our Backs* 4, no. 11 (November 1974), quoted in Jane Gerhard, *Desiring Revolution: Second-Wave Feminism and the Rewriting of American Sexual Thought* (New York: Columbia University Press, 2001), 150; and Jocelyn Olcott, "Cold War Conflicts and Cheap Cabaret: Sexual Politics at the 1975 United Nations International Women's Year Conference," *Gender and History* 22, no. 3 (November 2010): 733–54.

10. G. J. Barker-Benfield, *The Horrors of the Half-Known Life: Male Attitudes toward Women and Sexuality in Nineteenth-Century America* (1974; repr., New York: Routledge, 2000); and Stephen Nissenbaum, *Sex, Diet, and Debility in Jacksonian America: Sylvester Graham and Health Reform* (Westport, CT: Greenwood Press, 1980). The quote is from Bruce Dorsey, *Reforming Men and Women: Gender in the Antebellum City* (Ithaca, NY: Cornell University Press, 2002), 117–20.

11. Helen Horowitz coined the term *reform physiology* in *Rereading Sex: Battles over Sexual Knowledge and Suppression in Nineteenth-Century America* (New York: Knopf, 2002).

12. Sylvester Graham, *Lectures on the Science of Human Life*, vol. 2 (Boston: Marsh, Capen, Lyon, and Webb, 1839); *Health Journal and Advocate of Physiological Reform* (June 17, 1840); Richard H. Shryock, "Sylvester Graham and the Popular Health Movement, 1830–1870," *Mississippi Valley Historical Review* 18 (June 1931–March 1932): 172–83; and Thomas Le Duc, "Graham and Grahamites," *New York History* 20, no. 2 (April 1939): 189–91.

13. On the effect of meat on the genitals, Graham rose to celebrity during the first of "the cholera years," when *prevention* was the watchword. For a complete intellectual biography, see Nissenbaum, *Sex, Diet, and Debility*; on the medical context, see Charles E.

Rosenberg, *The Cholera Years: The United States in 1832, 1844, and 1866* (Chicago: University of Chicago Press, 1962).

14. *Edutainment* is a neologism, but nineteenth-century audience members described popular physiology lectures as both educational and entertaining. See, for example, Sarah Tilton to Catherine Tilton, July 30, 1841, American Science and Medicine Collection, box 1, CL; and letter fragment, Sarah M. Douglass to Rebecca White, n.d. [1857–58], Josiah White Papers, Haverford College.

15. Sylvester Graham, *A Lecture to Young Men on Chastity* (Providence: Weeden and Cory, 1834), 51; *New Bedford Gazette* (August 11, 1834); *Boston Morning Post* (March 5, 1837), quoted in *New York Spectator* (March 10, 1837); and *Boston Courier* (March 6, 1837).

16. Graham, *Lecture to Young Men*; and *Providence Patriot & Columbian Phenix* (November 22, 1834). On representations of intersexual people as monstrous, see Alice Dreger, *Hermaphrodites and the Medical Invention of Sex* (Cambridge, MA: Harvard University Press, 1998); and Elizabeth Reis, *Bodies in Doubt: An American History of Intersex* (Baltimore: Johns Hopkins University Press, 2009).

17. Graham's advice also contained racist elements; see Kyla Wazana Tompkins, *Racial Indigestion: Eating Bodies in the 19th Century* (New York: NYU Press, 2012). However, Graham's racist discourse emphasized cultural chauvinism over corporeal essentialism. See Graham, *Science of Human Life*. On the divergent strains of white racial logic during the antebellum period, see George M. Frederickson, *The Black Image in the White Mind: The Debate on Afro-American Character and Destiny, 1817–1914* (New York: Harper and Row, 1971); and Bruce Dain, *A Hideous Monster of the Mind: American Race Theory in the Early Republic* (Cambridge, MA: Harvard University Press, 2002). Black abolitionists seized the discursive opportunity created by physiological universalism (discussed below).

18. Ruth H. Bloch, *Gender and Morality in Anglo-American Culture, 1650–1800* (Berkeley: University of California Press, 2003); Thomas A. Foster, *Sex and the Eighteenth-Century Man: Massachusetts and the History of Sexuality in America* (Boston: Beacon Press, 2007); Mark E. Kann, *Taming Passions for the Public Good* (New York: NYU Press, 2013); and Martha Saxton, *Being Good: Women's Moral Values in Early America* (New York: Hill and Wang, 2003).

19. Mary Ryan, *Women in Public: Between Banners and Ballots, 1825–1880* (Baltimore: Johns Hopkins University Press, 1990); and Patricia Cline Cohen, Timothy Gilfoyle, and Helen Horowitz, *The Flash Press: Sporting Male Weeklies in 1840s New York* (Chicago: University of Chicago Press, 2008).

20. Foster, *Sex and the Eighteenth-Century Man*; and Sharon Block, *Rape and Sexual Power in Early America* (Chapel Hill: University of North Carolina Press, 2006). On the gradual racial segregation of northern public life, see Joanne Pope Melish, *Disowning Slavery: Gradual Emancipation and "Race" in New England, 1780–1860* (Ithaca, NY: Cornell University Press, 1998); John Saillant, "The Black Body Erotic and the Republican Body Politic, 1790–1820," *Journal of the History of Sexuality* 5, no. 3 (January 1995): 403–28; David Waldstreicher, *In the Midst of Perpetual Fetes: The Making of American Nationalism, 1776–1820* (Chapel Hill: University of North Carolina Press, 1997); Graham Russell Hodges, *Root and Branch: African Americans in New York and East Jersey, 1613–1863* (Chapel Hill: University of North Carolina Press, 1999); and Leslie M. Harris, *In the*

Shadow of Slavery: African Americans in New York City, 1626–1863 (Chicago: University of Chicago Press, 2003).

21. Graham, *Lecture to Young Men*, 20.

22. Mark E. Kann, *A Republic of Men: The American Founders, Gendered Language, and Patriarchal Politics* (New York: New York University Press, 1998); and Bloch, *Gender and Morality*.

23. Asenath Nicholson, *Nature's Own Book* (New York: W. S. Dorr, 1835), 11; *Boston Courier* (July 12, 1838); Edmund Quincy to Caroline Weston, Dedham, MA, July 9, 1840, Antislavery Collection, BPL; and Lewis Perry, *Radical Abolitionism: Anarchy and the Government of God in Antislavery Thought* (Ithaca, NY: Cornell University Press, 1973).

24. *New York Evangelist* (June 7, 1834); *AMR* (December 1835); APS, *Second Annual Report, June 1, 1838*, APS Publications (Boston: Light and Stearns, 1839), 22.

25. Carroll Smith-Rosenberg, "Beauty, the Beast, and the Militant Woman: A Case Study in Sex Roles and Social Stress in Jacksonian America," *American Quarterly* 23, no. 4 (October 1971): 562–84; Mary P. Ryan, "The Power of Women's Networks: A Case Study of Female Moral Reform in Antebellum America," in "Women and Power: Dimensions of Women's Historical Experience," special issue, *Feminist Studies* 5, no. 1 (Spring 1979): 66–85; Nancy A. Hewitt, *Women's Activism and Social Change: Rochester, New York, 1822–1872* (Ithaca, NY: Cornell University Press, 1984); Christine Stansell, *City of Women: Sex and Class in New York, 1789–1860* (New York: Knopf, 1986); Barbara Meil Hobson, *Uneasy Virtue: The Politics of Prostitution and the American Reform Tradition* (New York: Basic Books, 1987); Lori D. Ginzberg, *Women and the Work of Benevolence: Morality, Politics, and Class in the Nineteenth-Century United States* (New Haven, CT: Yale University Press, 1990); Marilyn Wood Hill, *Their Sisters' Keepers: Prostitution in New York City, 1830–1870* (Berkeley: University of California Press, 1993); and Daniel S. Wright, *The First of Causes to Our Sex: The Female Moral Reform Movement in the Antebellum Northeast, 1834–1848* (New York: Routledge, 2006).

26. *New England Spectator* (March 18, 1835); Constitution of the Oberlin Female Moral Reform Society (May 1835), Oberlin College Archives, RG 31-6-11 (Oberlin Community), box 1; *New York Evangelist* (May 21, 1836); and *AMR* (July 1, 1836).

27. Graham, *Lecture to Young Men*, 20.

28. *Pennsylvania Freeman* (November 20, 1845); Frederick Hollick, *The Origin of Life* (New York: T. W. Strong, 1845), 169–70; *Philadelphia Public Ledger and Daily Transcript* (April 4, 1846); and *Philadelphia Saturday Courier*, quoted in *Boston Investigator* (May 13, 1846).

29. William C. Woodbridge, *Annals of Education*, quoted in *Health Journal and Advocate of Physiological Reform* (April 1, 1840); and Mary Ann Johnson, "Organs of Generation," lecture to the Providence Physiological Society, April 11, 1851, minutes of the PPS, folder 1 (Minutes 1850.1–1853.2), PPS records, RIHS.

30. "Mrs. Douglass' Lectures," *Weekly Anglo-African* (July 23, 1859), quoted in Dorothy Sterling, ed., *We Are Your Sisters: Black Women in the Nineteenth Century* (New York: Norton, 1984), 129.

31. Rene Spitz, "Authority and Masturbation: Some Remarks on a Bibliographic Investigation," *Yearbook of Psychoanalysis* 9 (1953); E. H. Hare, "Masturbatory Insanity: The History of an Idea," *Journal of Mental Science* 108 (January 1962): 2–25; Barker-Benfield,

Horrors; R. P. Neuman, "Masturbation, Madness, and the Modern Concepts of Childhood and Adolescence," *Journal of Social History* 8, no. 3 (Spring 1975): 1–27; Nissenbaum, *Sex, Diet, and Debility;* Michael Stolberg, "Self-Pollution, Moral Reform, and the Venereal Trade: Notes on the Historical Sources and Context of Onania," *Journal of the History of Sexuality* 9, nos. 1–2 (January–April 2000): 37–61; and Thomas Laqueur, *Solitary Sex: A Cultural History of Masturbation* (New York: Zone Books, 2003).

32. *Huntress* (February 4, 1837; April 1, 1837; April 8, 1837; and April 22, 1837). For more on its editor, see Elizabeth J. Clapp, "'A Virago-Errant in Enchanted Armor?' Anne Royall's 1829 Trial as a Common Scold," *Journal of the Early Republic* 23, no. 2 (Summer 2003): 207–32.

33. Samuel B. Woodward, "State Lunatic Hospital at Worcester, Mass.," *BMSJ* (March 11, 1835); Samuel B. Woodward, *Reports and Other Documents of the State Lunatic Hospital at Worcester, Mass.* (Boston: Dutton and Wentworth, 1837); *State Lunatic Hospital at Worcester Records, 1833–1924,* vol. 1, AAS; William M. Awl, MD, *First Annual Report of the Directors of the Ohio Lunatic Asylum to the 38th General Assembly, Presented Dec. 5, 1839* (Columbus: s.n., 1839), CL; William M. Awl, MD, *Sixth Annual Report of the Ohio Lunatic Asylum, 1844* (Columbus: s.n., 1844), CL; *In Senate, January 12, 1842: Report of the Trustees of the State Lunatic Asylum with the Documents Accompanying the Same, Pursuant to the Act of the Legislature Passed May 26th, 1841* (New York: s.n., 1842), CL; *Charity Hospital* [New Orleans] *Lunatic Asylum Admission Book, 1841–48,* CL; John Galt, *Annual Report of the Eastern* [Virginia] *Lunatic Asylum* (Richmond: s.n., 1850); and John Galt, *Dr. Galt's Reports of the Physician and Superintendent of the Eastern Lunatic Asylum for the Years 1855–57, 1857–59, 1859–61* (Richmond: s.n., 1861), CL.

34. The tenets of reform became integrated into the "hygiene" curricula of late nineteenth-century schools and colleges in the postwar South. African American women activists who attended Spelman and other historically black colleges incorporated reform physiology into their Social Purity arguments. See Evelyn Brooks Higginbotham, *Righteous Discontent: The Women's Movement in the Black Baptist Church, 1880–1920* (Cambridge, MA: Harvard University Press, 1993), 71, 100. On antimasturbation advice in particular, see Michele Mitchell, *Righteous Propagation: African Americans and the Politics of Racial Destiny after Reconstruction* (Chapel Hill: University of North Carolina Press, 2004), 10, 83, 87, 96, 102–5, 132–33. On the Sanitary Commission and YMCA's antimasturbation program during the Civil War, see Horowitz, *Rereading Sex;* on the YWCA's antimasturbation sex education during the early twentieth century, see Mabel Ulrich, "Lectures at the National YWCA" (1915) and "Social Morality" (1917), record group 6, Program Subjects, subseries B, Health and Recreation, box 594, YWCA of America Archive, Sophia Smith Collection.

35. Michel Foucault, *The History of Sexuality,* vol. 1, *The Will to Knowledge,* trans. Robert Hurley (1978; repr., New York: Vintage, 1990); and Michel Foucault, *Birth of the Clinic* (1963; repr., New York: Routledge, 1989); Barker-Benfield, *Horrors;* Janice Irvine, *Disorders of Desire: Sex and Gender in Modern American Sexology* (Philadelphia: Temple University Press, 1990); and Jennifer Terry, *An American Obsession: Science, Medicine, and Homosexuality in Modern Society* (Chicago: University of Chicago Press, 1999).

36. James C. Mohr, *Abortion in America: The Origins and Evolution of National Policy* (New York: Oxford University Press, 1978); Morris J. Vogel and Charles E. Rosenberg,

eds., *The Therapeutic Revolution: Essays in the Social History of American Medicine* (Philadelphia: University of Pennsylvania Press, 1979); and Paul Starr, *The Social Transformation of American Medicine* (New York: Basic Books, 1982).

37. Throughout the 1830s and 1840s, regular physicians condemned popular lecturers on sex, including those against masturbation. See, for example, *BMSJ* (July 1, 1835; July 15, 1846; and December 10, 1845).

38. See *BMSJ* (April 8, 1846).

39. G. Stanley Hall, *Adolescence: Its Psychology and Relation to Physiology, Anthropology, Sociology, Sex, Crime, Religion, and Education*, vol. 2 (New York: Appleton, 1905); Gail Bederman, *Manliness and Civilization: A Cultural History of Gender and Race in the United States, 1880–1917* (Chicago: University of Chicago Press, 1995); Jeffrey P. Moran, *Teaching Sex: The Shaping of Adolescence in the 20th Century* (Cambridge, MA; Harvard University Press, 2000); Mary Wood Allen, MD, *What a Young Girl Ought to Know* (Philadelphia: Vir Publishing, 1905), 89; Sarah Webber, "The 'Unnecessary' Organ: Female Circumcision and Clitoridectomy, 1865–1995" (PhD diss., University of Nebraska Medical Center, 2005); and Sarah W. Rodriguez, "Rethinking the History of Female Circumcision and Clitoridectomy: American Medicine and Female Sexuality in the Late Nineteenth Century," *Journal of the History of Medicine and Allied Sciences* 63, no. 3 (July 2008): 323.

40. State Lunatic Hospital at Worcester Records, 1833–1924, vol. 1; *BMSJ* (March 25, 1835; and April 8, 1835); Woodward, *Reports and Other Documents*; Samuel B. Woodward, *Hints for the Young, on a Subject Relating to the Health of Body and Mind* (Boston: Weeks and Jordan, 1838); *Boston Post* (March 11, 1837); *American Annals of Education* (April 1838); William A. Alcott, *Health in Common Schools* (Boston: George W. Light, 1840), 27–28; *An American Seafarer in the Age of Sail: The Erotic Diaries of Philip C. Van Buskirk*, ed. Barry Burg (New Haven, CT: Yale University Press, 1994); and Terry, *American Obsession*.

41. Jonathan Ned Katz, *The Invention of Heterosexuality* (Chicago: University of Chicago Press, 1995), 13–14; and Christina Simmons, *Making Marriage Modern: Women's Sexuality from the Progressive Era to World War II* (New York: Oxford University Press, 2009). On the heteronormative work of marriage manuals, see Theodoor Van de Velde, *Ideal Marriage: Its Physiology and Technique* (New York: Random House, 1926); and Gerhard, *Desiring Revolution*.

42. Frederick Hollick, *The Marriage Guide* (New York: T. W. Strong, 1851), 151, 312–13, 344; and Russel Canfield, *Practical Physiology: Being a Synopsis of Lectures on Sexual Physiology* (Philadelphia: J. Wixson, 1850), 22.

43. Barbara Welter, "The Cult of True Womanhood," *American Quarterly* 18, no. 2 (Summer 1966): 152, 156; and Christopher Lasch, *Haven in a Heartless World: The Family Besieged* (New York: Basic Books, 1977).

44. Jennifer Manion, "Historic Heteroessentialism and Other Orderings in Early America," *Signs* 34, no. 4 (Summer 2009): 981–1003.

45. Barker-Benfield argued that, in reality, doctors believed that "a woman's physical capacity for sexual intercourse was unlimited, in direct contrast to a man's" and that they feared as a result that women's demands for sexual satisfaction would overwhelm and weaken men. *Horrors*, xxvii, 46, 277. Carl N. Degler thought Barker-Benfield had over-

stated the degree of consensus among medical writers who prescribed female passionlessness. Degler was also one of the earliest to note that antimasturbation advisors addressed women as well as men, but unlike the present study, he drew on postbellum sources. See Carl N. Degler, "What Ought to Be and What Was: Women's Sexuality in Nineteenth-Century America," *AHR* 79, no. 5 (December 1974): 1467–90.

46. Nancy F. Cott, "Passionlessness: An Interpretation of Victorian Sexual Ideology, 1790–1850," *Signs* 4, no. 2 (Winter 1978): 219–36. Population scholars have argued that white women drove the "demographic transition" that began in the generation after the Revolution by intentionally controlling their fertility, especially through periodic abstinence. Cott cited Daniel Scott Smith, "Family Limitation, Sexual Control, and Domestic Feminism in Victorian America," and Linda Gordon, "Voluntary Motherhood: The Beginnings of Feminist Birth Control Ideas in the United States," both in *Feminist Studies* 1, nos. 3–4 (Winter–Spring 1973): 40–57 and 5–22, respectively. See also Janet Farell Brodie, *Contraception and Abortion in 19th-Century America* (Ithaca, NY: Cornell University Press, 1994); and Susan Klepp, *Revolutionary Conceptions: Women, Fertility, and Family Limitation in America, 1760–1820* (Chapel Hill: University of North Carolina Press, 2009).

47. Mary Wollstonecraft, *A Vindication of the Rights of Woman*, ed. Miriam Brody (1792; repr., New York: Penguin, 2004), 6, 14–15, 21, 36, 100–101; Horowitz, *Rereading Sex*; Gail Bederman, "Revisiting Nashoba: Slavery, Utopia, and Frances Wright in America, 1818–1826," *American Literary History* 17, no. 3 (Fall 2005): 438–59; Lori D. Ginzburg, "'The Hearts of Your Readers Will Shudder': Fanny Wright, Infidelity, and American Freethought," *American Quarterly* 46, no. 2 (June 1994): 195–227; and Celia Morris, *Fanny Wright: Rebel in America* (Cambridge, MA: Harvard University Press, 1984).

48. Carroll Smith-Rosenberg, "The Female World of Love and Ritual," *Signs* 1 (1975): 1–29; Nancy F. Cott, *The Bonds of Womanhood: "Woman's Sphere" in New England, 1780–1835* (New Haven, CT: Yale University Press, 1977); and Cott, "Passionlessness," 233–34.

49. Lillian Faderman, *Surpassing the Love of Men: Romantic Friendship and Love between Women from the Renaissance to the Present* (New York: William Morrow, 1981); Leila J. Rupp, "Imagine My Surprise: Women's Relationships in Historical Perspective," *Frontiers* 5, no. 3 (1981); Martin Duberman, Martha Vicinus, and George Chauncey, eds., *Hidden from History: Reclaiming the Gay and Lesbian Past* (New York: Meridian, 1989); Marylynne Diggs, "Romantic Friends or a 'Different Race of Creatures'? The Representation of Lesbian Pathology in Nineteenth-Century America," *Feminist Studies* 21, no. 2 (Summer 1995): 317–40; Karen Hansen, "'No Kisses Is Like Youres': An Erotic Friendship between Two African-American Women during the Early Nineteenth Century," *Gender & History* 7 (August 1995): 153–82; and Martha Vicinus, *Intimate Friends: Women Who Loved Women, 1778–1928* (Chicago: University of Chicago Press, 2004).

50. Kathryn Kish Sklar, "All Hail to Pure Cold Water," in *Women and Health in America: Historical Readings*, ed. Judith Walker Leavitt (Madison: University of Wisconsin Press, 1984), 246–54.

51. Rachel Maines, *The Technology of Orgasm* (Baltimore: Johns Hopkins University Press, 1999).

52. Sklar, "All Hail," 252; T. C. Boyle, *The Road to Wellville* (New York: Penguin,

1994); and *Hysteria*, directed by Tanya Wexler (New York: Sony Pictures Classics, 2011, DVD).

53. Patients occasionally did complain about wet sheet packing and the rigorous exercise that constituted the bulk of the water-cure regimen. See, for example, B. S. Rotch to William Rotch Jr., Esq., 1846, Rotch-Lawrence Papers, MHS; and Sylvester Graham, undated account of treatment, GFP, CL.

54. Kathryn Kish Sklar, *Catherine Beecher: A Study in American Domesticity* (New York: Norton, 1976); Susan Cayleff, *Wash and Be Healed: The Water-Cure Movement and Women's Health* (Philadelphia: Temple University Press, 1987); and Jane B. Donegan, *Hydropathic Highway to Health: Women and Water-Cure in Antebellum America* (New York: Greenwood Press, 1986).

55. Hollick, *Origin of Life*, 76.

56. Mary S. Gove, *Lectures to Ladies on Anatomy and Physiology* (Boston: Saxton and Pierce, 1842), 226–27.

57. Joel Shew, *Hydropathic Family Physician* (New York: Fowler and Wells, 1854), 221. Sklar quoted Thomas Low Nichols on this very point in "All Hail," 252.

58. Cott, *Bonds of Womanhood*.

59. Angela Y. Davis, *Women, Race and Class* (1981; repr., New York: Vintage, 1983), 6, 23–24; and Jacqueline Dowd Hall, "'The Mind That Burns in Each Body': Women, Rape, and Racial Violence," in *Powers of Desire: The Politics of Sexuality*, ed. Ann Snitow, Christine Stansell, and Sharon Thompson (New York: Monthly Review Press, 1983).

60. Deborah Gray White, *Ar'n't I a Woman? Female Slaves in the Plantation South* (New York: Norton, 1985).

61. Paula Giddings, *When and Where I Enter: The Impact of Black Women on Race and Sex in America* (New York: Bantam, 1984); Elsa Barkley Brown, "What Has Happened Here: The Politics of Difference in Women's History and Feminist Politics," *Feminist Studies* 18 (Summer 1992): 298; and Nell Irvin Painter, "Of Lily, Linda Brent and Freud: A Non-exceptionalist Approach to Race, Class, and Gender in the Slave South," *Georgia Historical Quarterly* 76 (Summer 1992).

62. Crystal Feimster, "The Impact of Racial and Sexual Politics on Women's History," *Journal of American History* 99, no. 3 (December 2012): 822–26.

63. Mary P. Ryan, *Cradle of the Middle Class: The Family in Oneida County, New York, 1790–1865* (Cambridge: Cambridge University Press, 1981); Ryan, *Women in Public*; Stansell, *City of Women*; and Ginzberg, *Women and the Work of Benevolence*, 24.

64. Angela Y. Davis, *Women, Race and Class*; White, *Ar'n't I a Woman?*; Jacqueline Jones, *Labor of Love, Labor of Sorrow: Black Women, Work, and the Family, from Slavery to the Present* (New York: Basic Books, 1985); Stephanie Camp, *Closer to Freedom: Enslaved Women & Everyday Resistance in the Plantation South* (Chapel Hill: University of North Carolina Press, 2004); and Annette Gordon-Reed, *The Hemingses of Monticello: An American Family* (New York: Norton, 2008).

65. Melton A. McLaurin, *Celia, a Slave* (Athens: University of Georgia Press, 1991); Edward E. Baptist, "'Cuffy,' 'Fancy Maids,' and 'One-Eyed Men': Rape, Commodification and the Domestic Slave Trade in the United States," *AHR* 106, no. 5 (December 2001): 1619–50; Nell Irvin Painter, "Soul Murder and Slavery: Toward a Fully-Loaded Cost Ac-

counting," in *Southern History across the Color Line* (Chapel Hill: University of North Carolina Press, 2002); and Jennifer Morgan, *Laboring Women: Reproduction and Gender in New World Slavery* (Philadelphia: University of Pennsylvania Press, 2004).

66. Dorothy Sterling, ed., *We Are Your Sisters: Black Women in the Nineteenth Century* (New York: Norton, 1984); Marilyn Richardson, ed., *Maria W. Stewart, America's First Black Woman Political Writer: Essays and Speeches* (Bloomington: Indiana University Press, 1987); Frances Smith Foster, *Written by Herself: Literary Production by African American Women, 1746-1892* (Bloomington: Indiana University Press, 1992); Shirley J. Yee, *Black Women Abolitionists: A Study in Activism, 1828-1860* (Knoxville: University of Tennessee Press, 1992); Jean Fagan Yellin and John C. Van Horne, eds., *The Abolitionist Sisterhood: Women's Political Culture in Antebellum America* (Ithaca, NY: Cornell University Press, 1994); Carla Peterson, *Doers of the Word: African American Women Speakers and Writers in the North* (New York: Oxford University Press, 1995); Anne M. Boylan, *The Origins of Women's Activism: New York and Boston, 1797-1840* (Chapel Hill: University of North Carolina Press, 2000); Elizabeth McHenry, *Forgotten Readers: Recovering the Lost History of African American Literary Societies* (Durham, NC, and London: Duke University Press, 2002); and Martha S. Jones, *All Bound Up Together: The Woman Question in African American Public Culture* (Chapel Hill: University of North Carolina Press, 2007).

67. Hortense J. Spillers, "Interstices: A Small Drama of Words," in *Pleasure and Danger: Exploring Female Sexuality*, ed. Carol. S. Vance (New York: Pandora, 1989), 74.

68. Darlene Clark Hine, "Rape and the Inner Lives of Black Women in the Middle West: Preliminary Thoughts on the Culture of Dissemblance," *Signs* 14, no. 4 (Summer 1989): 912-20.

69. James Oliver Horton has found that free black women, often relegated to domestic labor, faced disproportionate sexual harassment and abuse by white employers. See "Freedom's Yoke: Gender Conventions among Antebellum Free Blacks," *Feminist Studies* 12, no. 1 (Spring 1986): 58. On northern stereotypes of black women, see Martha S. Jones, *All Bound Up Together*; Clare A. Lyons, *Sex among the Rabble: An Intimate History of Gender and Power in the Age of Revolution, Philadelphia, 1730-1830* (Chapel Hill: University of North Carolina Press, 2006); and Block, *Rape and Sexual Power*.

70. Angela Y. Davis, *Women, Race and Class*, 25; Hine, "Rape," 912; Jean Fagan Yellin, *Harriet Jacobs: A Life* (New York: Basic Books, 2004); Painter, "Of Lily"; Nell Irvin Painter, *Sojourner Truth: A Life, a Symbol* (New York: Norton, 1997); and Margaret Washington, *Sojourner Truth's America* (Urbana and Chicago: University of Illinois Press, 2009).

71. Higginbotham, *Righteous Discontent*, 191-92, 198.

72. Julie Winch, *Philadelphia's Black Elite: Activism, Accommodation, and the Struggle for Autonomy, 1787-1848* (Philadelphia: Temple University Press, 1993); Martha S. Jones, *All Bound Up Together*; Erica Armstrong Dunbar, *A Fragile Freedom: African American Women and Emancipation in the Antebellum City* (New Haven, CT: Yale University Press, 2008); and Jane E. Dabel, *A Respectable Woman: The Public Roles of African American Women in 19th-Century New York* (New York: New York University Press, 2008); and Erica Ball, *To Live an Antislavery Life: Personal Politics and the Antebellum Black Middle Class* (Athens: University of Georgia Press, 2012).

CHAPTER ONE

1. *New England Galaxy* (December 7, 1833); *New York Evening Star*, quoted in *Providence Patriot & Columbian Phenix* (January 4, 1834); and *Boston Weekly Reformer; or, the Herald of Union and Progress* (November 25, 1836).

2. *Providence Patriot* (January 4 and September 6, 1834); and *Emancipator and Journal of Public Morals* (July 1, 1834).

3. *Christian Mirror* (June 20, 1834).

4. *Daily Evening Transcript* (June 30, 1834); *Daily Evening Advertiser* (July 3, 1834); *Christian Mirror* (June 20 and 26, 1834); *New England Galaxy* (February 14, 1835); and *Liberator* (March 11, 1837; and April 7, 1837). Graham had contracted to lecture in Boston in 1834, but did not follow through until 1837; see Sylvester Graham, "To the Citizens of Northampton" (April 1, 1850), GFP, CL.

5. *Liberator* (March 11, 1837; March 24, 1837, emphasis in original; April 7, 1837; and September 29, 1837).

6. "Anti-Graham Riot," *Barre (MA) Gazette* (March 10, 1837); and *Boston Atlas*, quoted in *New York Spectator* (March 17, 1837).

7. "Anti-Grahamite," *Liberator* (March 11, 1837; and March 24, 1837); *Boston Morning Post* (March 5, 1837), quoted in *New York Spectator* (March 10, 1837); *Philadelphia Public Ledger and Daily Transcript* (March 9, 1837); and Lucia Weston (Boston) to Debra Weston (New Bedford), March 3, 183[7] (misdated 1835), Antislavery Collection, BPL, Ms.A.9.2.8.15.

8. Lucia Weston to Debra Weston, March 3, 183[7]; and *Boston Courier* (March 9, 1837). "Anti-Graham Riot"; *Liberator* (March 11, 1837; and April 7, 1837); *Boston Atlas*, quoted in the *New York Spectator* (March 17, 1837); Harriet Martineau, *Autobiography*, ed. Linda Peterson (n.p.: Broadview Press, 2007), 345n1; and Leonard L. Richards, *Gentlemen of Property and Standing: Anti-abolition Mobs in Jacksonian America* (New York: Oxford University Press, 1970).

9. A bookseller and abolitionist named Simeon Collins had hoped to publish Graham's lecture to women, noting how profitable his *Lecture to Young Men* was; in April 1837, he stopped writing about it. Simeon Collins to Cynthia Painter Collins, March 18, 1837, Collins Family Papers, box 1, folder 3, CL.

10. Stephen Nissenbaum, *Sex, Diet and Debility in Jacksonian America: Sylvester Graham and Health Reform* (Westport, CT: Greenwood Press, 1980), inspired this interpretation in E. Anthony Rotundo, *American Manhood: Transformations in Masculinity from the Revolution to the Modern Era* (New York: Basic Books, 1993); Bruce Dorsey, *Reforming Men and Women: Gender in the Antebellum City* (Ithaca, NY: Cornell University Press, 2002); Rodney Hessinger, *Seduced, Abandoned, and Reborn: Visions of Youth in Middle-Class America, 1780–1850* (Philadelphia: University of Pennsylvania Press, 2005); and Michael S. Kimmel, *Manhood in America: A Cultural History*, 2nd ed. (New York: Oxford University Press, 2006).

11. Galatians 3:28; Grahamite women made this scripture the masthead of the *Friend of Virtue* (Boston, 1838–39).

12. *Onania; or, The Heinous Sin of Self Pollution and All Its Frightful Consequences in Both Sexes, Considered*, 8th ed. (London: printed by Eliz. Rumball, for Thomas Crouch,

1723); and Thomas Laqueur, *Solitary Sex: A Cultural History of Masturbation* (New York: Zone Books, 2003).

13. Laqueur, *Solitary Sex*, 61, 200.

14. Juvenal, *The Sixteen Satires*, trans. Peter Green (1967; repr., New York: Penguin, 1998); Eva C. Keuls, *The Reign of the Phallus: Sexual Politics in Ancient Athens* (Berkeley and Los Angeles: University of California Press, 1985); and Leila Rupp, *Sapphistries: A Global History of Love between Women* (New York: New York University Press, 2009).

15. *Onania* (London, 1723), frontispiece.

16. Ibid., iii, vii, 114.

17. *A Supplement to the Onania, or the Heinous Sin of SELF-POLLUTION, and All Its Frightful Consequences, in the Two Sexes, Considered, &c.* (London: T. Crouch, 1723), 3. See especially the letters from Aan Myn Heer J.G., Hague, November 17, 1724, 118–19, and the author's replies to "The Afflicted Onan," November 26, 1722, 100–104, and Thomas T., London, September 2, 1725, 123–25, 150–51.

18. *Onania* (London, 1723), 164–66; on bathhouses as houses of assignation, see Laura Weigert, "Autonomy as Deviance: Sixteenth-Century Images of Witches and Prostitutes," in *Solitary Pleasures: The Historical, Literary, and Artistic Discourses of Autoeroticism*, ed. Paula Bennett and Vernon Rosario (New York: Routledge, 1995); and Kathleen M. Brown, *Foul Bodies: Cleanliness in Early America* (New Haven, CT: Yale University Press, 2009).

19. *Supplement to the Onania*, 2–3, 151–52, 155, 157–58, 159, 164, 165, 166–67; and Laqueur, *Solitary Sex*, 340.

20. *Onania* (London, 1723), vii, 82–100, 101–4; *Onania; or, The Heinous Sin of Self Pollution, and All Its Frightful Consequences, in Both Sexes, Considered* (Boston: John Phillips, 1724), 51–52, 57–61; and *Supplement to the Onania*, 34–35.

21. *Onania* (Boston, 1724).

22. Cotton Mather, *The Pure Nazarite* (Boston: Fleet for Phillips, 1723), 4–5, 7, 16. On the Puritan belief that the soul was feminine and thus permeable to evil spirits, see Elizabeth Reis, *Damned Women: Sinners and Witches in Puritan New England* (Ithaca, NY: Cornell University Press, 1997).

23. Rene Spitz, "Authority and Masturbation: Some Remarks on a Bibliographic Investigation," *Yearbook of Psychoanalysis* 9 (1953); E. H. Hare, "Masturbatory Insanity: The History of an Idea," *Journal of Mental Science* 108 (January 1962): 2–25; Michel Foucault, *The History of Sexuality*, vol. 1, *The Will to Knowledge*, trans. Robert Hurley (1978; repr., New York: Vintage, 1990); Michel Foucault, *Birth of the Clinic* (1963; repr., New York: Routledge, 1989); Patrick Singy, "Friction of the Genitals and Secularization of Morality," *Journal of the History of Sexuality* 12, no. 3 (July 2003): 345–64; and Laqueur, *Solitary Sex*, 42–45, 277–80.

24. Rousseau, *Émile; or, On Education* (originally published 1762); see esp. book 4. On *Émile* in America, see Linda Kerber, "The Republican Mother: Women and the Enlightenment—An American Perspective," *American Quarterly* 28, no. 2 (Summer 1976): 187–225; Jay Fliegelman, *Prodigals and Pilgrims: The American Revolution against Patriarchal Authority* (New York: Cambridge University Press, 1985); and Rosemarie Zagarri, "Morals, Manners, and the Republican Mother," *American Quarterly* 44, no. 2 (June 1992): 192–215. On Rousseau's impact on postrevolutionary France, including Moreau de la Sarthe's

patriarchal advice on female masturbation, see Sean M. Quinlan, "Physical and Moral Regeneration after the Terror: Medical Culture, Sensibility, and Family Politics in France, 1794–1804," *Social History* 29, no. 2 (May 2004): 139–64.

25. Tissot added that masturbating women became aloof to marriage and as warm toward other women as "the Second Sappho." "The Second Sappho" refers to Madeleine de Scudery (1607–1701), a writer who used the pseudonym *Sappho* and is considered the first bluestocking. S. A. D. Tissot, *Onanism; or, A Treatise upon the Disorders Produced by Masturbation; or, The Dangerous Effect of Secret and Excessive Venery*, trans. A. Hume, MD (London: printed for the translator, 1766), 12, 41–47, 71, 156–59.

26. Benjamin Rush, *Medical Inquiries & Observations upon the Diseases of the Mind* (1812; repr., New York: Hafner Publishing, 1962), 33.

27. Brian Carroll, "'I Indulged My Desire Too Freely': Sexuality, Spirituality, and the Sin of Self-Pollution in the Diary of Joseph Moody," *William and Mary Quarterly* 60, no. 1 (January 2003): 155–70.

28. Samuel Solomon, *A Guide to Health, or, Advice to both sexes; with an essay on a certain disease, seminal weakness and a destructive habit of a private nature: also an address to parents, tutors, and guardians of youth* (Stockport, UK: printed for the author, sold by Robert Bach of New York, 1800), 33–35; and Thomas A. Foster, *Sex and the Eighteenth-Century Man: Massachusetts and the History of Sexuality in America* (Boston: Beacon Press, 2007), 110, 112.

29. *Portland Courier*, quoted in *New York Spectator* (July 20, 1834); *New England Galaxy* (February 14, 1835); *Boston Courier* (March 6, 1837, emphasis in the original); and *Providence Patriot* (November 22, 1834).

30. Samuel Agnew, Harrisburg, PA, to Robert Vaux, March 16, 1831, GFP, box 1, folder 9.

31. D. Francis Condie to Sylvester Graham, April 13 and 16, 1832, and December 15, 1832, GFP, box 1, folders 9–10; and Sylvester Graham, Physiology Notes, GFP, box 3, folder 4.

32. Sylvester Graham, *Aesculapian Tablets of the Nineteenth Century* (Providence: Weeden and Cory, 1834), 16; Angelina E. Grimké to Sarah M. Grimké, November 8, 1831, WG MSS, CL; and Sylvester Graham, "History of Health" notebook (n.d., [1831–32]), GFP, CL; and Graham, "To the Citizens of Northampton."

33. Anonymous Quaker woman (Phebe Corlies?) to Sylvester Graham, May 22, 1832, and Graham, untitled journal, 1830s, GFP, box 1, folders 10–11.

34. *Address to the Master Mechanics, Journeymen, and Apprentices; Especially Intended for the State of Pennsylvania, by a Brother Mechanic* (Philadelphia: printed by T.W. Ustick, No. 3 Franklin Place, 1832).

35. *Microcosm, American and Gazette* (October 5, 1833).

36. Flora Northrup, *The Record of a Century, 1834–1934* (New York: American Female Guardian Society and Home for the Friendless, 1934), 15; and "Moral Reform in Providence," *AMR* (April 1, 1836). While historians tend to focus on the New York Female Moral Reform Society split with the Female Benevolent Society as the origin of female moral reform, Northrup and local newspapers show women organizing outside New York prior to creation of the New York Female Moral Reform Society. For more on the feminization of the movement, see Daniel S. Wright, *The First of Causes to Our Sex: The Female Moral Reform Movement in the Antebellum Northeast, 1834–1848* (New York: Routledge, 2006).

37. *FOV* (October 1838).

38. *Christian Mirror* (June 26, 1834).

39. Frances Wright, *Course of Popular Lectures* (New York: Office of the Free Enquirer, 1829).

40. Robert Dale Owen, *Moral Physiology* (New York: Wright and Owen, 1831).

41. Charles Knowlton, *Fruits of Philosophy: The Private Companion of Married People* (New York: published by the author, 1832). Russel Canfield, who plagiarized *Fruits of Philosophy* in his *Practical Physiology*, lectured to women on sex, marriage, and physiology in Philadelphia during the early 1830s and likely crossed paths with Sylvester Graham. Canfield compiled and published his lectures to women and men between 1830 and 1832 in 1832 (allegedly at the request of female audience members), but no copy of his book has survived. Russell Canfield, *Temple of Reason* (May 23, 1835; May 30, 1835; and October 10, 1835). Graham blamed atheists for instigating the Portland riots. See Sylvester Graham, Lecture Notes, 1831–47, back flap, AAS.

42. *Microcosm, American and Gazette* (January 18, 1834); Sylvester Graham, *A Lecture to Young Men on Chastity* (Providence: Weeden and Cory, 1834), 170; and "The Sin of Onan," *Illuminator* (April 6, 1836). Historians have interpreted women's interest in popular physiology in this light. See Linda Gordon, "Voluntary Motherhood: The Beginnings of Feminist Birth Control Ideas in the United States," *Feminist Studies* 1, nos. 3–4 (Winter–Spring 1973): 5–22; Regina Markell Morantz, "Nineteenth Century Health Reform and Women: A Program of Self Help," in *Medicine without Doctors: Home Health Care in American History*, ed. Guenter B. Risse (New York: Science History Publications, 1977), 73; and Janet Farrell Brodie, *Contraception and Abortion in 19th-Century America* (Ithaca, NY: Cornell University Press, 1994).

43. Susan Klepp, *Revolutionary Conceptions: Women, Fertility, and Family Limitation in America, 1760–1820* (Chapel Hill: University of North Carolina Press, 2009).

44. Sylvester Graham, undated handwritten notes [1830s], GFP, CL, box 3, folder 5.

45. Sylvester Graham, undated handwritten notes [1830s], GFP, CL.

46. Angelina E. Grimké to Sarah M. Grimké, November 8, 1831, WG MSS, box 2; Simeon Collins to Cynthia Painter Collins, March 18, 1837, and Sylvester Graham to Cynthia Painter Collins, March 24, 1837, Collins Family Papers, box 1, folder 3, CL.

47. Graham, *Lecture to Young Men*, 20.

48. Sylvester Graham, Journal, 1830s, GFP, box 1, folder 11, CL; Graham, Lecture Notes, 1831–47, octavo vol., n.p., AAS; anonymous testimonial in Mary S. Gove, *Lectures to Ladies on Anatomy and Physiology* (Boston: Saxton and Pierce, 1842), 229.

49. Graham, Lecture Notes, 1831–47, folio vol., AAS, 328–31, 335; Graham, *Lecture to Young Men*, 111; and Linda K. Kerber, *Women of the Republic: Intellect and Ideology in Revolutionary America* (Chapel Hill: University of North Carolina Press, 1997).

50. Percentage is based on 148 signers of a petition defending the lecture appearing in *Liberator* (March 11, 1837), using US federal census data, 1840, 1850, and 1860. For more detail, see April Haynes, "Riotous Flesh: Gender, Physiology, and the Solitary Vice" (PhD diss., University of California, Santa Barbara, 2009), 155–56.

51. *Portland Courier*, quoted in *New York Spectator* (July 20, 1834). Examples of married, single, and teenage attendance can be found in *Liberator* (March 11, 1837) and *Boston Morning Post* (March 6, 1837).

52. Graham, *Lecture to Young Men*, 151; Sylvester Graham, Lecture Notes, 328–31,

335; and Sylvester Graham, unsigned medical notebook, GFP, box 3, folder 6. The association between female masturbation, nymphomania, and lesbianism gathered momentum during the late nineteenth and early twentieth centuries. See Carol Groneman, *Nymphomania: A History* (New York: Norton, 2000); Leila Rupp, *A Desired Past: A Short History of Same-Sex Love in America* (Chicago: University of Chicago Press, 1999); and Jennifer Terry, *An American Obsession: Science, Medicine and Homosexuality in Modern Society* (Chicago: University of Chicago Press, 1999).

53. Jean DuBois, *The Secret Habits of the Female Sex* (New York: sold by the booksellers generally, 1848); Roger Thompson, *Unfit for Modest Ears: A Study of Graphic, Obscene, and Bawdy Works Written or Published in England in the Second Half of the Seventeenth Century* (Totowa, NJ: Rowman and Littlefield, 1979); Lynn Hunt, *The Invention of Pornography: Obscenity and the Origins of Modern Identity, 1500–1800* (New York: Zone Books, 1993); and Laqueur, *Solitary Sex*.

54. Patricia Cline Cohen, *The Murder of Helen Jewett: The Life and Death of a Prostitute in Nineteenth-Century New York* (New York: Knopf, 1998); and Sharon Block, *Rape and Sexual Power in Early America* (Chapel Hill: University of North Carolina Press, 2006).

55. *Boston Post* (March 6, 1838), emphasis in the original.

56. *Liberator* (March 11, March 24, and April 7, 1837).

57. For class diversity within the lectures, see *Workingman's Advocate* (July 2, 1831), and the testimonials published in Graham, *Aesculapian Tablets*. Original letters, collected in the GFP, CL, authenticate the testimonials.

58. Graham, Lecture Notes, 1831–1847, folio vol., back flap.

59. *The Abolitionist; or, Record of the New England Anti-slavery Society*, edited by a committee (Boston: Garrison and Knapp, 1833), 95.

60. Otis split the rest of his life between New York and Louisiana. He edited the *New Orleans Picayune*, and even fought for the Confederacy as a cannoneer in 1862 before returning to New York to edit the "copperhead" *New York Express*. *Lynchburg Virginian*, quoted in *Workingman's Advocate* (August 22, 1835); *Liberator* (September 19, 1835); *Boston Courier* (August 16, 1838); *Liberator* (September 14, 1838); *Illuminator* (December 2, 1835); *Spirit of the Times* (February 20, 1836; May 21, 1836; October 22, 1836; April 15, 1837; and June 17, 1837); "Death of James F. Otis, the Journalist," *New York Times* (February 10, 1867); Benjamin Blake, Minor, LLD, *Southern Literary Messenger, 1834–1864* (New York: Neale Publishing Company, 1905), 41, 49.

61. *Federal Census of 1870, Maine City Directories: Portland, 1831, 1834, 1837*, online database (Provo, UT: Generations Network, 2005), available from http://ancestry.com, accessed April 15, 2009; Charles Mussey et al., defendants, "Covenant Broken," Portland, Washington County District Court, February 1840, location 12-325, vol. 1:469, p. 325, in *York County Court of Common Pleas (1696–1760), Kennebec County Supreme Court (1799–1854), and Washington County District Court (1839–46)*, quoted in *Maine Court Records, 1696–1854*, online database (Provo, UT: Generations Network, 2003), available from http://ancestry.com, accessed April 15, 2009; *General Catalogue of Bowdoin College and the Medical School of Maine, 1794–1894* (Brunswick, ME: Bowdoin College, 1894), 157; *Letter from the Treasurer of the State to the President of the Senate and the Speaker of the House of Representatives* (Portland, ME: printed by Todd and Smith, printers to the

state, December 31, 1825), 8, 23; Clarence Hale, Esq., city solicitor, *The Charter and Ordinances of the City of Portland, together with Acts of the Legislature, Relating to the City, and to Municipal Matters* (Portland, ME: Dressler, McLellan, 1881), 604; William W. Story, recorder of the court, *Reports of Cases Argued and Determined in the Circuit Court of the United States, for the First Circuit*, vol. 3 (Boston: Charles C. Little and James Brown, 1847), 660–76; *Register of the Kentucky State Historical Society* (1930): 30; *Liberator* (February 16, 1838); "Maine Anti-Slavery Society," *Liberator* (November 12, 1836); *Collections and Proceedings of the Maine Historical Society*, 2nd ser., vol. 3 (Portland: Maine Historical Society, 1892), 255–56. On brothel real estate, see Timothy J. Gilfoyle, *City of Eros: New York City, Prostitution, and the Commercialization of Sex, 1790–1920* (New York: Norton, 1992); and Judith Schafer, *Brothels, Depravity, and Abandoned Women: Illegal Sex in Antebellum New Orleans* (Baton Rouge: Louisiana State University Press, 2009).

62. *Microcosm, American and Gazette* (December 28, 1833). Nissenbaum argues that disgruntled butchers and bakers instigated the mobs based on economic self-interest, an idea contained in the biographical note on Graham written by an anonymous descendant; see *Sex, Diet & Debility*, box 3, folder 8, GFP. On working-class men who parodied, appropriated, and rejected bourgeois respectability in urban environments, see Paul A. Gilje, *The Road to Mobocracy: Popular Disorder in New York City, 1763–1834* (Chapel Hill: University of North Carolina Press, 1987); Patricia Cline Cohen, "Unregulated Youth: Masculinity and Murder in the 1830s City," *Radical History Review* 52 (1992): 33–52; and Dell Upton, *Another City: Urban Life and Urban Spaces in the New American Republic* (New Haven, CT: Yale University Press, 2008).

63. Patricia Cline Cohen, Timothy Gilfoyle, and Helen Horowitz, *The Flash Press: Sporting Male Weeklies in 1840s New York* (Chicago: University of Chicago Press, 2008).

64. John Neal and James W. Miller, "Bachelors' Journal," *Yankee and Boston Literary Gazette* (September 24, 1828); and "Tabitha," *Yankee and Boston Literary Gazette* (September 3, 1828).

65. *New England Galaxy* (February 14, 1835); and *Boston Pearl and Galaxy* (April 21, 1838).

66. On brothel riots, see Christine Stansell, *City of Women: Sex and Class in New York, 1789–1860* (1982; repr., New York: Knopf, 1986); and Cohen, *Murder of Helen Jewett*.

67. *Providence Patriot, Columbian Phenix* (September 6, 1834; and September 20, 1834); and *Atkinson's Saturday Evening Post* (October 6, 1838).

68. *Boston Post* (February 17, 1837); and *North American Review*, quoted in *New Bedford Mercury* (October 12, 1838).

69. *New Bedford Mercury* (July 25, 1834); and *Boston Morning Transcript* (October 18, 1834). On gender indeterminacy as monstrous, see Anne G. Myles, "From Monster to Martyr: Re-presenting Mary Dyer," *Early American Literature* 36, no. 1 (2001): 1–30; and Elizabeth Reis, *Bodies in Doubt: An American History of Intersex* (Baltimore: Johns Hopkins University Press, 2009).

70. For occasional emission as a necessary deterrent to sexual abuse, see M. L. Bush, *What Is Love? Richard Carlile's Philosophy of Sex* (London: Verso, 1998). There are many examples of the anti-Catholic rhetoric of sexual deviance in the United States; see esp. George Bourne, *Lorette: The History of Louise, Daughter of a Canadian Nun: Exhibiting the Interior of Female Convents* (New York: Wm. A. Mercein, 1833); and Maria Monk, *Awful*

Disclosures by Maria Monk of the Hotel Dieu Nunnery of Montreal (New York: Howe and Bates, 1836). On "sodomites" as male monsters, see Jonathan Ned Katz, *Love Stories: Sex between Men before Homosexuality* (Chicago: University of Chicago Press, 2001); and Cohen, Gilfoyle, and Horowitz, *Flash Press*, 195–97.

71. *Daily Evening Advertiser* (July 3, 1834); and *Portland Courier*, quoted in *New York Spectator* (July 20, 1834).

72. *Illuminator* (October 14, 1835; and May 18, 1836); and *Illuminator*, quoted in *Huntress* (April 1, 1837).

73. J. N. Bolles, *Solitary Vice Considered* (New York: printed by the author, 1834).

74. *Zion's Herald* (July 15, 1835); *Liberator* (December 15, 1837); and "A New Work," *Trumpet and Universalist Magazine* (January 28, 1837).

75. Stephanie M. H. Camp, "The Pleasures of Resistance: Enslaved Women and Body Politics in the Plantation South, 1830–1861," in *New Studies in the History of American Slavery*, ed. Edward E. Baptist and Stephanie M. H. Camp, 87–124 (Athens: University of Georgia Press, 2006).

76. See *Illuminator* (October 21, 1835; and February 24, April 6, April 20, and May 18, 1836); *AMR* (January 1, 1836); *FOV* (January 1, 1838); "Reflections of the Past," *AMR* (February 1, 1841); and *Huntress* (April 1 and April 22, 1837).

77. D. C. Lansing and J. R. McDowall to Theodore Dwight Weld, March 29, 1834, in *Letters of Theodore D. Weld and Angelina Grimké Weld and Sarah Grimké*, ed. Gilbert H. Barnes and Dwight L. Dumond (New York: Appleton-Century, 1934), 136.

78. "Over-delicacy" is contrasted with "true delicacy" in Samuel Richardson, *Clarissa; or, The History of a Young Lady* (London: printed for the author, 1748); and "false delicacy" reaches full flower in Hugh Kelly, *False Delicacy: A Comedy* (London: R. Baldwin, 1768).

79. *Christian Mirror* (June 26, 1834).

80. *Portland Courier*, quoted in *New York Spectator* (July 20, 1834); *Christian Mirror* (June 26, 1834); and *AMR* (April 1, 1836).

81. *Portland Courier*, quoted in *Daily Evening Transcript* (June 30, 1834); *New York Spectator* (July 20, 1834); "New York City Female Moral Reform Society," *New York Evangelist* (May 23, 1835); *AMR* (September 1835; April 1, 1836; and June 1, 1836); and "Recollections of the Past," *AMR* (March 15, 1841).

82. *Illuminator*, quoted in *Liberator* (March 18, 1837).

83. *Liberator* (March 11, 1837). On women and petitioning in antebellum social movements, see Nancy Isenberg, *Sex and Citizenship in Antebellum America* (Chapel Hill: University of North Carolina Press, 1998); Judith Wellman, "Women and Radical Reform in Upstate New York: A Profile of Grassroots Women Activists," in *Clio Was a Woman: Studies in the History of American Women*, 113–27 (Washington, DC: Howard University, 1980); and Susan Zaeske, *Signatures of Citizenship: Petitioning, Antislavery, & Women's Political Identity* (Chapel Hill: University of North Carolina Press, 2003).

84. *Microcosm, American and Gazette* (December 14, 1833), quoted in *Illuminator* (October 21, 1835); *Hampshire Gazette*, quoted in *New Bedford (MA) Mercury* (September 25, 1835); and *Zion's Herald* (September 30, 1835).

85. "Mr. Graham's Reply," in April 7, [1837], folder 4, LPS record book, 1837–40, Codman-Butterfield Papers, MHS.

86. Nancy Cott, *Public Vows: A History of Marriage and the Nation* (Cambridge, MA: Harvard University Press, 2000); Sylvia D. Hoffert, *When Hens Crow: The Woman's Rights Movement in Antebellum America* (Bloomington: Indiana University Press, 1995); and Isenberg, *Sex and Citizenship*.

87. *Providence Patriot and Columbian Phenix* (July 5, 1834).

CHAPTER TWO

1. Lucia Weston (Boston) to Debra Weston (New Bedford), March 3, 183[7] (misdated 1835), Antislavery Collection, BPL, Ms.A.9.2.8.15; *Boston Courier* (March 9, 1837); "Anti-Graham Riot," *Barre (MA) Gazette* (March 10, 1837); *Liberator* (March 11, 1837; and April 7, 1837); *Boston Atlas*, quoted in *New York Spectator* (March 17, 1837); Harriet Martineau, *Autobiography*, ed. Linda Peterson (n.p.: Broadview Press, 2007), 345n1; and Leonard L. Richards, *Gentlemen of Property and Standing: Anti-abolition Mobs in Jacksonian America* (New York: Oxford University Press, 1970).

2. Carla Peterson, *Doers of the Word: African American Women Speakers and Writers in the North* (New York: Oxford University Press, 1995).

3. *Liberator* (March 11, 1837; and March 24, 1837); and *Pittsburgh Manufacturer*, quoted in *Liberator* (April 21, 1837).

4. Leslie M. Harris, "From Abolitionist Amalgamators to 'Rulers of the Five Points': The Discourse of Interracial Sex and Reform in Antebellum New York City," in *Sex, Love, Race: Crossing Boundaries in North American History*, ed. Martha Hodes (New York: NYU Press, 1999). See also Richards, *Gentlemen of Property and Standing*; Paul A. Gilje, *The Road to Mobocracy: Popular Disorder in New York City, 1763–1834* (Chapel Hill: University of North Carolina Press, 1987); and David Grimsted, *American Mobbing, 1828–1861* (New York: Oxford University Press, 1998).

5. Richards, *Gentlemen of Property and Standing*, 27–29.

6. *New York Commercial Advertiser*, quoted in *New Bedford Mercury* (July 25, 1834); *Courier and Enquirer* (March 11, 1834), quoted in *Liberator* (April 5, 1834); *Courier and Enquirer* (May 21, 1834), quoted in *United States Catholic Miscellany* (July 26, 1834); and *Pittsburgh Manufacturer*, quoted in *Liberator* (April 21, 1837).

7. *Bay State Democrat* (May 12, 1840); and William Lloyd Garrison to Helen Garrison, May 15, 1840, *Letters of William Lloyd Garrison*, ed. Walter M. Merrill (Cambridge, MA: Harvard University Press, 1971), 2:612.

8. *New England Spectator* (March 18, 1835); *Constitution of the Oberlin Female Moral Reform Society* (May 1835), Oberlin College Archives, RG 31-6-11 (Oberlin Community), box 1; *New York Evangelist* (May 21, 1836); and *AMR* (July 1, 1836).

9. JPD, "For the *Western Christian Advocate*: Mr. Brown's Lecture, July 7, 1834," *Western Christian Advocate* (July 25, 1835).

10. Timothy J. Gilfoyle, *City of Eros: New York City, Prostitution, and the Commercialization of Sex, 1790–1920* (New York: Norton, 1992).

11. *Man* (July 14, 1834).

12. Lewis Tappan to Charles Grandison Finney, February 28, 1832, Finney MSS, Oberlin College Archives; *Man* (July 14, 1834); "Bishop Onderdonk's Letter to the Rev. Peter

Williams," *Liberator* (July 26, 1834). On antiblack violence and the disproportionate destruction of black households, see *Journal of Commerce*, quoted in *Christian Watchman* (July 18, 1834). For a comparison of St. Philips and A.M.E. Zion, see Kyle Timothy Bulthuis, "Four Steeples over the City Streets: Trinity Episcopal, St. Philip's Episcopal, John Street Methodist, and African Methodist Episcopal Zion Churches in New York City, 1760–1840" (PhD diss., University of California, Davis, 2006). For more on the politics of the early A.M.E. Zion Church, see Benjamin Quarles, *Black Abolitionists* (New York: Oxford University Press, 1969); and William J. Walls, *The African Methodist Episcopal Zion Church: Reality of the Black Church* (Charlotte, NC: Zion Publishing Clearinghouse, 1974).

13. Margaret Washington, *Sojourner Truth's America* (Urbana and Chicago: University of Illinois Press, 2009), 91–97.

14. *Freedom's Journal* (July 18, 1828); and Erica Armstrong Dunbar, *A Fragile Freedom: African American Women and Emancipation in the Antebellum City* (New Haven, CT: Yale University Press, 2008).

15. *Courier and Enquirer* (May 21, 1834), quoted in *United States Catholic Miscellany* (July 26, 1834).

16. *Free Enquirer* (March 8, 1835).

17. New York city had four other female moral reform societies in 1835, all organized through churches and likely all white; of these, the largest counted 106 members, followed by 60 in the next largest and 45 in the smallest. Zion Female Moral Reform Society outnumbered all of them. See *First Annual Report of the Female Moral Reform Society of the City of New York, Presented May 1835, with the Constitution, List of Officers, Names of Auxiliaries &c.* (New York, 1835), AAS; and *AMR* (May 1, 1837).

18. Eliza Coker recalled these discussions in a history of the Zion Female Moral Reform Society for *AMR* (May 1, 1837); for earlier documentation of the society's existence, see *New York Evangelist* (May 9, 1835). Zion Female Moral Reform Society seems to have been most active between 1835 and 1839. Although I have not seen formal evidence of its dissolution, an 1839 fire destroyed the church building and may have suspended the group's activities indefinitely. *AMR* (May 1, 1837; August 15, 1837; and June 1, 1838); and *New York Spectator* (September 26, 1839). By 1844, Zion's church had moved to a new building and resumed its role as a space for community organizing; see *New York Herald* (May 4, 1844).

19. Darlene Clark Hine, "Rape and the Inner Lives of Black Women in the Middle West: Preliminary Thoughts on the Culture of Dissemblance," *Signs* 14, no. 4 (Summer 1989): 912–20.

20. "Countenancing Mobs," *AMR* (September 1835); "A Wretch and His Victims," *AMR* (December 1835); "Daring Outrages upon the Press," *AMR* (July 15, 1836); "Moral Courage of the Ladies," *AMR* (January 15, 1837); "Premium for Crime," *AMR* (March 15, 1837); "Country Visitors' Report," *AMR* (December 1, 1837); Elijah Demond, *The Sin of Lewdness: A Discourse Delivered to the Church and Congregation in Holliston, Mass. March 13, 1836* (Boston: New England Spectator, 1836); Mary Ann B. Brown, *An Address on Moral Reform, before the Worcester Female Moral Reform Society, October 22, 1839* (Worcester, MA: Aegis Office, W and J Butterfield, 1839); *FOV* (September 1838); and Margaret Prior, *Walks of Usefulness; or, Reminiscences of Mrs. Margaret Prior* (New York: American Female Moral Reform Society, 1848).

21. Alonzo Lewis, "Prospectus for the Lynn Mirror," quoted in *Liberator* (January 22, 1831); *New York Evangelist* (May 23, 1835); and *AMR* (March 1, 1836; August 15, 1836; and March 15, 1837).

22. *Protestant* (January 16, 1830); *AMR* (June 15, 1838); *FOV* (September 1838; and November 15, 1842); and *AMR* (October 15, 1844).

23. Walls, *African Methodist Episcopal Zion Church*; Graham Russell Hodges, *Root and Branch: African Americans in New York and East Jersey, 1613–1863* (Chapel Hill: University of North Carolina Press, 1999); and Leslie M. Harris, *In the Shadow of Slavery: African Americans in New York City, 1626–1863* (Chicago: University of Chicago Press, 2003).

24. *AMR* (May 1, 1837); and *North Star* (May 19, 1848).

25. A Puritan, *The Abrogation of the Seventh Commandment, by the American Churches* (New York: David Ruggles, 47 Howard Street, March 4, 1835), in *Early Negro Writing, 1760–1837*, ed. Dorothy Porter (Boston: Beacon Press, 1971), 479. While Dwight Dumond and Carol Lasser have attributed *Abrogation* to George Bourne, scholars of black abolitionism have long credited Ruggles with authorship. See, for example, Graham Russell Gao Hodges, *David Ruggles: A Radical Black Abolitionist and the Underground Railroad in New York City* (Chapel Hill: University of North Carolina Press, 2010); and Dorothy Porter, "David Ruggles, Apostle of Human Rights," *Journal of Negro History* 28, no. 1 (January 1943): 23–50. Ruggles was also known to white moral reformers as coeditor of the *Emancipator*. As far as I know, Ruggles was the only African American member of the Seventh Commandment Society. For more on his relationship with moral reformers, see David Ruggles, "Appeals to the Colored Citizens of New York and Elsewhere in Behalf of the Press, by David Ruggles, a Man of Color," in *Early Negro Writing, 1760–1837*, ed. Dorothy Porter, 637–55 (Boston: Beacon Press, 1971). Originally published in the *Emancipator and Journal of Public Morals* (January 13, 1835; January 20, 1835; January 27, 1835; February 3, 1835; February 10, 1835; and February 17, 1835); *New York Evangelist* (May 9, 1835); and *AMR* (May 1, 1837).

26. David Ruggles, *Reese Dissected* (1834; repr., New York: William Stuart, 1838), 14; and Puritan [Ruggles], *Abrogation*, 479.

27. Puritan [Ruggles], *Abrogation*, 479.

28. Ibid., 478, 483; and *AMR* (January and February 1835; May 1835; and October 1835).

29. Ronald Walters, "The Erotic South: Civilization and Sexuality in American Abolitionism," *American Quarterly* 25, no. 2 (May 1973): 177–201.

30. Olaudah Equiano, *The Interesting Narrative of the Life of Olaudah Equiano, or Gustavus Vassa, the African, Written by Himself*, ed. Vincent Carretta (London, 1789; repr., New York: Penguin, 2003), 104; and Marilyn Richardson, ed., *Maria W. Stewart, America's First Black Woman Political Writer: Essays and Speeches* (Bloomington: Indiana University Press, 1987), 31.

31. White abolitionist men followed suit, enjoining white women to join the antislavery movement precisely because they shared with enslaved women and men an interest in eradicating licentiousness. George Bourne, who had previously defined the sin of slavery primarily in terms of its violation of the eighth commandment (thou shalt not steal), began to address its breach of the seventh commandment in 1834. See George Bourne, *Picture of Slavery in the United States of America* (Middletown, CT: Edwin Hunt, 1834); and James A. Thome, *Address to the Females of Ohio Delivered at the State Anti-slavery*

Anniversary (Cincinnati: Ohio Anti-slavery Society, 1836). For more on the uses to which white women put the licentiousness of slavery, see Carol Lasser, "Voyeuristic Abolitionism: Sex, Gender, and the Transformation of Antislavery Rhetoric," *Journal of the Early Republic* 28 (Spring 2008): 83.

32. James Forten Jr., *An Address Delivered before the Ladies Antislavery Society of Philadelphia, on the Evening of April 14, 1836* (Philadelphia: Merrihew and Gunn, No. 7 Carter's Alley, 1836); William Wells Brown, "A Lecture delivered before the FASS of Salem, at Lyceum Hall, November 14, 1847," reported by Henry M. Parkhurst, phonographic reporter, Boston, 1847; NYFMRS 4th Annual Report, AMR (June 1, 1838); Harriet Jacobs, *Incidents in the Life of a Slave Girl, Written by Herself*, ed. Jean Fagan Yellin (Cambridge, MA: Harvard University Press, 2000), 51, 76. While Jacobs's editor, Lydia Maria Child, also used the word *licentiousness* in reference to slavery, it would be a mistake to assume that Child chose this word for Jacobs. As Jean Fagan Yellin has shown, Child reported that she "altered" very few of Jacobs's original words. See Lydia Maria Child, *An Appeal in Favor of That Class of Americans Called Africans* (1833; repr., New York: 1836), 184, 119, 193; and Jean Fagan Yellin, *Harriet Jacobs: A Life* (New York: Basic Books, 2004), 141.

33. *An Appeal to the Women of the Nominally Free States, Issued by an Antislavery Convention of American Women. Held by Adjournment from the 9th to the 12th of May, 1837*, 2nd ed. (Boston: Isaac Knapp, 1838), 15.

34. "A Few Facts," AMR (April 1835).

35. Harriet Martineau, *Society in America*, vol. 1 (New York: Saunders and Otley, 1837); and Walters, "Erotic South."

36. *New York Evangelist* (December 6, 1834); AMR (March 15, 1839); and FOV (June 15, 1840).

37. AMR (June 1, 1838).

38. "Warning to Domestics," AMR (May 1835); "The Sequel," AMR (March 1, 1836); Sharon Block, *Rape and Sexual Power in Early America* (Chapel Hill: University of North Carolina Press, 2006), 27; and Hannah Rosen, *Terror in the Heart of Freedom: Citizenship, Sexual Violence, and the Meaning of Race in the Postemancipation South* (Chapel Hill: University of North Carolina Press, 2009), 68–83. Regarding the constraints on black women's resistance to rape, see also Melton A. McLaurin, *Celia, A Slave* (New York: HarperCollins, 1991); Nell Irvin Painter, "Soul Murder and Slavery: Toward a Fully Loaded Cost Accounting," in *Southern History across the Color Line* (Chapel Hill: University of North Carolina Press, 2002); and Edward E. Baptist, "'Cuffy,' 'Fancy Maids,' and 'One-Eyed Men': Rape, Commodification, and the Domestic Slave Trade in the United States," AHR 106, no. 5 (December 2001): 1619–50.

39. AMR (April 1835 and May 1835).

40. Jacqueline Jones, *Labor of Love, Labor of Sorrow: Black Women, Work, and the Family, from Slavery to the Present* (New York: Basic Books, 1985); and James Oliver Horton, "Freedom's Yoke: Gender Conventions among Antebellum Free Blacks," *Feminist Studies* 12, no. 1 (Spring 1986): 58.

41. AMR (July 15, 1837).

42. *New England Spectator* (March 4, 1835).

43. *Boston Atlas*, quoted in Boston Female Anti-slavery Society, *Right & Wrong in Boston, No. 1* (Boston: published by Isaac Knapp, No. 25 Cornhill, 1836); and *Report of*

the BFASS, with a Concise Statement of Events, Previous and Subsequent to the Annual Meeting of 1835, 2nd ed. (Boston: Henry E. Benson, 1836), 9–10, 12, 14, 18.

44. AMR (June 1, 1837; and June 1, 1838); and Liberator (March 22, 1839).

45. Liberator (March 22, 1839).

46. Christine Stansell, City of Women: Sex and Class in New York, 1789–1860 (1982; repr., New York: Knopf, 1986); and Patricia Cline Cohen, The Murder of Helen Jewett: The Life and Death of a Prostitute in Nineteenth-Century New York (New York: Knopf, 1998).

47. AMR (April 1835).

48. Nancy Prince, A Narrative of the Life and Travels of Mrs. Nancy Prince (Boston: published by the author, 1850); and Dorothy Sterling, ed., We Are Your Sisters: Black Women in the Nineteenth Century (New York: Norton, 1984), 222.

49. Prince, Narrative, 9–10.

50. Frances Smith Foster, Written by Herself: Literary Production by African American Women, 1746–1892 (Bloomington: Indiana University Press, 1992), 86.

51. Bourne, Picture of Slavery; Sarah M. Grimké, "Narrative and Testimony of Sarah M. Grimké," National Reformer (March 1839); and Thome, Address. Nor was this all rhetorical. See Jacobs, Incidents; Painter, "Soul Murder"; and Thavolia Glymph, Out of the House of Bondage: The Transformation of the Plantation Household (New York: Cambridge University Press, 2008).

52. Hazel V. Carby, Reconstructing Womanhood: The Emergence of the Afro-American Woman Novelist (New York: Oxford University Press, 1987), 43.

53. "Moral Reform," New York Evangelist (December 6, 1834); and New York Evangelist (June 14, 1834).

54. Deborah Gray White, Ar'n't I a Woman? Female Slaves in the Plantation South (New York: Norton, 1985).

55. AMR (November 1, 1838).

56. Sarah M. Grimké, in Letters on the Equality of the Sexes and the Condition of Woman, addressed to Mary S. Parker, president of the Boston Female Antislavery Society (Boston: Isaac Knapp, 1838), 4, 53–54, 87, emphasis in the original.

57. Sarah M. Grimké, in Letters on the Equality of the Sexes, 16, 123; Gerda Lerner, The Grimké Sisters: Pioneers for Women's Rights and Abolition (1967; repr., Chapel Hill: University of North Carolina Press, 2004); Aileen Kraditor, Means and Ends in American Abolitionism: Garrison and His Critics on Strategy and Tactics, 1834–1850 (New York: Vintage Books, 1970); and Kathryn Kish Sklar, Women's Rights Emerges within the Antislavery Movement (New York: Palgrave Macmillan, 2000).

58. Angelina E. Grimké diary, June 4, June 21, July 23, and September 8, 1829 (emphasis added), in Walking by Faith: The Diary of Angelina Grimké, 1828–1835, ed. Charles Wilbanks (Columbia: University of South Carolina Press, 2003). Between 1831 and 1833—the period just after Angelina's move to Philadelphia—the diary makes no mention of slavery. It records her religious turmoil, search for a vocation, conflicted courtship with Edward Bettles, then her grief and guilt after his death. One undated [1833] letter to Thomas Smith Grimké responds to the British Abolition Act of 1833 by stating that American slavery "must be abolished" but says that "only time can answer" whether this will be accomplished by peaceful legislation or violent insurrection. WG MSS, box 1, CL.

59. Sarah Mapps Douglass to William Bassett, March 3, 1839, quoted in Sarah M.

Grimké to Elizabeth Pease, April 13, 1839, WG MSS, box 6, CL. Douglass is most familiar to historians for having protested the segregated "Negro Pew" in the Arch Street meeting of the Philadelphia Society of Friends. See, for example, Margaret Hope Bacon, *Sarah Mapps Douglass: Faithful Attender of Quaker Meeting: View from the Back Bench* (Philadelphia: Quaker Press of Friends General Conference, 2003); Bruce Dorsey, *Reforming Men and Women: Gender in the Antebellum City* (Ithaca, NY: Cornell University Press, 2002), 176; Lerner, *Grimké Sisters*, 100–121, 192–93; Ryan P. Jordan, *Slavery and the Meetinghouse: The Quakers and the Abolitionist Dilemma, 1820–1864* (Bloomington: Indiana University Press, 2007); and Carol Faulkner, *Lucretia Mott's Heresy: Abolition and Women's Rights in Nineteenth-Century America* (Philadelphia: University of Pennsylvania Press, 2011).

60. *Colored American* (February 17, 1837; March 25, 1837; and April 1, 1837); *Liberator* (June 21, 1834; and July 2, 1836); *Colored American* (August 26, 1837; and August 25, 1838); and *National Reformer* (September 1838 and October 1838). For other interpretations of the American Moral Reform Society, see Martha S. Jones, *All Bound Up Together: The Woman Question in African American Public Culture* (Chapel Hill: University of North Carolina Press, 2007); Quarles, *Black Abolitionists*; Harry Reed, *Platform for Change: The Foundations of the Northern Free Black Community, 1775–1865* (Lansing: Michigan State University Press, 1994); C. Peter Ripley, ed., *Black Abolitionist Papers* (Chapel Hill: University of North Carolina Press, 1991); Julie Winch, *Philadelphia's Black Elite: Activism, Accommodation and the Struggle for Autonomy, 1787–1848* (Philadelphia: Temple University Press, 1993); and R. J. Young, *Antebellum Black Activists: Race, Gender and Self* (New York: Garland, 1996).

61. *Minutes and Proceedings of the First Annual Meeting of the American Moral Reform Society, Held at Philadelphia. In the Presbyterian Church in Seventh Street, below Shippen, from the 14th to the 19th of August, 1837*, Afro-American History Series, ed. Maxwell Whiteman, Historic Publication no. 244, 22 (Philadelphia: Historic Publications, 1969); and *National Reformer* (August–September 1838; October 1838; and November 1838).

62. The Philadelphia Female Moral Reform Society may have included women of color, but it only reprinted these white officers' names in its annual reports. *AMR* (June 1, 1838; and January 15, 1839). Mott also addressed the American Moral Reform Society in 1837, a year before the women's organization formed; see Angelina E. Grimké to Jane Smith, August 26, 1837, WG MSS, CL. For more on Mott's interracialism, see Faulkner, *Lucretia Mott's Heresy*. On the Grimkés' preference for the American Moral Reform Society, see *Minutes and Proceedings of the First Annual Meeting of the American Moral Reform Society*, 22; Angelina E. Grimké to Jane Smith, August 26, 1837, box 4, WG MSS, CL; and *National Reformer* (August–September 1838).

63. Angelina E. Grimké to Sarah Mapps Douglass, April 3, 1837, and Angelina E. Grimké to Jane Smith, June 27, July 2, and August 10, 1837, WG MSS, box 4, CL.

64. Sarah M. Grimké and Angelina E. Grimké to Sarah Mapps Douglass, April 3, 1837, WG MSS, box 4, CL.

65. Angelina E. Grimké and Sarah M. Grimké to Jane Smith, March 22, 1837, WG MSS, box 4, CL.

66. Angelina E. Grimké and Sarah M. Grimké to Sarah Mapps Douglass, March 22, 1837, WG MSS, box 3, CL; Sarah M. Grimké and Angelina E. Grimké to Sarah Mapps Doug-

lass, April 3, 1837, and Angelina E. Grimké to Jane Smith, April 17, 1837, WG MSS, box 4, CL; Sarah Mapps Douglass to Abby Kelley, May 18, 1838, AK collection, AAS; and Sarah Forten to Angelina E. Grimké, April 15, 1837, in Barnes and Dumond, 379–82.

67. The New York Female Moral Reform Society held its annual meeting on May 1, 1837, and its third quarterly meeting on May 11, 1837. *AMR* (May 1, 1837). Out of seventy-one delegates, nineteen (26.8 percent) held or would hold offices in moral reform societies: Mary S. Parker (BFMRS), Lucretia Mott (PFMRS), Grace Douglass (AMRS), Louisa Whipple (Dunbarton FMRS), Sarah G. Buffum (Fall River FMRS), Lucy Parker (BFMRS), Eliza Pope (Dorchester FMRS), Ruby Knight (Peru FMRS), Lydia Fuller (Boston FMRS), M. Irena Treadwell (NYFMRS), Mary Smith (Marion FMRS), Juliana A. Tappan (NYFMRS), Mary O. B. Pennimen (NYFMRS), Margaret Prior (NYFMRS), Azuba Whittlesey (NYFMRS), Mrs. A. J. Lane (AFMRS), Grace Martyn (NYFMRS), Angelina Grimké (honorary member of NYFMRS), and Sarah Grimké (honorary member of NYFMRS).

68. Dorothy Sterling, ed., *Turning the World Upside Down: The Antislavery Convention of American Women Held in New York City, May 9–12, 1837* (New York: Feminist Press at CUNY, 1987). For more on the Cassey-Douglass friendship, see Philip Lapsansky, "Afro-Americana: In a Garden of Radical Gentility," *Annual Report of the LCP*, 1998, presented at the annual meeting, May 1999. Julia Williams was a former student of Prudence Crandall's and a current member of the Boston Female Anti-slavery Society. *Letters of William Lloyd Garrison*, 2:260; and *AMR* (June 1, 1837).

69. After the convention, Angelina Grimké republished the *Appeal* under her own name, believing it would be taken more seriously given her growing celebrity. See Sarah M. Grimké and Angelina E. Grimké to Theodore D. Weld, November 30, 1837, quoted in Barnes and Dumond, 448.

70. Sterling, *Turning the World Upside Down*, 10; *Appeal to the Women of the Nominally Free States*, 14; and Angelina E. Grimké to Jane Smith, May 20, 1837, WG MSS, box 4, CL.

71. "Licentious Men Most to Blame," *AMR* (December 1835); *AMR* (February 8, 1836); Sarah M. Grimké, in *Letters on the Equality of the Sexes*, 87, 122; and Sarah M. Grimké, "What Are the Duties of Woman at the Present Time?" *AMR* (January 1, 1838).

72. Sarah M. Grimké to L.T.Y., *FOV* (February 1, 1838); and Barnes and Dumond, 51–54.

73. Angelina E. Grimké to Jane Smith, July 17, 1837, WG MSS, box 4, CL.

74. This distinctive piece of what Gerda Lerner calls Grimké's "feminist Bible criticism" privileged the creation account of Genesis 1:27, in which God simultaneously created the first man and woman, over Genesis 2:21–24, in which God created Eve out of Adam's rib. Prince, *Narrative*, 36–37; and Lerner, *Grimké Sisters*, xviii. On Grimké's Boston FMRS lecture, see *AMR* (August 1, 1837).

75. Quoted in Shirley J. Yee, *Black Women Abolitionists: A Study in Activism, 1828–1860* (Knoxville: University of Tennessee Press, 1992), 144.

76. Martha S. Jones, *All Bound Up Together*.

77. For more on debates over Grimké in the moral reform press, see Daniel S. Wright, *The First of Causes to Our Sex: The Female Moral Reform Movement in the Antebellum Northeast, 1834–1848* (New York: Routledge, 2006), 138–39.

78. The AAS's bound vols. 1–5 (1835–38) bear evidence of Ingraham's ownership. Book-plates establish her ownership of vols. 1–2 (1835–36) and 3–4 (1837–38).

79. "To the Members of the Moral Reform Convention, Salem, May 3, 1838," *AMR* (June 1, 1838); and *AMR* (March 15, 1837).

80. "New Haven, Conn.," *AMR* (December 1835); "Peterboro Constitution," *AMR* (May 15, 1836); "The Moral Reform Society and Its Auxiliaries," *AMR* (May 1, 1837); "New Alstead," *AMR* (July 15, 1837); *AMR* (June 1, 1838); *FOV* (February 1, 1838); and *Health Journal and Advocate of Physiological Reform* (June 17, 1840).

81. March 27, 1839, minutes, *Constitution and Record of the Grafton Female Moral Reform Community*, Grafton city records, 1838–62, AAS; "Peterboro Constitution"; and "An Efficient Auxiliary," *AMR* (July 1, 1837).

82. Mary Ann B. Brown, *Address on Moral Reform*, 5; *AMR* (November 1, 1838); and Lerner, *Grimké Sisters*.

83. *AMR* (August 15, 1844).

84. *AMR* (June 1, 1844; and October 15, 1844).

CHAPTER THREE

1. [Mary Gove], *Solitary Vice: An Address to Parents, and Those Who Have Care of Children* (Portland, ME: printed at the Journal Office, 1839), 135, extracted from her serialized articles in *FOV*, beginning with *FOV* (July 1838). An abridged version appeared in Gove's compilation of her *Lectures to Ladies on Anatomy and Physiology* (Boston: Saxton and Pierce, 1842), confirming that she delivered it orally before publishing it in the moral reform press.

2. *FOV* (February 15, 1840; and June 15, 1840). In 1841, the American Female Moral Reform Society claimed to have 555 auxiliary societies with between forty thousand and fifty thousand members. *AMR* (June 1, 1841). See also Daniel S. Wright, *The First of Causes to Our Sex: The Female Moral Reform Movement in the Antebellum Northeast, 1834–1848* (New York: Routledge, 2006), 3.

3. May 16, 1837, minutes, in LPS record book, 1837–40, Codman-Butterfield Papers, MHS.

4. *AMR* (October 1, 1844).

5. "Rescue" had been the male-dominated, philanthropic model of 1800–1830, from which the New York Female Moral Reform Society initially distinguished itself by seeking "prevention." See Clare A. Lyons, *Sex among the Rabble: An Intimate History of Gender and Power in the Age of Revolution, Philadelphia, 1730–1830* (Chapel Hill: University of North Carolina Press, 2006); Barbara Meil Hobson, *Uneasy Virtue: The Politics of Prostitution and the American Reform Tradition* (New York: Basic Books, 1987); and Larry Whiteaker, *Seduction, Prostitution and Moral Reform in New York, 1830–1860* (New York: Garland Publishers, 1997). On the distinction between rescue and prevention, see Daniel S. Wright, *First of Causes*.

6. Here I am referring to the first wave of physiological societies, 1837–41, as opposed to the second wave of the 1840s and 1850s. The Ladies' Physiological Society of Boston, founded in 1837, for example, should not be confused with the Ladies Physiological Institute of Boston and Vicinity, founded in 1850, which will be discussed in chapter 5 below.

7. "Resolutions of the Friends of Dr. Graham," *Boston Morning Post* (December 31, 1836); *Constitution of the American Physiology Society*, APS Publications (Boston: George W.

Light, 1838), 3–36; *Health Journal and Advocate of Physiological Reform* (April 15, 1840). On the Alcott-Graham rivalry, see *Graham Journal of Health and Longevity* (March 30, 1839); and *Health Journal and Advocate of Physiological Reform* (May 22, 1841).

8. Prosopography based on 148 LPS members and Graham-defense signers, using US federal census data 1840, 1850, and 1860. For more detail, see April Haynes, "Riotous Flesh: Gender, Physiology, and the Solitary Vice" (PhD diss., University of California, Santa Barbara, 2009), 152.

9. APS minutes, 1837–39, throughout, Ms. S-530, MHS.

10. April 6, 1837, May 16, 1837, and July 9, 1839, minutes, in LPS record book, 1837–40, Codman-Butterfield Papers, MHS; and Rebecca Codman to the *Health Journal and Advocate of Physiological Reform* (August 5, 1840).

11. Simeon Collins to Cynthia Painter Collins, March 24, 1837, Collins Family Papers, box 1, folder 3, CL; and *Graham Journal of Health and Longevity* (April 4, 1837).

12. Simeon Collins to Cynthia Painter Collins, March 18, 1837; Sylvester Graham to Cynthia Painter Collins, March 24, 1837, Collins Family Papers, box 1, folder 3, CL; and M. M. Bartlett to Simeon Collins, March 29, 1837, Collins Family Papers, CL.

13. APS, *Second Annual Report, June 1, 1838*, APS Publications (Boston: Light and Stearns, 1839), 19; and March 13, 1838, and April 10, 1838, minutes, in LPS record book, 1837–40, Codman-Butterfield Papers, MHS.

14. July 10, 1838, minutes, in LPS record book, 1837–40, Codman-Butterfield Papers, MHS.

15. Mary S. Gove, "To Parents, Guardians, and Those Who Have the Care of Children," *FOV* (July 1838); July 10, 1838, May 16, 1837, and August 7, 1838, minutes, in LPS record book, 1837–40, Codman-Butterfield Papers, MHS; and "Graham in Petticoats," *Boston Courier* (August 23, 1838). For more on Gove's career and sexual philosophy, see Patricia Cline Cohen, "Sex and Sexuality: The Public, the Private, and the Spirit Worlds," *Journal of the Early American Republic* 24, no. 2 (Summer 2004): 310–18; Jean L. Silver-Isenstadt, *Shameless: The Visionary Life of Mary Gove Nichols* (Baltimore: Johns Hopkins University Press, 2002); "Female Associations," *Moral Reformer and Teacher on the Human Constitution* (May 1836); and *Graham Journal of Health and Longevity* (February 2, 1839; March 30, 1839; and April 13, 1839).

16. October 8, 1839, minutes, in LPS record book, 1837–40, Codman-Butterfield Papers, MHS; and *Graham Journal of Health and Longevity* (March 2, 1839).

17. "Woman, the Hope of Our Cause," *Graham Journal* (November 9, 1839); and APS minutes, February 6, 1839, and July 27, 1839, MHS.

18. June 14, [1839], folder 4, in LPS record book, 1837–40, Codman-Butterfield Papers, MHS. Nancy Hobart Prince should not be confused with Nancy Gardner Prince.

19. *FOV* (January 15, 1840); and April 10, 1838, minutes, in LPS record book, 1837–40, Codman-Butterfield Papers, MHS.

20. *Health Journal and Advocate of Physiological Reform* (July 15, 1840); February 12, 1839, minutes, in LPS record book, 1837–40, Codman-Butterfield Papers, MHS. On the Boston Female Anti-slavery Society's 1839 split, see Maria Weston Chapman, *Right and Wrong in Massachusetts* (Boston: Dow and Jackson, 1839); Debra Gold Hansen, *Strained Sisterhood: Gender and Class in the Boston Female Antislavery Society* (Amherst: University of Massachusetts Press, 1993); Debra Gold Hansen, "The Boston Female Anti-slavery

Society and the Limits of Gender Politics," in *The Abolitionist Sisterhood: Women's Political Culture in Antebellum America*, ed. Jean Fagan Yellin and John C. Van Horne (Ithaca, NY: Cornell University Press, 1994), 50; Julie Roy Jeffrey, *The Great Silent Army of Abolitionism: Ordinary Women in the Antislavery Movement* (Chapel Hill: University of North Carolina Press, 1998); Aileen S. Kraditor, *Means and Ends in American Abolitionism: Garrison and His Critics on Strategy and Tactics, 1834–1850* (New York: Vintage Books, 1970); and Bruce Laurie, *Beyond Garrison: Antislavery and Social Reform* (New York: Cambridge University Press, 2005).

21. *New York Evangelist* (November 15, 1834); and *AMR* (October 1835; February 1, 1837; August 1, 1843; and October 1, 1843).

22. APS, *Second Annual Report*, 14–16, 25; and *FOV* (July 1838).

23. *AMR* (March 15, 1837).

24. Ibid.; "Quarterly Meeting of the Grafton Female Moral Reform Society," December 26, 1839, *Constitution and Record of the Grafton Female Moral Reform Community*, Grafton city records, 1838–62, AAS; and *Eleventh Annual Report of the Grafton Female Moral Reform Society*, Grafton Female Moral Reform Society minutes, 1849, Grafton City Records, 1838–62, AAS.

25. *FOV* (July 1838); and *AMR* (April 1, 1839).

26. Daniel S. Wright, *First of Causes to Our Sex*, 121.

27. Sylvester Graham, *A Lecture to Young Men on Chastity* (Providence: Weeden and Cory, 1834); John R. McDowall [Asenath Nicholson], *The Memoir and Select Remains of the Late John R. McDowall, the Martyr of the Seventh Commandment* (New York: Leavitt, Lord, 1838); Samuel B. Woodward, *Hints for the Young, on a Subject Relating to the Health of Body and Mind, from the "Boston Medical and Surgical Journal," with Additions by the Author* (Boston: Weeks, Jordan, 1838); *AMR* (September 2, 1839); and *FOV* (November 1, 1839). Samuel B. Woodward, the superintendent of the Massachusetts State Lunatic Asylum at Worcester, quantified cases of masturbatory insanity throughout the 1830s. See chapter 5, below.

28. Gove, *Lectures to Ladies*, 226–28.

29. Ibid., 230–31.

30. Ibid., 222.

31. *FOV* (October 1, 1841).

32. *AMR* (May 15, 1837); Fourteenth Annual Meeting, *Constitution and Record of the Grafton Female Moral Reform Society*, Grafton city records, 1838–62, AAS; and *FOV* (June 15, 1841).

33. Eve Kosokfsky Sedgwick, "Jane Austen and the Masturbating Girl," *Critical Inquiry* 17, no. 4 (Summer 1991): 834. "Another Voice from Woman," *Health Journal* (March 26, 1842); Carroll Smith-Rosenberg, "The Female World of Love and Ritual: Relations between Women in Nineteenth-Century America," in *Disorderly Conduct: Visions of Gender in Victorian America*, 53–76 (New York: Knopf, 1985); and *Constitution and Record of the Grafton Female Moral Reform Society*, Grafton city records, 1838–62, AAS.

34. *AMR* (August 15, 1837; and June 1, 1838).

35. *FOV* (June 1838, emphasis in the original).

36. *AMR* (June 1, 1838); *FOV* (June 1838); and Elizabeth Cady Stanton, *History of Woman Suffrage* (New York: Fowler and Wells, 1881), 337–38.

37. *AMR* (June 1, 1839).

38. William J. Walls, *The African Methodist Episcopal Zion Church: Reality of the Black Church* (Charlotte, NC: Zion Publishing Clearinghouse, 1974); and Martha Saxton, *Being Good: Women's Moral Values in Early America* (New York: Hill and Wang, 2003), 228.

39. Jas. A. Thome and J. Horace Kimball, *Emancipation in the West Indies: A Six Months Tour in Antigua, Barbadoes, and Jamaica in the Year 1837* (New York: American Anti-slavery Society, 1838), 320.

40. *AMR* (September 1, 1841); Nancy Prince, *A Narrative of the Life and Travels of Mrs. Nancy Prince* (Boston: published by the author, 1850), 36–37, 45, 50; Elizabeth Cady Stanton, Susan B. Anthony, and Matilda Joselyn Gage, eds., *History of Woman Suffrage*, vol. 1, *1848–1861* (New York: Fowler and Wells, 1889), 384. Prince was unable to raise the needed funds. She later opened an employment agency for African American girls and women in Boston. See Jean Fagan Yellin, *Harriet Jacobs: A Life* (New York: Basic Books, 2004), 77.

41. "Moral Reform," *Friends' Review* (January 6, 1849).

42. Ibid. On Hetty Burr, see Julie Winch, *The Elite of Our People: Joseph Willson's Sketches of Black Upper-Class Life in Antebellum Philadelphia* (University Park: Pennsylvania State University Press, 2000), 123n11. On Hetty Reckless, see Shirley J. Yee, *Black Women Abolitionists: A Study in Activism, 1828–1860* (Knoxville: University of Tennessee Press, 1992), 97–99; and Gayle T. Tate, *Unknown Tongues: Black Women's Political Activism in the Antebellum Era* (East Lansing: Michigan State University Press, 2003), 212–13.

43. Committee for Improving the Condition of Free Blacks, minutebook, February 14, 1837–November 17, 1853, June 24, 1846, p. 84, Pennsylvania Abolition Society records, HSP.

44. *FOV* (August 15, 1841); and "The Moral Reform Retreat," *Friend: A Religious and Literary Journal* (November 6, 1847).

45. *AMR* (February 1, 1844).

46. *AMR* (November 15, 1838).

47. *AMR* (September 16, 1844).

48. *AMR* (February 1, 1845).

49. *AMR* (October 1, 1844).

50. *AMR* (October 1, 1845).

51. *AMR* (October 1, 1843); *FOV* (July 1, 1846); and Lori D. Ginzberg, *Women and the Work of Benevolence: Morality, Politics, and Class in the Nineteenth-Century United States* (New Haven, CT: Yale University Press, 1990), 119–28.

52. *AMR* (October 1, 1843); and *FOV* (July 1, 1846).

53. *Constitution and Report of the Managers of the Rosine Association, with a List of the Annual Subscribers and Contributors* (Philadelphia: printed by Merrihew and Thompson, No. 7 Carter's Alley, 1848), 4, HSP.

54. Committee for Improving the Condition of Free Blacks, minutebook, February 14, 1837–November 17, 1853, October 10, 1845, p. 70, Pennsylvania Abolition Society records, HSP.

55. *Constitution and Report of the Managers of the Rosine Association*; and Marcia Carlisle, "Disorderly City, Disorderly Women: Prostitution in Ante-bellum Philadelphia," *Pennsylvania Magazine of History and Biography* 110, no. 4 (October 1986): 549–68.

56. *AMR* (July 1, 1846).

57. *AMR* (June 1, 1838). On Green's relationship with the American Female Moral Reform Society, see *AMR* (June 1, 1838). On his relationship with the New England Female Moral Reform Society, see *FOV* (April 15, 1844). On his on his relationship with the Holliston Female Moral Reform Society, see *FOV* (November 15, 1842). On funds moral reformers contributed to the seminary, see *AMR* (July 1, 1841; September 16, 1844; and May 15, 1841).

58. Hopkinton Town Record, Maternal Association box, 1842–49, August 31, 1842, minutes. On Eaton's lecture tour, see *FOV* (June 1, 1841).

59. "Sandwich Islands Anatomy," *Graham Journal of Health and Longevity* (May 1838); *Missionary Herald* (1840); Calvin Cutter, *Physiology . . . for Schools & Families* (Boston: Robert S. Davis, 1844), 38; Calvin Cutter, *Female Guide: Containing Facts & Info upon the Effects of Masturbation and the Causes . . . for Females Exclusively* (West Brookfield, MA: Charles A. Mirick, 1844), 31; "The Editor's Table," *Christian Reflector* (February 26, 1846); *Trumpet and Universalist Magazine* (February 28, 1846); *Liberator* (July 3, 1846); *Zion's Herald and Wesleyan Journal* (December 9, 1846); *New York Evangelist* (August 5, 1847); *Connecticut Common School Journal and Annals of Education* (December 4, 1851); *Massachusetts Teacher* (October 1852); *Missionary Herald* (February 1857); *Missionary Herald* (December 1867); and Michael Sappol, *A Traffic of Dead Bodies: Anatomy and Embodied Social Identity in Nineteenth-Century America* (Princeton, NJ: Princeton University Press, 2002), 187.

60. *New England Spectator* (April 27, 1836); Sylvester Graham, Lecture Notes, 1831–47, AAS; Sylvester Graham, *Lectures on the Science of Human Life*, vol. 2 (Boston: Marsh, Capen, Lyon, and Webb, 1839), 190–99; *AMR* (March 1, 1841; and February 1, 1844); *FOV* (October 15, 1845); *Oberlin Evangelist* (August 15, 1849); and *FOV* (August 1, 1855).

61. *AMR* (November 15, 1838).

62. *AMR* (October 15, 1841; and August 15, 1844).

CHAPTER FOUR

1. Although Gove's new credibility was short lived—she would later be denounced as a free lover—she provides an especially striking example of the growing respectability of women's physiology during the 1840s. *New York Herald* (April 29 and May 7, 1839); G. H. Ballou (Lynn) to Abby Kelley, September 8, 1839, Abby Kelley Foster Papers, AAS; and "Lectures to Ladies on Anatomy and Physiology," *BMSJ* (March 16, 1842). See Jean L. Silver-Isenstadt, *Shameless: The Visionary Life of Mary Gove Nichols* (Baltimore: Johns Hopkins University Press, 2002).

2. Hollick arrived at 39,000 by multiplying 196 by 200 (39,200); he had delivered 196 lectures in Philadelphia between 1845 and 1846 and estimated an average attendance of about 200. *Philadelphia Public Ledger and Daily Transcript* (May 5, 1846); Frederick Hollick, *The Origin of Life* (New York: T. W. Strong, 1845), x; and Michael Sappol, *A Traffic of Dead Bodies: Anatomy and Embodied Social Identity in Nineteenth-Century America* (Princeton, NJ: Princeton University Press, 2002), 199–200. Hollick's works were still being copied posthumously in 1902 and proliferated so widely that they are to this day widely available at antiquarian bookstores, yard sales, and on eBay.

3. Ellen Carol DuBois and Linda Gordon, "Seeking Ecstasy on the Battlefield: Danger and Pleasure in Nineteenth-Century Feminist Sexual Thought," in *Pleasure and Danger: Exploring Female Sexuality*, ed. Carol Vance, 31–49 (New York: Pandora, 1989).

4. For more on the popular health movement, see John Haller, *The People's Doctors: Samuel Thomson and the American Botanical Movement, 1790–1860* (Carbondale: Southern Illinois University Press, 2000); Paul Starr, *The Social Transformation of American Medicine* (New York: Basic Books, 1982); Morris J. Vogel and Charles E. Rosenberg, eds., *The Therapeutic Revolution: Essays in the Social History of American Medicine* (Philadelphia: University of Pennsylvania Press, 1979); Sappol, *Traffic of Dead Bodies*, 275–90; Helen Horowitz, *Rereading Sex: Battles over Sexual Knowledge and Suppression in Nineteenth-Century America* (New York: Knopf, 2002), 209–47; and Patricia Cline Cohen, Timothy Gilfoyle, and Helen Horowitz, *The Flash Press: Sporting Male Weeklies in 1840s New York* (Chicago: University of Chicago Press, 2008).

5. *Life in Boston & New York* (November 22, 1856).

6. Hollick, *Origin of Life*, 226–28; and Jonathan Ned Katz, *The Invention of Heterosexuality* (Chicago: University of Chicago Press, 1995).

7. Lori D. Ginzberg, *Women and the Work of Benevolence: Morality, Politics, and Class in the Nineteenth-Century United States* (New Haven, CT: Yale University Press, 1990), 98–132.

8. *Philadelphia Public Ledger and Daily Transcript* (April 4, 1846).

9. Robert Owen (1771–1858) was the founder of British socialism and father of Robert Dale Owen. The British secular movement agitated for the disestablishment of the Church of England during the early nineteenth century. For more on Owen and the British secular movement, see John Edwin McGee, *A History of the British Secular Movement* (Girard, KA: Haldeman-Julius, 1948); and Barbara Taylor, *Eve and the New Jerusalem* (Cambridge, MA: Harvard University Press, 1993).

10. "Charles Arthur Hollick," *Bulletin of the Botanical Club* 60, no. 8, in Charles Arthur Hollick Papers, box 1, folder 1.27 38.2H, Staten Island Institute of Arts and Sciences; Frederick Hollick and John Brindley, "Public Discussion on Socialism, Held at the New Theatre, Leicester, on the Evenings of Tuesday and Wednesday, April 14th and 15th, 1840 between Mr. Brindley and Mr. Hollick, Socialist Missionary," *Leicester Journal* (April 17, 1840); Robert Owen, *The Book of the New Moral World* (New York: Gilbert Vale, 1845); and *Daily Chronicle* (April 2, 1846). For a more detailed discussion of Hollick's biography, see April Haynes, "The Trials of Frederick Hollick: Obscenity, Sex Education, and Medical Democracy in the Antebellum United States," *Journal of the History of Sexuality* 12, no. 2 (October 2003): 543–74.

11. Dr. F. Hollick, "Opening Address," *People's Medical Journal and Home Doctor: A Monthly Journal, Devoted to the Dissemination of Popular Information on Anatomy, Physiology, the Laws of Health and the Cure of Disease* (July 1853).

12. Hollick gave a retrospective of his career in the preface to an 1878 edition of *Origin of Life*, and many of the details have been confirmed by Christopher Hoolihan's bibliographic research. See Christopher Hoolihan, *An Annotated Catalogue of the Edward C. Atwater Collection of American Popular Medicine and Health Reform*, 3 vols. (Rochester, NY: University of Rochester Press, 2008), 3:355–56; and "Original resolutions adopted by the women of Philadelphia who attended lectures of Frederick Hollick, MD, during the

years 1844, 1845 (these resolutions were followed, in 1846, by the presentation of a gold medal), presented by Charles Arthur Hollick," box 1, folder 1, Charles Arthur Hollick Papers, Staten Island Institute of Arts and Sciences. On Fanny Wright's sexual physiology lectures to women, see Horowitz, *Rereading Sex*, 54–56.

13. Lydia Maria Child, "Letter XI, April 7th, 1844," in *Letters from New York*, 11th ed. (New York: C. S. Francis, 1850); and Lydia Maria Child, "Letter from New York, No. 11," *United States Gazette* (May 5, 1846).

14. *Pennsylvania Freeman* (February 27, 1845); *Philadelphia Public Ledger and Daily Transcript* (May 5, 1846); and Lydia Maria Child, *Letters from New York*, 2nd ser. (New York: C. S. Francis, 1846), 110–12. See also Child, *Letters from New York* (11th ed.), 110–12.

15. Hollick, *Origin of Life*, xxi–xxii, 243; and Frederick Hollick, *The Marriage Guide* (New York: T. W. Strong, 1851), 136, 178–79, 312–13, 344, 368, 382–83.

16. Frederick Hollick, *A Popular Treatise on Venereal Diseases, Their Cure and Prevention, for Private Use, with Colored Plates* (New York: T. W. Strong, 1852), 27; Hollick, *Origin of Life*, 207; and Hollick, *Marriage Guide*, 320, 334.

17. Though flawed by miscalculations, the rhythm method that Hollick promoted offered one key advantage to women: it did not rely entirely on the male partner to be effective. See Janet Farrell Brodie, *Contraception and Abortion in 19th-Century America* (Ithaca, NY: Cornell University Press, 1994), 115.

18. Hollick, *Marriage Guide*, 344–46.

19. Ibid., 290–93, 296, 344.

20. Frederick Hollick, *Diseases of Woman*, 53rd ed. (New York: T. W. Strong, 1855); and Hollick, *Origin of Life*, 246–47.

21. Ronald Walters, *Primers for Prudery: Sexual Advice to Victorian America* (Englewood Cliffs, NJ: Prentice Hall, 1973). More recently, Michael Sappol's *A Traffic of Dead Bodies* interprets Hollick's graphic representations of syphilis and gonorrhea as didactic in tone; however, sporting men could find recipes for self-cures and ads for prophylactics in the pages of his books. An entrepreneur and a libertarian, Hollick intended to sell sporting men tools to abet their sexual freedom—not scare them straight, as it were.

22. Hollick, *Origin of Life*, 236; *People's Monthly Medical Journal* (March 1854); and Michel Foucault, *The History of Sexuality*, vol. 1, *The Will to Knowledge*, trans. Robert Hurley (1978; repr., New York: Vintage, 1990). On the connection between the masturbator and the homosexual, see also Roy Porter, "Love, Sex, and Madness in Eighteenth-Century England," *Social Research* 53, no. 2 (Summer 1986): 211–42. On marriage manuals as primers for heteronormativity, see esp. Theodoor Van de Velde, *Ideal Marriage: Its Physiology and Technique* (New York: Random House, 1926); and Jane Gerhard, *Desiring Revolution: Second-Wave Feminism and the Rewriting of American Sexual Thought* (New York: Columbia University Press, 2001).

23. Hollick, *Origin of Life*, xv.

24. "Cato" (pseud.), *Daily Chronicle* (March 5, 1846).

25. *North American* (March 3, 5, 10, and 11, 1846); and *Daily Chronicle* (March 6 and April 2, 1846).

26. William Darrah Kelley later became one of the architects of the Republican Party. The Progressive reformer Florence Kelley was his daughter. See "The Philadelphia Quarter

Sessions—April 20," *National Police Gazette* (April 25, 1846); and Hollick, *Origin of Life*, 75, 165, 235, 245.

27. Donna Dennis, *Licentious Gotham: Erotic Publishing and Its Prosecution in Nineteenth-Century New York* (Cambridge, MA: Harvard University Press, 2009); and Horowitz, *Rereading Sex*.

28. *United States Gazette* (March 16, 1846); *Daily Chronicle* (March 17, 1846); and *Philadelphia Public Ledger and Daily Transcript* (April 27, 1846).

29. *Philadelphia Public Ledger and Daily Transcript* (March 24, 1846); *United States Gazette* (March 24, 1846; and April 21, 1846); *Daily Chronicle* (April 21, 1846); and "Philadelphia Quarter Sessions," 283.

30. "Hollick's Lectures," *Daily Chronicle* (March 20, 1846); "Dr. Hollick's Statement," *Daily Chronicle* (April 2, 1846); *North American* (March 5, 1846); and "HOLLICK LECTURES," *North American* (March 11, 1846). In this lecture advertisement, Hollick promised to inform attendees of these "operations" in order to avoid them; such reversals were conventional in antebellum abortion advertising. He later named "the smallest amount of opium" and "ergot of rye" as powerful abortifacients that women could easily obtain. See Hollick, *Origin of Life*, 153; and Hollick, *Marriage Guide*, 220, 260, 297.

31. Hollick, *Origin of Life*, xviii–xix. Hollick's contemporary Paulina Wright Davis (discussed in chapter 5) told the same story as a way to underline the false delicacy of women who could not stand to look upon the female body. In both cases, the lecture made a case for her or his own importance—they were "acquainting" women with their own bodies. See Alice Felt Tyler, "Paulina Kellogg Wright Davis," *Notable American Women, 1607–1950*, ed. Edward T. James, Janet Wilson James, and Paul S. Boyer (Cambridge, MA: Belknap Press of Harvard University Press, 1971), 1:444–45; and Lynne Derbyshire, "Paulina Kellogg Wright Davis (1813–1876): Activist, Organizer, Publisher, Lecturer," in *Women Public Speakers in the United States, 1800–1925: A Bio-critical Sourcebook*, ed. Karlyn Kohrs Campbell (Westport, CT: Greenwood Press, 1993), 309.

32. Graham had illustrated his lectures to women with anatomical transparencies. See *Pittsburgh Manufacturer*, quoted in *Liberator* (April 21, 1837); manikins were recommended to moral reformers in *AMR* (December 1, 1843).

33. "Original resolutions adopted by the women of Philadelphia." For more on Mary Grew, see Ira V. Brown, *Mary Grew: Abolitionist and Feminist* (London: Associated University Press, 1992).

34. *AMR* (April 15, 1839; and June 1, 1839); Philadelphia Female Anti-slavery Society minutes, 1835–43, HSP; "Original resolutions adopted by the women of Philadelphia", Angelina Grimké Weld to Theodore Dwight Weld, May 20, 1846, WG MSS, CL; *Pennsylvania Freeman* (March 12, 1846; and August 20, 1846); Antiwar petition, *Philadelphia Public Ledger and Daily Transcript* (June 16, 1846); semiannual report of the managers of the Rosine Association (Philadelphia, October 7, 1848); and *Una* (July 1853 and November 1854).

35. Grew and Ellis signed all three petitions: women's petitions published in *Philadelphia Public Ledger and Daily Transcript* (April 4, 1846); *United States Gazette* (March 8, 1846; and April 17, 1846); Andrew J. King, "The Law of Slander in Early Antebellum America," *American Journal of Legal History* 35, no. 1 (January 1991): 1–43. On women's signatures as citizenship claims, see Lori D. Ginzberg, *Untidy Origins: A Story of Woman's Rights*

in *Antebellum New York* (Chapel Hill: University of North Carolina Press, 2005); Nancy Isenberg, *Sex and Citizenship in Antebellum America* (Chapel Hill: University of North Carolina Press, 1998); and Susan Zaeske, *Signatures of Citizenship: Petitioning, Antislavery, & Women's Political Identity* (Chapel Hill: University of North Carolina Press, 2003).

36. "To the Pure All Things Are Pure," *North American* (March 10, 1846). *Pennsylvania Freeman* (March 12, 1846); *Philadelphia Public Ledger and Daily Transcript* (April 4, 1846 and April 18, 1846); and *United States Gazette* (April 27, 1846).

37. Hollick, *Origin of Life*, x, 249.

38. Ibid., 248–49; *Daily Chronicle* (March 6, 1846); "To the Pure All Things Are Pure"; and *United States Gazette* (May 30, 1846).

39. *Philadelphia Public Ledger and Daily Transcript* (May 3, 1846); and Charles J. Hempel, *Homeopathic Guide in All Diseases of the Urinary & Sexual Organs* (New York: Radde, 1855), College of Physicians, Philadelphia. The successful English proprietor Samuel Solomon made a short-lived attempt to capture the American market with his "Balm of Gilead" in 1800, only to find a general lack of interest. Samuel Solomon, *A Guide to Health, or, Advice to both sexes; with an essay on a certain disease, seminal weakness and a destructive habit of a private nature: also an address to parents, tutors, and guardians of youth* (Stockport, UK: printed for the author, sold by Robert Bach of New York, 1800). On the English proprietary market, see Thomas Laqueur, *Solitary Sex: A Cultural History of Masturbation* (New York: Zone Books, 2003); *Onania; or, The Heinous Sin of Self Pollution and All Its Frightful Consequences in Both Sexes, Considered*, 8th ed. (London: printed by Eliz. Rumball, for Thomas Crouch, 1723); and *A Supplement to the Onania, or the Heinous Sin of SELF-POLLUTION, and All Its Frightful Consequences, in the Two Sexes, Considered, &c.* (London: T. Crouch, 1723).

40. "Let No False Delicacy Prevent You," *Philadelphia Public Ledger and Daily Transcript* (March 1852); Mme. Kinkelin "To Respectable Females," *Daily Chronicle* (February 13, 1841); "By Indulging in a Secret Habit," *Philadelphia Public Ledger and Daily Transcript* (May 3, 1846); Philadelphia tax lists, 1863–64, HSP; and US federal census, Philadelphia, 1850, 1880 (Ancestry.com).

41. *United States Gazette* (March 23, 1846); *Philadelphia Public Ledger and Daily Transcript* (June 9, 1846); and Hollick, *Marriage Guide*, 446.

42. Hollick, *Marriage Guide*, 141–42, 446; "A Parent," *North American* (March 11, 1846); "Hollick's Lectures"; "Dr. Hollick's Statement," *Daily Chronicle* (April 2, 1846); and Rachel Maines, *The Technology of Orgasm* (Baltimore: Johns Hopkins University Press, 1999).

43. "Original resolutions adopted by the women of Philadelphia"; Harriet Hyman Alonso, *Growing Up Abolitionist: The Story of the Garrison Children* (Amherst: University of Massachusetts Press, 2002), 61, 115, 129; Ira V. Brown, *Mary Grew*; and Julie Roy Jeffrey, *The Great Silent Army of Abolitionism: Ordinary Women in the Antislavery Movement* (Chapel Hill: University of North Carolina Press, 1998), 60, 69, 74, 89, 211.

44. The passionless reading relies on a particular emphasis: "*Love* is spiritual, only *passion* is sexual." I propose, as an alternative: "Love is spiritual, *only* passion is sexual." See Ira V. Brown, *Mary Grew*, 56; Carroll Smith Rosenberg, "The Female World of Love and Ritual: Relations between Women in Nineteenth-Century America," *Signs* 1, no. 1 (Autumn 1975): 1–29; and Nancy F. Cott, "Passionlessness: An Interpretation of Victo-

rian Sexual Ideology, 1790–1850," *Signs* 4, no. 2 (Winter 1978): 233–34. See also Marylynne Diggs, "Romantic Friends or a 'Different Race of Creatures'? The Representation of Lesbian Pathology in Nineteenth-Century America," *Feminist Studies* 21, no. 2 (Summer 1995): 317–40; Lillian Faderman, *Surpassing the Love of Men: Romantic Friendship and Love between Women from the Renaissance to the Present* (New York: William Morrow, 1981); and Martha Vicinus, *Intimate Friends: Women who Loved Women, 1778–1928* (Chicago: University of Chicago Press, 2004).

45. *Pennsylvania Freeman* (February 27, 1845; and March 12, 1846).

46. "Philadelphia Quarter Sessions," 283.

47. *Philadelphia Public Ledger and Daily Transcript* (April 23, 1846); "Doctor Hollick's Book—and Russell Jarvis' Recommendation of It," *Daily Chronicle* (April 27, 1846); and "Philadelphia Quarter Sessions," 283.

48. *United States Gazette* (April 21, 1846); and *Daily Chronicle* (April 21, 1846). "See it for himself": "Philadelphia Quarter Sessions," 283; and *United States Gazette* (April 27, 1846).

49. *Philadelphia Public Ledger and Daily Transcript* (April 2, 1846; and April 4, 1846); *United States Gazette* (March 31, 1846; and April 2–9, 1846); *Philadelphia Public Ledger and Daily Transcript* (April 17, 1846); Hollick, *Origin of Life*, xxxii; and *Pennsylvania Freeman* (March 12, 1846).

50. *United States Gazette* (May 14, 1846; March 16, 1846; and May 5, 1846).

51. US federal census, Philadelphia, New Market Ward, 1850, 1860 (Ancestry.com); "Fire Department," *Philadelphia Album and Ladies' Literary Portfolio* (March 22, 1834); state assembly: *Atkinson's Saturday Evening Post* (October 8, 1836); postmaster: *New York Evangelist* (November 21, 1844); Freemason: *American Masonic Register and Literary Companion* (March 1845); Mexican War: "Aid for the Volunteers," *Christian Observer* (December 18, 1846); 1850 election to House of Representatives: *National Era* (October 17, 1850); supported by workingmen, "popular education": "Political Portraits with Pen and Pencil: Thomas B. Florence," *United States Magazine, and Democratic Review* (February 1851); and "rubicund-faced": "Hollick's Lectures," *Daily Chronicle* (March 20, 1846).

In 1850, Florence went to Congress. One of the last proslavery northerners to hold office in the years immediately preceding the Civil War, Florence earned the ire of abolitionists through his involvement in the Christiana affair of 1851 and by helping to kill the Wilmot Proviso in 1854. He was joined in local Democratic politics by another "Friend of Dr. Hollick" named John Dolby Jr. "Treason in Pennsylvania, 1851," *Liberator* (December 5, 1851); end of congressional career: "Political News," *Saturday Evening Post* (September 8, 1860). For details on the Christiana riot, see Thomas P. Slaughter, *Bloody Dawn: The Christiana Riot and Racial Violence in the Antebellum North* (New York: Oxford University Press, 1991).

52. *United States Gazette* (May 5, 1846; and May 7, 1846); and "Hollick's Lectures," *Daily Chronicle* (March 20, 1846).

53. Leopold Deslandes, *De l'onanisme et des autres abus vénériens: Considérés dans leurs rapports avec la santé* (Paris: A. Lelange, 1835; 1st American ed., 1839); and Jerome V. C. Smith, "Extent and Evils of Masturbation Exposed," quoted in *Graham Journal of Health and Longevity* (February 2, 1839).

54. *Third Annual Report of the APS* (Boston: George W. Light, 1 Cornhill, 1839), 8; and Jean Dubois, *The Secret Habits of the Female Sex* (New York: sold by the booksellers generally, 1848).The original release date of this work is not known. On Dubois, see Brodie, *Contraception and Abortion*, 207, 320; and Dennis, *Licentious Gotham*.

55. *Awful Disclosures of Maria Monk, of the Hotel Dieu Nunnery of Montreal* (Philadelphia: T. B. Peterson, 1836). T. B. Peterson's 1846 book list was published in *Philadelphia Public Ledger and Daily Transcript* (May 1, 1846). *The Life of Helen Jewett, Illustrated*, by the editor of the *New York National Police Gazette*, Peterson's Popular Series of 50 Cent Novels (Philadelphia: T. B. Peterson and Brothers, 1878).

56. Frederick Hollick, *An Inquiry into the Rights, Duties, and Destinies, of the Different Varieties of the Human Race, with a View to a Proper Consideration of the Subjects of Slavery, Abolition, Amalgamation, and Aboriginal Rights* (New York: printed by W. B. and T. Smith, 1843), 3, 10, 27–29.

57. *New York Scorpion* (June 23, 1849), courtesy of Patricia Cline Cohen.

58. Here the *Scorpion* poked fun at Hollick's claims of working-class solidarity in order to expose him as a confidence man, but there is some evidence that he might have taken such a trip: Hollick reprinted undated lecture notices from southern cities in the preface to *Origin of Life* (1878 ed.). On northern circulation of *Rights, Duties, and Destinies*, see "The Magazines," *Pathfinder* (March 4, 1843).

59. Hollick, *Origin of Life*, 247, 265.

60. Hollick, *Marriage Guide*, 36, 42. On Baartman, see Clifton C. Crais and Pamela Scully, *Sara Baartman and the Hottentot Venus: A Ghost Story and a Biography* (Princeton, NJ: Princeton University Press, 2009); Anne Fausto-Sterling, "Gender, Race and Nation: The Comparative Anatomy of 'Hottentot' Women in Europe, 1815–17," in *Deviant Bodies: Critical Perspectives on Difference in Science and Popular Culture*, ed. Jennifer Terry and Jacqueline Urla (Bloomington: Indiana University Press, 1995); Sander Gilman, "Black Bodies, White Bodies: Toward an Iconography of Female Sexuality in Late Nineteenth-Century Art, Medicine, and Literature," in *"Race," Writing and Difference*, ed. Henry Louis Gates Jr., 223–61 (Chicago: University of Chicago Press, 1986); Rachel Holmes, *African Queen: The Real Life of the Hottentot Venus* (New York: Random House, 2007); and Londa Schiebinger, *Nature's Body: Gender in the Making of Modern Science* (Boston: Beacon Press, 1993). On embodied inscriptions of deviance, see Jennifer Morgan, *Laboring Women: Gender and New World Slavery* (Philadelphia: University of Pennsylvania Press, 2004); Siobhan Somerville, *Queering the Color Line: Race and the Invention of Homosexuality in American Culture* (Durham, NC: Duke University Press, 2000); and Jennifer Terry, *An American Obsession: Science, Medicine, and Homosexuality in Modern Society* (Chicago: University of Chicago Press, 1999).

61. Philadelphia Female Anti-slavery Society resolutions, 1838, quoted in Dorothy Sterling, ed., *We Are Your Sisters: Black Women in the Nineteenth Century* (New York: Norton, 1984), 115; *AMR* (June 1, 1839); Ronald Walters, "The Erotic South: Civilization and Sexuality in American Abolitionism," *American Quarterly* 25, no. 2 (May 1973): 177–201; and Carol Lasser, "Voyeuristic Abolitionism: Sex, Gender, and the Transformation of Antislavery Rhetoric," *Journal of the Early Republic* 28 (Spring 2008): 83.

62. *Philadelphia Public Ledger and Daily Transcript* (May 1, 1846; May 19, 1846; May 29, 1846; and July 1, 1846); *Philadelphia Galaxy*, quoted in *Boston Investigator* (March 10,

1847); *Boston Daily Atlas* (February 2, 1848; and February 28, 1848); and "Literary Notices," *Godey's Lady's Book & Magazine* (February 1861).

63. *BMSJ* (March 16, 1842; and December 10, 1845). On midcentury masturbation, see Estelle B. Freedman, "Sexuality in Nineteenth-Century America: Behavior, Ideology, and Politics," in "The Promise of American History: Progress and Prospects," *Reviews in American History* 10, no. 4 (December 1982): 196-215; R. P. Neuman, "Masturbation, Madness, and the Modern Concepts of Childhood and Adolescence," *Journal of Social History* 8, no. 3 (Spring 1975): 1-27; and Charles Rosenberg, "Sexuality, Class and Role in 19th-Century America," *American Quarterly* 25, no. 2 (May 1973): 131-53.

CHAPTER FIVE

1. Davison specifically mentioned watercolors, maps, a library, and an anatomy book. I have speculated that one of the paintings might have been a botanical alphabet, based on Douglass's didactic use of the language of flowers. It is also likely that Douglass foregrounded African geography and history in her curriculum since she taught Africa-bound missionaries, and, at the time of this visit, her brother Robert actively collaborated with the black abolitionist Martin Delany in formulating an emigration plan. Sarah Douglass had long insisted that African Americans should work for change in the United States and remained wary of emigration, but by the 1850s her brother's travels had awakened a transnational sense of social justice that made her "deeply interested in Africa." *African Repository* (January 1859); Amy Matilda Cassey album, 24, LCP; Mary Anne Dickerson album, 75-76, LCP; Anna Maria Davison diaries, 1847-60, vols. 2-7, BPL; letter fragment, Sarah M. Douglass to Rebecca White, n.d. [1857-58], Josiah White Papers, Haverford College; and *Weekly Anglo-African* (May 12, 1861). On the language of flowers, see also Erica R. Armstrong, "A Mental and Moral Feast: Reading, Writing, and Sentimentality in Black Philadelphia," *Journal of Women's History* 16, no. 1 (2004): 78-103; and Dorri Rabung Beam, "The Flower of Black Female Sexuality in Pauline Hopkins's *Winona*," in *Recovering the Black Female Body: Self-Representations by African American Women*, ed. Michael Bennett and Vanessa D. Dickerson (New Brunswick, NJ: Rutgers University Press, 2000), 71-72.

2. The daughter of Josiah White, a wealthy Quaker, and sister of Hannah White Richardson, Rebecca participated in Philadelphia Female Anti-slavery Society, Rosine Association, and Female Medical College of Pennsylvania events. Like Douglass, the White sisters also taught African American students in nearby schools; moreover, they possessed both capital and clout among white philanthropists. *Friends' Intelligencer* (June 4, 1853); *Friends' Review: A Religious, Literary and Miscellaneous Journal* (June 10, 1854); Anna Maria Davison diaries, 1847-60, vols. 2 (1847-50), 3 (1853-54), and 5 (1857-58); and *Constitution and Report of the Managers of the Rosine Association, with a List of the Annual Subscribers and Contributors* (Philadelphia: printed by Merrihew and Thompson, No. 7 Carter's Alley, 1848).

3. *Liberator* (July 7, 1832; and July 28, 1832); *Colored American* (December 2, 1837); *North Star* (February 24, 1849); *Friends' Intelligencer* (June 4, 1853); *Friends' Review* (June 10, 1854); and Jean Soderlund, "Priorities and Power: The Philadelphia Female Anti-Slavery Society," in *The Abolitionist Sisterhood: Women's Political Culture in Antebellum*

America, ed. Jean Fagan Yellin and John C. Van Horne, 67–87 (Ithaca, NY: Cornell University Press, 1994).

4. Martha S. Jones, *All Bound Up Together: The Woman Question in African American Public Culture* (Chapel Hill: University of North Carolina Press, 2007).

5. Mary Kelley, *Learning to Stand and Speak: Women, Education, and Public Life in America's Republic* (Chapel Hill: University of North Carolina Press, 2006).

6. "Mrs. Douglass' Lectures," *Weekly Anglo-African* (July 23, 1859).

7. *North Star* (February 24, 1849); *Friends' Intelligencer* (June 4, 1853); and *Friends' Review* (June 10, 1854).

8. *North Star* (July 6, 1849); Frederick Douglass (to whom Sarah Mapps Douglass was not related), "Address Delivered by Fred'Rick Douglass, before the Literary Societies of the Western Reserve College, at Commencement, July 12, 1854," *Frederick Douglass' Paper* (July 21, 1854); Anna Maria Davison diary, vol. 7 (1859–60), BPL; and Ryan P. Jordan, *Slavery and the Meetinghouse: The Quakers and the Abolitionist Dilemma, 1820–1864* (Bloomington: Indiana University Press, 2007), 79.

9. On the politics of the Female Literary Association, see Carla Peterson, *Theorizing African American Women Speakers and Writers in the Antebellum North* (New York: Oxford University Press, 1995); Emma Jones Lapsansky, "The World the Agitators Made: The Counterculture of Agitation in Urban Philadelphia," in *The Abolitionist Sisterhood: Women's Political Culture in Antebellum America*, ed. Jean Fagan Yellin and John C. Van Horne (Ithaca, NY: Cornell University Press, 1994), 91–100; Elizabeth McHenry, *Forgotten Readers: Recovering the Lost History of African American Literary Societies* (Durham, NC, and London: Duke University Press, 2002); and Julie Winch, "'You Have Talents—Only Cultivate Them,'" in *The Abolitionist Sisterhood: Women's Political Culture in Antebellum America*, ed. Jean Fagan Yellin and John C. Van Horne, 101–18 (Ithaca, NY: Cornell University Press, 1994).

10. "Ella" (pseud. [Sarah Mapps Douglass]), "Letter to a Brother," *Liberator* (March 24, 1832); "Zillah" (pseud. [Sarah Mapps Douglass]), "The Female Literary Association," in *Liberator* (June 30, 1832); "Sophanisba" (pseud.), "Extract from a Letter," *Liberator* (July 14, 1832); and "Zillah," *Liberator* (July 28, 1832).

11. Sarah Mapps Douglass was teaching in New York in 1833, but joined upon her return. Margaret Hope Bacon, *Sarah Mapps Douglass: Faithful Attender of Quaker Meeting: View from the Back Bench* (Philadelphia: Quaker Press of Friends General Conference, 2003), 9; and Dorothy Sterling, ed., *We Are Your Sisters: Black Women in the Nineteenth Century* (New York: Norton, 1984), 131.

12. "Constitution of the Afric-American Female Intelligence Society of Boston," *Liberator* (January 7, 1832). For more on the Afric-American Female Intelligence Society, see Anne M. Boylan, *The Origins of Women's Activism: New York and Boston, 1797–1840* (Chapel Hill: University of North Carolina Press, 2000), 225; McHenry, *Forgotten Readers*, 69–76; and C. Peter Ripley, ed., *Black Abolitionist Papers* (Chapel Hill: University of North Carolina Press, 1991), 225.

13. Lavinia Hilton, *Liberator* (May 5, 1832), and "Address and Constitution of the Phoenix Society of New York, and of the Auxiliary Ward Associations," quoted in *Early Negro Writing, 1760–1837*, ed. Dorothy Porter (Boston: Beacon Press, 1971), 123–26, 141–45.

14. *Emancipator* (December 21, 1833); *Colored American* (March 4, 1837); and Amina Gautier, "African American Women's Writings in the Woman's Building Library," *Libraries and the Cultural Record* 41, no. 1 (Winter 2006): 55–81.

15. *Colored American* (December 2, 1837).

16. Sarah Moore Grimké to Jane Smith, April 11, 1837, box 3, WG MSS, CL; Sarah Moore Grimké to Sarah Mapps Douglass, July 16 and October 25, 1848, and Sarah Moore Grimké to Sarah Mapps Douglass, September 25, 1850, box 9, WG MSS, CL; Sarah Moore Grimké to Sarah Mapps Douglass, December 22, [1857], box 23, WG MSS, CL; and Sarah Moore Grimké to Anne Smith, April 11, 1842, quoted in *Letters of Theodore D. Weld and Angelina Grimké Weld and Sarah Grimké*, ed. Gilbert H. Barnes and Dwight L. Dumond (New York: Appleton-Century, 1934), 939.

17. The PAS Board of Education specifically employed Charlotte Van Dine, Elizabeth Appo, and Emeline Curtis; May 11 and July 6, 1848, April 12 and June 14, 1849, *Annual Report for 1849*, PAS Board of Education minutes (229), PAS records, HSP. For the names of other African American teachers in Philadelphia during this period, see the PAS's "Statistical Inquiry into the Status of the People of Color in Philadelphia," PAS records, HSP. The Lombard Street Infant School is the main example of the emphasis on very young children who learned the alphabet, sewing, and embroidery. See, for example, November 27, 1843, minutes, Committee for the Improvement of Colored People (41), PAS records, HSP. Tensions between white abolitionists and black teachers persisted there, particularly over disciplinary matters. See February 14, 1840, June 13, 1850, September 26, 1850, and November 5, 1850, minutes, PAS Board of Education (245, 252, 255), PAS records, HSP.

18. *Liberator* (June 9, 1832), quoted in *Early Negro Writing, 1760–1837*, ed. Dorothy Porter (Boston: Beacon Press, 1971), 127–28; and *National Anti-slavery Standard* (March–November 1842). For two different interpretations of the conflict, see Soderlund, "Priorities and Power"; and Carol Faulkner, *Lucretia Mott's Heresy: Abolition and Women's Rights in Nineteenth-Century America* (Philadelphia: University of Pennsylvania Press, 2011), 113.

19. Sarah Moore Grimké to Sarah Mapps Douglass, September 25, 1849, box 9, WG MSS, CL; Angelina Grimké Weld to Harriot K. Hunt, n.d. [1853], box 10, WG MSS, CL; and April 10, 1851, minutes, PAS Board of Education, HSP.

20. Miriam R. Levin, *Defining Women's Scientific Enterprise: Mount Holyoke Faculty and the Rise of American Science* (Lebanon, NH: University Press of New England, 2005); and Fanny Jackson Coppin, *Reminiscences on School Life and Hints on Teaching* (Philadelphia: A. M. E. Book Concern, 1913).

21. *Una* (February 1, 1853, and January 1855). Although Sarah Grimké sent "love to dear sister Wright" in a letter to Douglass, few of Douglass's own letters mention Wright as an individual. Douglass did refer the White sisters to Wright's ideas in the *Una*. Sarah Mapps Douglass to Rebecca White, May 28, 1855, Josiah White Papers, Haverford College.

22. Henrietta Sargent to Angelina Grimké Weld, February 8, 1839, box 6, WG MSS, CL; and William Bassett to Abby Kelley, November 6, 1839, Abby Kelley Foster Papers, AAS.

23. Sarah M. Grimké to Sarah Mapps Douglass, February 15, 1839, box 6, WG MSS CL; Sarah M. Grimké to Jane Smith, December 24, 1843, box 8, WG MSS, CL; Sarah M. Grimké to Sarah Mapps Douglass, February 19, 1845, WG MSS, CL; Sarah Grimké to Sarah Mapps Douglass, September 25, 1849, WG MSS, CL; and Sarah Mapps Douglass to Sarah Grimké,

August 1, 1853, quoted in Marie Lindhorst, "Sarah Mapps Douglass: The Emergence of an African American Educator/Activist in Nineteenth Century Philadelphia" (PhD diss., Pennsylvania State University, Education Policy Studies, 1995), 173.

24. Sarah M. Grimké to Sarah Mapps Douglass, June 19, 1855, box 23, WG MSS, CL; Sarah M. Grimké to Sarah Mapps Douglass, n.d. [1855], box 23, WG MSS, CL; and Sterling, *We Are Your Sisters*, 129–32.

25. Early in their friendship, Douglass wrote to Grimké that she was attending lectures by J. Simmons, a teacher who lectured before the Philadelphia Lyceum—comprised mainly of scholars and teachers, "especially females." The lyceum met every Saturday and included lectures on anatomy and physiology. Sarah M. Grimké to Sarah Mapps Douglass, February 22, 1837, in *Letters of Theodore D. Weld and Angelina Grimké Weld and Sarah Grimké*, ed. Gilbert H. Barnes and Dwight L. Dumond (New York: Appleton-Century, 1934), 1:363; and "Report of the Philadelphia Lyceum, May 5, 1837," in *American Monthly Magazine* (August 1837).

26. At less than ten cents per attendee, Douglass must have admitted listeners who could not afford tickets. Letter fragment, Sarah M. Douglass to Rebecca White, n.d. [1855], 5 Mo.28.55, Josiah White Papers, Haverford College; and "Mrs. Douglass' Lectures," *Weekly Anglo-African* (July 23, 1859), quoted in Dorothy Sterling, ed., *We Are Your Sisters: Black Women in the Nineteenth Century* (New York: Norton, 1984), 129.

27. Julie Winch, review of *Black Women Abolitionists*, by Shirley Yee, in *Journal of American History* 80, no. 2 (September 1993): 667–68; December 25, 1843, Committee for the Improvement of the Colored People minutes (47), PAS, HSP; and letter fragment, Sarah M. Douglass to Rebecca White, n.d. [1855], Josiah White Papers, Haverford College.

28. Bacon, *Sarah Mapps Douglass*, 24; and Lindhorst, "Sarah Mapps Douglass," 174.

29. *Proceedings of the Worcester Woman's Rights Convention, 1850* (Boston: Prentiss and Sawyer, 1851).

30. Bruce Fye, *The Development of American Physiology: Scientific Medicine in the 19th Century* (Baltimore: Johns Hopkins University Press, 1987). On the New England Female Medical College, see *The Male Midwife and the Female Doctor: The Gynecology Controversy in Nineteenth-Century America*, ed. Charles Rosenberg and Carroll Smith-Rosenberg (repr., North Stratford, NH: Ayer, 1999); Arleen Tuchman, *Science Has No Sex: The Life of Marie Zakrzewska, M.D.* (Chapel Hill: University of North Carolina Press, 2006); and Frederick C. Waite, *History of the New England Female Medical College* (Boston: Boston University School of Medicine, 1950). For more on the Female Medical College of Pennsylvania, see Steven Peitzmann, *A New and Untried Course: Woman's Medical College and Medical College of Pennsylvania, 1850–1998* (New Brunswick, NJ: Rutgers University Press, 2000); Regina Markell Morantz-Sanchez, *Sympathy and Science: Women Physicians in American Medicine* (New York: Oxford University Press, 1985); and Susan Wells, *Out of the Dead House: Nineteenth-Century Women Physicians and the Writing of Medicine* (Madison: University of Wisconsin Press, 2001).

31. Elizabeth Blackwell, *The Laws of Life, with Special Reference to the Physical Education of Girls* (New York: George P. Putnam, 1852); and Harriot K. Hunt, *Glances and Glimpses; or, Fifty Years Social, Including Twenty Years Professional Life* (Boston: John P. Jewett, 1856).

32. Ann Preston to Lavinia Passmore, October 8, 1843, Ann Preston, Deceased Alumnae Files, folder 1; "Correspondence to and from Ann Preston," Medical College of Pennsylvania / Hahnemann Archives; Mary Gove, "Lectures to Ladies on Anatomy and Physiology," *Daily Chronicle* (February 18, 1841); Ann Preston to Hannah Darlington, Baltimore, April 2, 1852, Deceased Alumnae Files, Medical College of Pennsylvania / Hahnemann Archives; and *To Ladies* (Philadelphia: n.p., 1860), broadside, Deceased Alumnae Files, folders 1-2, Medical College of Pennsylvania / Hahnemann Archives.

33. Sarah M. Grimké to Sarah Mapps Douglass, August 1, 1853, and Joseph S. Longshore to Sarah M. Grimké, January 31, 1854, box 10, WG MSS, CL.

34. Letter fragment, Sarah M. Douglass to Rebecca White, n.d. [1857-58], Josiah White Papers, Haverford College.

35. The white Hollick defenders and Philadelphia Female Anti-slavery Society members who attended the Female Medical College of Pennsylvania alongside Douglass included Olive Bacon, Margaret Jones Burleigh, Amy Cassey, Hannah Ellis, Susanna Ellis, Mary Grew, Rebecca Hallowell, Susanna Sartain, Susan Stackhouse, Harriet P. Webb, and Sarah J. Webb. Medical College of Pennsylvania / Hahnemann student catalog, 1851-52, 1857-58; Deceased Alumnae Files and Hollick defenders' signatures in "Original Resolutions," Charles Arthur Hollick Papers; *Philadelphia Public Ledger and Daily Transcript* (April 4, 1846); *United States Gazette* (March 8, 1846; and April 17, 1846); and *Constitution and Report*. See also Ira V. Brown, *Mary Grew: Abolitionist and Feminist* (London: Associated University Press, 1992), 100, 116.

36. Letter fragment, Sarah M. Douglass to Rebecca White, n.d. [1857-58], Josiah White Papers, Haverford College.

37. *Una* (February 1, 1853; October 1853; and August 1855).

38. Linda Gordon, "Voluntary Motherhood: The Beginnings of Feminist Birth Control Ideology in the U.S.," in *Clio's Consciousness Raised*, ed. Mary Hartmann and Lois Banner (New York: Harper Torchbook, 1974); and Thomas Low Nichols, *Esoteric Anthropology* (Cincinnati: Valentine Nicholson, 1853), 151-53.

39. Sarah M. Grimké to Harriot Hunt, n.d. (1850?), box 9, and June 28, 1857, box 11, WG MSS, CL. Harriot Hunt had learned homeopathy from a British woman named Mott during the early 1830s; in 1838, she stayed with May Gove at her boardinghouse in Lynn and afterward incorporated reform physiology into her own lectures. See Harriot K. Hunt, *Glances and Glimpses*, 139-40; and *Daily Chronicle* (February 18, 1841).

40. Mary Gove Nichols and Thomas Low Nichols, *Marriage: Its History, Character, and Results* (New York: T. L. Nichols, 1854), 202-3, 207; Angelina Grimké Weld to Harriot K. Hunt, n.d. [1853], box 10, WG MSS, CL; and Harriot K. Hunt, *Glances and Glimpses*, 384.

41. Nichols and Nichols, *Marriage*, 202; and Nichols, *Esoteric Anthropology*, 200.

42. Elizabeth Blackwell, *Essays in Medical Sociology*, vol. 2 (London: Ernest Bell, 1902), 16, 22, 28, 34-35, 38-39, 42; and Nichols, *Esoteric Anthropology*, 202, 397.

43. Nichols was extremely unusual in this regard: most antebellum writers promoted heterosexual intercourse by contrasting it with masturbation, but explicit references to sodomy were rare and overwhelmingly negative. See Nichols, *Esoteric Anthropology*, 399.

44. Ibid., 151, 200-201, 398-402; and Blackwell, *Essays*, 23, 56.

45. Anna Longshore Potts documented the content of her lectures to ladies later in the century. See Anna Longshore Potts, "Correspondence," *Medical Press* (March 11, 1885); and Anna Longshore Potts, *Discourses to Women on Medical Subjects* (London and San Diego: published by the author, 1896).

46. Beecher explained that "Miss Blackwell" had converted her to physiology reform when they met at an exercise cure. See Catherine Beecher, *Letters to the People on Health and Happiness* (New York: Harper and Brothers, 1855), 91, 124–25, 163, 211–12.

47. Phrenology was the study of the personality by study of the skull; phrenologists attributed human behavior to several "faculties" of the brain that they claimed to measure by the shape of the skull. Fowler located the faculty of amativeness in the cerebellum. The quote is from Orson Squire Fowler, *Fowler's Practical Phrenology* (New York: Fowler and Fowler, 1840); he made the connection to a spiritual "love principle" in *Love and Parentage* (New York: Fowler and Wells, 1844). The phrase *love principle* was originally used by the Swedish mystic Emanuel Swedenborg (not necessarily in a sexual sense), to whom utopians and spiritualists of the mid-nineteenth century increasingly looked for inspiration. For more on phrenology, see Roger Cooter, *The Cultural Meaning of Popular Science: Phrenology and the Organization of Consent in Nineteenth Century Britain* (New York: Cambridge University Press, 1984); Daniel Patrick Thurs, *Science Talk: Changing Notions of Science in American Popular Culture* (New Brunswick, NJ: Rutgers University Press, 2007); and Stephen Tomlinson, *Head Masters: Phrenology, Secular Education, and Nineteenth-Century Social Thought* (Tuscaloosa: University of Alabama Press, 2005).

48. Fowler, *Love and Parentage*, 76; and Orson Squire Fowler, *Amativeness; or, Evils and Remedies of Excessive and Perverted Sexuality* (New York: Fowler & Wells, 1844), 20, 48, 73.

49. Jonathan Ned Katz, *Invention of Heterosexuality* (Chicago: University of Chicago Press, 1995).

50. Fowler, *Love and Parentage*, 68, 122; and Fowler, *Amativeness*, 27.

51. Fowler, *Love and Parentage*, 59.

52. Harriot K. Hunt, *Glances and Glimpses*, 73, 324–25; and *FOV* (April 1, 1858).

53. While Social Purity advocates did not all support women's political rights, the late nineteenth-century movement for woman suffrage—despite significant divisions over race, class, and strategy—generally supported stricter laws against prostitution and "white slavery." John D'Emilio and Estelle B. Freedman, *Intimate Matters: A History of Sexuality in America* (Chicago: University of Chicago Press, 1997).

54. *Pennsylvania Freeman* (March 11, 1847); Paulina Wright Davis, "Lecture to Providence Physiological Society, January 20, 1853," Providence Physiological Society Records, folder 1 (Mss 649); and *Una* (September 1854).

55. June 10, 1850, June 12, 1850, and September 30, 1853, secretary's reports and board meetings, retrospective in (box 2), p. 29, "Printed Material by and about LPI," Ladies Physiological Institute of Boston and Vicinity, 1848–1966, SL, Radcliffe Institute for Advanced Study, 1922–23; and Harriot K. Hunt, *Glances and Glimpses*, 168. For a more thorough examination of the LPI, see Martha H. Verbrugge, *Able-Bodied Womanhood: Personal Health and Social Change in Nineteenth-Century Boston* (New York: Oxford University Press, 1988).

56. Secretary's reports, February 11, 1852, LPI, 1848-1966, SL; and December 2, 1852, and February 10, 1853, minutes, PPS, RIHS.

57. *Second Annual Report*, LPI minutes, 1850, and secretary's reports and board meetings, 1850-51, LPI, SL; Frederick Hollick, *The Marriage Guide* (New York: T. W. Strong, 1851), 443; and May 22, 1851, minutes, PPS, RIHS.

58. April 11, 1851, minutes of the PPS, folder 1 (Minutes 1850.1-1853.2), PPS records, RIHS; and *Second Annual Report*, LPI minutes, 1850.

59. Sarah M. Grimké to Sarah Mapps Douglass, June 19, 1855, quoted in Sterling, *We Are Your Sisters*, 132.

60. Sarah M. Grimké to Harriot K. Hunt, March 8, 1855, box 18, WG MSS, CL; and Angelina Grimké Weld and Sarah M. Grimké to Harriot K. Hunt, n.d., box 18, WG MSS, CL.

61. Sarah M. Grimké introduced Harriot K. Hunt to Sarah M. Douglass in a letter of September 25, 1849, box 9, WG MSS, CL; Angelina and Sarah asked Harriot K. Hunt to forward her book to Sarah M. Douglass, n.d. [1855], box 18, WG MSS, CL; Sarah M. Douglass forwarded it to Rebecca White (May 30, 1855), Josiah White Papers, Haverford College.

62. Letter fragment, Sarah M. Douglass to Rebecca White, n.d. [1857-58], Josiah White Papers, Haverford College.

63. *Weekly Anglo-African* (November 1860), quoted in Sterling, *We Are Your Sisters*, 129.

64. Blackwell, *Essays*, 34.

65. Although antimasturbation writers had long included mental disorders as one of the outcomes of masturbation, the term *masturbatory insanity* was not coined until 1868 (by the British alienist Henry Maudsley). Henry Maudsley, "Illustrations of a Variety of Insanity," *Journal of Mental Science* (1868), cited in *The Anatomy of Madness: Essays in the History of Psychiatry*, ed. W. F. Bynum, Roy Porter, and Michael Shepherd, vol. 3 (London: Taylor and Francis, 2005). See also E. H. Hare, "Masturbatory Insanity: The History of an Idea," *Journal of Mental Science* 108 (January 1962); and Patrick Singy, "Friction of the Genitals and Secularization of Morality," *Journal of the History of Sexuality* 12, no. 3 (July 2003): 345-64.

66. *BMSJ* (March 11, 1835); Samuel B. Woodward, *Hints for the Young, on a Subject Relating to the Health of Body and Mind, from the "Boston Medical and Surgical Journal," with Additions by the Author* (Boston: Weeks, Jordan, 1838), 23, 42-43; Mary S. Gove, "To Parents, Guardians, and Those Who Have the Care of Children," *FOV* (July 1838); *FOV* (December 1838; and December 16, 1839); *Health Journal and Advocate of Physiological Reform* (April 6, 1840); "Human Physiology," *AMR* (December 1, 1838); Philadelphia Female Moral Reform Society, *AMR* (January 15, 1839); "Impurity in Schools," *FOV* (February 1839); and "Resolutions," *FOV* (January 15, 1840). On moral treatment, see Gerald N. Grob, *Mental Institutions in America* (New York: Free Press, 1973); and Benjamin Reiss, *Theaters of Madness: Nineteenth-Century Insane Asylums and American Culture* (Chicago: University of Chicago Press, 2008).

67. Mary Ann Johnson, "Organs of Generation," lecture to the Providence Physiological Society, April 11, 1851, minutes of the PPS, folder 1 (Minutes 1850.1-1853.2), PPS records, RIHS.

68. Horace Mann, *Report of the Secretary of the Board of Education on the Subject of School Houses* (March 29, 1838), MHS; Mary S. Gove, "To Parents, Guardians, and Those

Who Have Care of Children," *FOV* (July 1838); "Human Physiology," *AMR* (December 1, 1838); Philadelphia Female Moral Reform Society, *AMR* (January 15, 1839); "Impurity in Schools," *FOV* (February 1839); "Resolutions at the Fourth Quarterly Meeting of the New England Female Moral Reform Society," *FOV* (January 15, 1840); "Boston Female Medical School," *FOV* (May 15, 1851); Horace Mann, *Mass. School Board 11th Annual Report* (Boston: s.n., 1848), 112–13; and Massachusetts Board of Education, *Twelfth Annual School Report* (Boston: s.n., 1849), 47–49.

69. Samuel Gregory, *Eighth Annual Report of the NEFMC* (Boston: published by the trustees of the New England Female Medical College, 1857), 15, MHS.

70. *AMR* (July 1, 1846).

71. Deceased Alumnae Filebox, 1850–55, folder 1, "Class Lists," Medical College of Pennsylvania / Hahnemann Archives; *Twenty-Second Annual Catalogue and Report of the NEFMC* (Boston: published by the trustees of the New England Female Medical College, 1870), 14, MHS; and Mary H. Stinson, "Work of Women Physicians in Asia," *Medical and Surgical Reporter* (May 17, 1884).

72. Massachusetts Board of Education, *Ninth Annual Report* (Boston: s.n., 1846), 33–34; Massachusetts Board of Education, *Twelfth Annual School Report*, 21; and *Eighth Annual Report of the NEFMC* (Boston: published by the trustees of the New England Female Medical College, 1857), 8, 15.

73. William C. Woodbridge, *Annals of Education*, quoted in *Health Journal and Advocate of Physiological Reform* (April 1, 1840); *Report of the Female Medical Education Society, for Its Third Year* (Boston: published by the Female Medical Education Society, 1852), 14; and *Sixth Annual Report of the Female Medical Education Society and the NEFMC* (Boston: s.n., 1855), 16.

74. *Seventh Annual Report of the New England Female Medical College* (Boston: Female Education Society, 1856), 13–15; and April 29, 1854, minutes, LPI, SL.

75. School returns—Sturbridge, *Massachusetts Board of Education Annual Report* (Boston: s.n., 1852), 85; Plymouth—*19th Massachusetts Board of Education Annual Report* (Boston: s.n., 1856); and Boston and Boxford—*Committee Reports on Physical and Moral Education*, in *21st Massachusetts Board of Education Annual Report* (Boston: s.n., 1858), 6, 126–27.

76. Jeffrey P. Moran, *Teaching Sex: The Shaping of Adolescence in the 20th Century* (Cambridge, MA; Harvard University Press, 2000); and Christina Simmons, *Making Marriage Modern: Women's Sexuality from the Progressive Era to World War II* (New York: Oxford University Press, 2009).

77. *Report of the Annual Examination of the Public Schools, of the City of Boston, 1853*, quoted in Frederick Hollick, *People's Medical Journal and Home Doctor* (February 1854). The maternal argument for girls' physiological education was still being made in 1867. See, for example, *The Massachusetts Teacher*, vol. 20 (Boston: published by the Massachusetts Teachers' Association, 1867), 41–42. On gendered Institute for Colored Youth curriculum, see *Friends' Review: A Religious, Literary and Miscellaneous Journal* (May 21, 1859).

78. Letter fragment, Sarah M. Douglass to Rebecca White, n.d. [1857–58], Josiah White Papers, Haverford College.

79. *Resolutions*, 1879, quoted in Bacon, *Sarah Mapps Douglass*, 176, emphasis added.

80. William Lloyd Garrison called Cutter "a public benefactor" and brought his *Anatomy and Physiology* to the particular attention of abolitionist "parents and teachers." He would later fight with free soil migrants to Kansas and join the Union army as a surgeon at the age of fifty-three. Cutter graduated Dartmouth in 1832, after which he lectured to the public on anatomy and physiology. He also supported the asylum reform movement. See *New Hampshire Statesman and State Journal* (August 25, 1832; and September 17, 1836); *Anatomy & Physiology! The Lecture of Drs. Cutter at the Hall, This Evening . . .*, broadside (n.p., 1839); *Dover Gazette and Strafford Advertiser* (January 22, 1842); William C. Woodbridge, quoted in Calvin Cutter, *The Female Guide* (West Brookfield, MA: Charles Mirick, 1844), 31; Calvin Cutter, *Anatomy and Physiology* (Boston: Benjamin Mussey, 1846, 1848); *Ohio Medical and Surgical Journal* (September 1, 1851); *Catalogue of the Library in the Reading Room of the Institute for Colored Youth* (Philadelphia: printed by Joseph Rakeshaw, 1853), HSP; Eunice Powers Cutter, *Human and Comparative Anatomy, Physiology, and Hygiene* (New York: Clark, Austin and Powers, 1854); and *Daily Inter Ocean* (May 12, 1893).

81. William Alcott, *The House I Live In* (Boston: Light and Stearns, 1837); Edward Carpenter, *Elements of Physiology* (Philadelphia: Lea and Blanchard, 1846); *Old Textbooks* (Pittsburgh: University of Pittsburgh Press, 1961), 306–7; and Christopher Hoolihan, *An Annotated Catalogue of the Edward C. Atwater Collection of American Popular Medicine and Health Reform*, 3 vols. (Rochester, NY: University of Rochester Press, 2008), 3:180–81.

82. Sarah Douglass to Charles K. Whipple, April 26, 1841, BPL; Sarah M. Douglass to Rebecca White, February 9, 1862, and Sarah M. Douglass to Rebecca White, October 29, 1860, Josiah White Papers, Haverford College; Bacon, *Sarah Mapps Douglass*, 24; and Gayle T. Tate, *Unknown Tongues: Black Women's Political Activism in the Antebellum Era* (East Lansing: Michigan State University Press, 2003), 192–93.

83. Davison diary, vol. 7 (1859–60).

84. Beam, "Flower of Black Female Sexuality," 71–72.

85. Charles P. Bronson, *Abstract of Elocution & Music* (New York: Henry Oliphant, 1842).

86. Erica Armstrong Dunbar, *A Fragile Freedom: African American Women and Emancipation in the Antebellum City* (New Haven, CT: Yale University Press, 2008); and Erica Ball, *To Live an Antislavery Life: Personal Politics and the Antebellum Black Middle Class* (Athens: University of Georgia Press, 2012).

87. Refined nineteenth-century women communicated emotions that were difficult to discuss openly by depicting flowers that represented specific messages. Mrs. L. Burke, *The Illustrated Language of Flowers* (London: Routledge and Farrington; New York: s.n., 18 Beekman Street, 1856), 17; and Davison diary, vol. 7 (1859–60).

88. Letter fragment, Sarah M. Douglass to Rebecca White, n.d. [1857–58], Josiah White Papers, Haverford College; and Amy Matilda Cassey album, 24, LCP.

89. J.J., "Worthy of Encouragement," *Liberator* (December 2, 1859); and Bacon, *Sarah Mapps Douglass*, 32.

90. Dana Nelson, *National Manhood: Capitalist Citizenship and the Imagined Fraternity of White Men* (Durham, NC: Duke University Press, 1998).

91. Michael Sappol, *A Traffic of Dead Bodies: Anatomy and Embodied Social Identity in Nineteenth-Century America* (Princeton, NJ: Princeton University Press, 2002).

92. *American Phrenological Journal* (January 1, 1841); *North American Medical and Surgical Journal* (July 1830); "Illustrated System of Human Anatomy, Special, General, and Microscopic," *BMSJ* (January 17, 1849); "Sketches of Eminent Living Physicians, No. X: Samuel George Morton," *BMSJ* (August 22, 1849); Dana Nelson, "No Cold or Empty Heart: Polygenesis, Scientific Professionalism, and the Unfinished Business of Male Sentimentalism," *Differences: A Journal of Feminist Cultural Studies* 11, no. 3 (1999): 29–56; and Ann Fabian, *The Skull Collectors: Race, Science, and America's Unburied Dead* (Chicago: University of Chicago Press, 2010).

93. On craniology before Morton, see Bruce Dain, *A Hideous Monster of the Mind: American Race Theory in the Early Republic* (Cambridge, MA: Harvard University Press, 2002); Winthrop Jordan, *White over Black: American Attitudes toward the Negro, 1550–1812* (Chapel Hill: University of North Carolina Press, 1968); Nell Irvin Painter, *The History of White People* (New York: Norton, 2010); Londa Schiebinger, *Nature's Body: Gender in the Making of Modern Science* (Boston: Beacon Press, 1993); "Miscellany," *American Phrenological Journal* (July 1, 1839); and Alexander Saxton, *The Rise and Fall of the White Republic: Class Politics and Mass Culture in Nineteenth-Century America* (New York: Verso, 1990). On black responses to environmentalism, see Patrick Rael, "A Common Nature, A United Destiny: African American Responses to Racial Science from the Revolution to the Civil War," in *Prophets of Protest: Reconsidering the History of American Abolitionism*, ed. Timothy Patrick McCarthy and John Stauffer, 183–99 (New York: New Press, 2006); and Dain, *Hideous Monster of the Mind*.

94. Frederick Hollick, *An Inquiry into the Rights, Duties, and Destinies, of the Different Varieties of the Human Race, with a View to a Proper Consideration of the Subjects of Slavery, Abolition, Amalgamation, and Aboriginal Rights* (New York: printed by W. B. and T. Smith, 1843); Josiah Nott, "The Mulatto, a Hybrid—Probable Extermination of the Two Races If the Whites and Blacks Are Allowed to Intermarry," *American Journal of the Medical Sciences* (1843); "Mr. Combe's Second Course of Lectures," *American Phrenological Journal* (May 1, 1839); "Mr. Morton makes his acknowledgements to Dr. McDowell, a gentleman whom our readers may remember as formerly attached to the colony of Liberia," *Christian Examiner* (May 1840). Aegyptica used cranial evidence to argue that Egypt had been a slaveholding society governed by whites; Samuel George Morton, *Crania Aegyptica* (Philadelphia: American Philosophical Society, 1844). See also Reginald Horsman, *Josiah Nott of Mobile: Southerner, Physician, Racial Theorist* (Baton Rouge: Louisiana State University Press, 1987).

95. On decorporealization, see Carla L. Peterson, "Foreword: Eccentric Bodies," in *Recovering the Black Female Body: Self-Representations by African American Women*, ed. Michael Bennett and Vanessa D. Dickerson (New Brunswick, NJ: Rutgers University Press, 2001). On James McCune Smith, see John Stauffer, *The Works of James McCune Smith: Black Intellectual and Abolitionist* (New York: Oxford University Press, 2006); and John Stauffer, *The Black Hearts of Men: Radical Abolitionists and the Transformation of Race* (Cambridge, MA: Harvard University Press, 2004).

96. "Phrenology," *Colored American* (September 23, 1837); *National Reformer* (March 5, 1839); and Frederick Douglass, "Address Delivered by Fred'Rick Douglass." For more on

black responses to Morton, see Dain, *Hideous Monster of the Mind*; and Nancy Leys Stepan and Sander Gilman, "Appropriating the Idioms of Science: The Rejection of Scientific Racism," in *The Bounds of Race: Perspectives on Hegemony and Resistance*, ed. Dominick LaCapra (Ithaca, NY: Cornell University Press, 1991).

97. W.J.B., "To Correspondents," *American Phrenological Journal* (June 1858).

98. Sarah M. Douglass to Rebecca White, February 9, 1862, Josiah White Papers, Haverford College.

EPILOGUE

1. Sarah M. Grimké to Sarah Mapps Douglass, January 27, 1859, box 11, WG MSS, CL.

2. Angelina Grimké Weld to Theodore Grimké Weld, n.d., Sarah Grimké to Theodore Grimké Weld, n.d. [ca. March 1860], and May 21, 1860; Elbridge Jefferson Cutler to Theodore Dwight Weld, n.d. [1860]; Sarah M. Grimké to Gerrit Smith, January 3, 1862; C. H. Farnham to Charles Stuart Weld, n.d. [1892]; Anna Weld to Sarah Hamilton, January 7, 1895, WG MSS, CL; and C. H. Bolles, Electrical Institute, *McElroy's Directory* (Philadelphia: Biddle, 1863).

3. Angelina Grimké Weld to Theodore Dwight Weld, n.d. [1843], WG MSS, box 7, CL; C. A. Coleman to Angelina Grimké Weld, July 4, 1860; Sarah M. Grimké to Theodore Grimké Weld, July 7, 1860; C. A. Coleman to Sarah M. Grimké, July 17, 1860; and Theodore Dwight Weld to Theodore Grimké Weld, July 26, 1860, WG MSS, box 12, CL.

4. Claude-François Lallemand, *A Practical Treatise on the Causes, Symptoms, and, Treatment of Spermatorrhea*, trans. Henry J. McDougall (Philadelphia: Blanchard and Lea, 1853). See also Robert Darby, *A Surgical Temptation: The Demonization of the Foreskin and the Rise of Circumcision in Britain* (Chicago: University of Chicago Press, 2013), 174–75.

5. Sarah Moore Grimké to Sarah Wattles, December 27, 1858, WG MSS, box 11, CL; Sarah Moore Grimké to Sarah Wattles, August 12, 1855, WG MSS, box 10, CL; and Sarah Grimké to Lizzie Smith Miller, June 1, 1873, WG MSS, box 14, CL.

6. Letter fragment, Sarah M. Grimké to Sarah Mapps Douglass, n.d. [ca. 1864], uncatalogued addition, WG MSS, CL.

7. Sarah M. Grimké to Sarah Mapps Douglass, undated fragment [ca. 1864–66], WG MSS, box 23, CL; and Eliza Farnham, *Woman and Her Era* (New York: Andrew Jackson Davis, 1864), 72, 95.

8. Sarah Moore Grimké to Sarah Mapps Douglass, May 26, 1868, WG MSS, box 14, CL.

9. Sarah Grimké to Sarah Mapps Douglass, December 1, 1869, and Sarah Mapps Douglass to Angelina Grimké Weld, December 26, 1873, WG MSS, box 15, CL. The postbellum dispute over the Fifteenth Amendment is well known. See Eleanor Flexner, *Century of Struggle: The Woman's Rights Movement in the United States* (Boston: Belknap Press, 1996); Louis Newman, *White Women's Rights: The Racial Origins of Feminism in the United States* (New York: Oxford University Press, 1999); and Lori Ginzberg, *Elizabeth Cady Stanton: An American Life* (New York: Hill and Wang, 2010). For more on Social Purity, as distinct from the female moral reform movement of the 1830s–1840s, see David J. Pivar, *Purity Crusade: Sexual Morality and Social Control, 1868–1900* (Westport, CT: Greenwood, 1973); and Mary E. Odem, *Delinquent Daughters: Protecting and Policing Adolescent Female Sexuality in the United States, 1885–1920* (Chapel Hill: University

of North Carolina Press, 1995). Relations between African American and white reform women reached a nadir in 1893, when Francis Willard of the Woman's Christian Temperance Union refused to support Ida B. Wells's antilynching campaign for fear of alienating southern white women from Social Purity. The conflict over lynching was especially significant since white men purported to act in defense of white feminine purity. See Jacqueline Jones Royster, *Southern Horrors and Other Writings: The Antilynching Campaign of Ida B. Wells, 1892–1900* (Boston: Bedford / St. Martin's, 1996); and Crystal Feimster, *Southern Horrors: Women and the Politics of Rape and Lynching* (Cambridge, MA: Harvard University Press, 2011).

10. *Health Journal and Advocate of Physiological Reform* (April 1, 1840).

11. "The Sexual System and Nervous Disorders," *Medical Gazette* (October 22, 1870); "Masturbation and Insanity," *Medical and Surgical Reporter* (May 2, 1874); "Relation of the Sexual Functions to Mental Disorders of Women," *Medical and Surgical Review* (November 22, 1890); "Early Treatment of the Insane," *Medical and Surgical Reporter* (August 26, 1893); "Secretary's Report," *National Citizen and Ballot Box* (April 1880); *Report of the International Council of Women Assembled by the National Woman Suffrage Association, Washington D.C., March 25–April 1, 1888* (Washington, DC: published for National American Woman Suffrage Association by Rufus H. Darby, printer, 1888), 169–73; Mary Putnam Jacobi, "Woman in Medicine," in *Woman's Work in America*, ed. Annie (Nathan) Meyer, chap. 7, 139–205 (New York: Henry Holt, 1891); Lillie Devereux Blake, "Address by Lillie Devereaux Blake of New York," in *The World's Congress of Representative Women*, vol. 1, ed. May Wright Sewall (Chicago: Rand McNally, 1894), 430–32; and Regina Markell Morantz-Sanchez, *Sympathy and Science: Women Physicians in American Medicine* (New York: Oxford University Press, 1985).

12. Clara Barrus, "Insanity in Young Women," in *Annual Report of the Managers of the Middletown State Homeopathic Hospital* (Middletown, NY: s.n., 1893), 131.

13. Clara Barrus, MD, "Gynecological Disorders and Their Relation to Insanity," *American Journal of Insanity* (1894–95); and Barrus, "Insanity in Young Women," 128, 131, 140. On clitoridectomy, see G. J. Barker-Benfield, *The Horrors of the Half-Known Life: Male Attitudes toward Women and Sexuality in Nineteenth-Century America* (1974; repr., New York: Routledge, 2000); Robert Darby, "A Compromising and Unpublishable Mutilation: Clitoridectomy and Circumcision in the 1860s," in *A Surgical Temptation: The Demonization of the Foreskin and the Rise of Circumcision in Britain* (Chicago: University of Chicago Press, 2013), 143; and Sarah W. Rodriguez, "Rethinking the History of Female Circumcision and Clitoridectomy: American Medicine and Female Sexuality in the Late Nineteenth Century," *Journal of the History of Medicine and Allied Sciences* 63, no. 3 (July 2008): 323–47.

14. Havelock Ellis cited Barrus's "Insanity in Young Women," *Journal of Nervous and Mental Disease* (June 1896), in *Autoeroticism* (1899; repr., Philadelphia: E. A. Davis, 1910), 252.

15. Ellis, *Autoeroticism*, 164.

16. Ibid., 245, 261–63, 271, 274; and Havelock Ellis, "The Love Rights of Woman," *Birth Control Review* 2, no. 5 (June 1918). For critiques of Ellis, see Jennifer Terry, *An American Obsession: Science, Medicine, and Homosexuality in Modern Society* (Chicago: University of Chicago Press, 1999); and Julian Carter, "Normality, Whiteness, Authorship:

Evolutionary Sexology and the Primitive Pervert," in *Science and Homosexualities*, ed. Vernon Rosario, 89–97 (New York: Routledge, 1997).

17. Ellis, "Love Rights," was published in the United Kingdom as *The Erotic Rights of Women*, which was also the phrase invoked throughout the text. Havelock Ellis, *The Erotic Rights of Women and the Objects of Marriage* (London: British Society for the Study of Sex Psychology, 1910).

18. Handwritten petition of a Portland group, 1915, quoted in Linda Gordon, *The Moral Property of Women: A History of Birth Control Politics in America* (Urbana and Chicago: University of Illinois Press, 2002), 153. Evidence regarding activities throughout the national network of grassroots organizations, including the titles of sexological works its members read, can also be found in *Birth Control Review* (1917–18).

19. The evidence of improved mental health often included decreased "nervousness" and "tension"; respondents also cited "psychological reading" and mentioned Ellis by name. Katharine Bement Davis, *Factors in the Sex Life of Twenty-Two Hundred Women* (New York: Harper, 1929), 110, 112, 129, 135–38, 140–41, 145, 164.

20. The survey report also established a clear connection between masturbation and the birth control movement: in narrating the reasons various women "use" masturbation, Davis always noted the individual's history of contraceptive use. This detail suggests an enduring connection between these two "erotic rights" of women. Katharine Bement Davis, *Factors in the Sex Life*, 95–96, 168–75. On the distinction between aspirational and statistical norms in the mutually reinforcing discourses of whiteness and sexual normativity, see Julian Carter, *The Heart of Whiteness: Normal Sexuality and Race in America, 1880–1940* (Durham, NC: Duke University Press, 2007), 22.

21. Michele Mitchell, *Righteous Propagation: African Americans and the Politics of Racial Destiny after Reconstruction* (Chapel Hill: University of North Carolina Press, 2004), 9–13, 84, 102.

22. See, for example, Theodoor Van de Velde, *Ideal Marriage: Its Physiology and Technique* (New York: Random House, 1926); and Marie Bonaparte, *Female Sexuality* (1951; repr., New York: International Universities Press, 1973). For one of many feminist responses, see Michael Gordon and Penelope J. Shankweiler, "Different Equals Less: Female Sexuality in Recent Marriage Manuals," *Journal of Marriage and the Family* 33, no. 3 (1971): 459–66.

23. Shulamith Firestone, *The Dialectics of Sex: The Case for Feminist Revolution* (New York: Bantam, 1970), 97.

24. Dodson, *Liberating Masturbation*, 21.

25. Ibid., 21, 30–31, 34, 38, 40 41.

26. Like Graham, Dodson advised abandoning "coffee, sugar, steaks and alcohol"; unlike Graham, she restricted herself to "raw vegetables, fruits, nuts, seeds, sprouts and herbs." Ibid., 30, 38.

27. Firestone, *Dialectics of Sex*, 96–97; Shere Hite, *The Hite Report: A Nationwide Study on Female Sexuality* (New York: Seven Stories Press, 1976), 63; and Lonnie Barbach, *Women Discover Orgasm: A Therapist's Guide to a New Treatment Approach* (New York: Free Press, 1980), 77.

28. Barbach, *Women Discover Orgasm*, 22, 29, 31, 111, 121; and Karen Sandler, "My First Orgasm" (1974), in *Dear Sisters: Dispatches from the Women's Liberation Movement*, ed. Rosalyn Baxandall (New York: Basic Books, 2001), 165.

29. There is a parallel "male orgasmic disorder," but as Jerome Wakefield has pointed out, the criteria are much less likely to apply to men. See Jerome Wakefield, "Female Primary Orgasmic Dysfunction: Masters and Johnson versus *DSM-II-R* on Diagnosis and Incidence," *Journal of Sex Research* 24 (1988): 363–77; and American Psychiatric Association, *DSM-5* (Arlington, VA: American Psychiatric Publishing, 2013), 432. On related diagnoses, see Janice M. Irvine, "Regulated Passions: The Invention of Inhibited Sexual Desire and Sexual Addiction," in *Deviant Bodies*, ed. Jennifer Terry and Jacqueline Urla (Bloomington: Indiana University Press, 1995).

30. Hortense J. Spillers, "Interstices: A Small Drama of Words," in *Pleasure and Danger: Exploring Female Sexuality*, ed. Carol. S. Vance (New York: Pandora, 1989), 76, 78–79, 96.

31. Ellen Carol DuBois and Linda Gordon, "Seeking Ecstasy on the Battlefield: Danger and Pleasure in Nineteenth-Century Feminist Sexual Thought," in *Pleasure and Danger: Exploring Female Sexuality*, ed. Carol Vance, 31–49 (New York: Pandora, 1989).

32. Katha Pollitt, "Why Do So Many Leftists Want Sex Work to Be the New Normal?" *Nation* (April 14, 2014).

33. Gina Kolata, "The Rule Dr. Elders Forgot: America Still Keeps Onan in the Closet," *New York Times* (December 18, 1994); and "After the Storm, Still No Calm," *New York Times* (October 24, 1996). For more recent discussions, see Thomas Laqueur, *Solitary Sex: A Cultural History of Masturbation* (New York: Zone Books, 2003), 416; and Janice M. Irvine, *Talk about Sex: The Battles over Sex Education in the United States* (Berkeley: University of California Press, 2004).

34. Jeffrey P. Moran, *Teaching Sex: The Shaping of Adolescence in the 20th Century* (Cambridge, MA; Harvard University Press, 2000); Irvine, *Talk about Sex*; Alexandra Lord, *Condom Nation: The U.S. Government's Sex Education Campaign from WWI to the Internet* (Baltimore: Johns Hopkins University Press, 2010); and Jessica Valenti, *The Purity Myth: How America's Obsession with Virginity Is Hurting Young Women* (Berkeley, CA: Seal Press, 2009).

35. Passionparties.com, accessed November 16, 2013; and interviews with Joanne Webb and BeAnne Sisemore, in *Passion and Power: The Technology of Orgasm*, directed by Wendy Slick and Emiko Omori (First Run Features, 2008), DVD.

INDEX

Page numbers in italics refer to figures.

abolitionist movement: African American women in, 10–11, 55, 56–57, 58–80, 127, 133; in Boston, 54, 56–57, 68–69; false delicacy and, 58, 72–73; goals, 9; Hollick and, 126–29; libertine republicans and, 46; licentiousness and, 62–65, 79–80; in New York, 59–62; split with moral reform, 95–101, 105, 142, 175; white southerners and, 15, 96–97; women's rights and, 25, 83, 105, 125–26, 147
abortion, 117, 120, 154, 213n30
Adelphic Union (Boston), 56–57
adultery: African American women's campaign against, 73–74; McDowall's crusade against, 37; slavery and, 21, 58–59, 62–65, 71, 79–80, 95, 147
Advocate and Family Guardian, 101
Advocate of Moral Reform, 38, 62, 63, 66, 74, 76–77, 78, 90, 91–92, 94, 99–100, 101, 150
Afric-American Female Intelligence Society, 136
African American Progressives, 172–73
African American women: amalgamation riots targeting, 59–62, 68, 75; anatomical texts' depictions, 110, 128–29, 157, 162; contributions to sexual thought, 11, 23–25, 72, 106, 175–76; empowerment, 135–36, 161–62; enslaved, 96–97, 139; excluded from Rosine Association, 102–3, 142; false delicacy applied to slavery's defenders by, 10–11, 58; Graham and, 55; in moral reform movement, 11, 12, 23–24, 55, 56–80, 83, 94–101, 106; passionlessness as viewed by, 20–23, 55, 102–3; peer-education groups, 136–37; politics of respectability, 24, 55, 60–61, 140, 172–73; postbellum women's movements and, 167–68, 173; postbellum southern black colleges' hygiene curricula, 172–73, 187n34; rescue of, 98–99; self-definition in black feminist thought, 2–3, 4; sex education for, 132–37, 154–58, 217n2; sexual excess blamed on, 13, 61, 65, 128–29, 130, 157, 162; sexual harassment of, 24, 66–67, 191n69; slaveholders' depredations, 21, 65, 96–97; uplift movement, 98–99. *See also specific names*
African Methodist Episcopal Zion Church, 10–11, 58–62, 74
AIDS, 176–77
Alcott, William Andrus: *The House I Live In*, 104, 154; women speakers condemned by, 87; *Young Man's Guide*, 51, 84–85
Alexander, Charles, 115–17, 119–21
amalgamation: cartoon, 70; discourse, 55, 57, 59, 64, 68–69, 127; riots and, 10–11, 57–58, 59–62, 64–65, 66, 68, 75, 160
amative indulgence, philosophy of, 108, 110–11, 112, 116–17, 128, 130, 134, 141, 146, 147–48, 166, 171, 176–77. *See also* love principle concept
amativeness, 145–46, 148, 154, 166, 222n47
American Anti-slavery Society, 60

231

American Board of Commissioners of Foreign Missions, 103
American Colonization Society, 125, 160
American Female Moral Reform Society, 96, 97, 99–101, 206n2
American Moral Reform Society, 73–74, 76
American Phrenological Journal, 161
American Physiological Society, 84–90
American Psychiatric Association, 174–75
American Seventh Commandment Society, 37, 63–64, 201n25, 201n31
anatomy museums, 108
anti-Catholic sentiment, 50, 126, 197–98n70
antilynching campaign, 228n9
antislavery movement. *See* abolitionist movement
aphrodisiacs, 17, 112
Appeal to the Women of the Nominally Free States, The, 75, 205n68
Appo, Elizabeth, 219n17
asylums for mentally ill, 13, 15, 130, 150–51, 170, 208n27
Awful Disclosures of Maria Monk, 126

Baartman, Sara, 128, 129
Bachelor's Journal, 47
Bacon, Olive, 118, 221n35
Bailey, Eleanor Eliza, 111
Balinville, Henri de, 128
Ball, Erica, 157
Bambara, Toni Cade, 2–3
Bangor, Maine, 88
Barbach, Lonnie, 174
Barker-Benfield, G. J., 17–18
Barrus, Clara, 170–71
Beam, Dorri, 155
Beecher, Catherine, 145, 166, 222n46
Bell, John, 36
Beman, Jehiel C., 76
Benfield, Barker, 188–89n45
Bennett, Sarah Ingraham, 205n78. *See also* Ingraham, Sarah R.
birth control movement, 168, 229n20
Blackwell, Elizabeth, 140–41, 144, 222n46
Blasland, Mehitable, 89
Block, Sharon, 67
Bodysex Workshops, 173, 177
Bogle, Amelia, 139–40
Bolles, C. H., 163
Bolles, J. N., 37; *Solitary Vice Considered*, 51–52

Boody, Henry H., 45, 47
Boston, Massachusetts: Ladies' Physiological Institute, 147–48, 152, 154, 206n6; Ladies' Physiological Society, 11–12, 81–82, 83–90, 95, 105, 206n6; rioters confronted by women in, 84; riots over Graham lectures, 27–28, 35, 45, 47–48, 52, 54, 56–58, 75, 84, 85, 90; women's activism, 54, 68
Boston Female Anti-slavery Society, 56, 59, 68, 89, 205n68
Boston Female Moral Reform Society, 54, 56, 68–71, 76, 90–91
Boston Medical and Surgical Journal, 107, 130
Boston Women's Health Collective, 2, 3–4
Boston Yankee, 47
botanical art, 155–58
Bourne, George, 201n25
Bowers, Margaret, 136
Boxford, Massachusetts, 152
Boyle, T. C., *The Road to Wellville*, 19
British Abolition Act of 1833, 203n58
Brown, Anna, 118
Brown, Elsa Barkley, 21
Brown, Isaac Baker, 170–71
Brown, Mary Ann, 79–80
Brown, William Wells, 65
Buffum, Sarah G., 205n67
Bunting, Elizabeth, 118
Burleigh, Margaret Jones, 122, 221n35
Burnett, Stella Kneeland, 104
Burr, Esther, 118
Burr, Hetty, 72, 96, 98–99, 136, 137
Burr, Nancy Gardner, 11
Burrus, Kandi, 177
Butler, Elizabeth, 136

Cambell, David, 87, 89–90
Cambell, Sylvia, 84, 87, 89–90
Camp, Stephanie, 51–52
Canfield, Russel, 39; *Practical Physiology*, 195n41
Carby, Hazel, 70
Carlisle, Richard, 111
Carpenter, William, *Elements of Physiology*, 154
Cassey, Amy Matilda, 75, 136, 155, 221n35
Catholic views on masturbation, 32
celibacy: anti-Catholicism and, 50; dangers associated with, 32, 37, 50, 141; masculinity and, 33, 48–52, 105

Chatham Chapel (New York), 59–61, 73, 75
Cheney University of Pennsylvania, 138
Child, Lydia Maria, 75, 110, 126, 127, 202n32; *Letters from New York*, 111–12
Cincinnati, Ohio, 67
Clark, McDonald, 40–41
Clarkson, J. G., 116
Clay, Edward, cartoon, 70
clerical abolitionists, 89, 95
Clinton, Bill, 176–77
Clinton, New York, 99–100
Clinton Hall (New York), 36
clitoral orgasm, 1–2, 20, 113, 144–45, 173
clitoridectomy, 16, 170–71
Codman, John, 85
Codman, Randolph, 45, 46, 47
Codman, Rebecca, 85, 89
coitus interruptus, 39–40
Coker, Eliza, 61, 65, 75, 200n18
Cole, Rebecca, 158
Coleman, C. A., 164
Colesworthy, Daniel, 51–52
Collins, Cynthia, 41, 86
Collins, Simeon, 86, 192n9
Colored American, 160–61
Combe, George, 160
Commercial Advertiser, 59
Committee of Vigilance, 63–64
Condee, Andalucia, 103, 104
Condie, D. Francis, 36
Cornish, Samuel, 73, 76
corsets, 35–36, 91
Cott, Nancy F., 18–19, 189n46
Courier & Enquirer, 57, 59
coverture, 143
Crandall, Prudence, 205n68
Curtis, Emeline, 219n17
Cutler, Hannah C., 56
Cutter, Calvin, 153–55, 156
Cutter, Eunice P., 154
Cutter's Anatomy, 153–55, 156
Cuvier, Georges, 128

Daily Chronicle, 115, 120, 123, 125
Davis, Angela, 20–21
Davis, Katharine Bement, 172, 173
Davis, Paulina Wright, 12, 90, 99–100, 105, 110, 138–39, 143, 147, 148, 162, 169–70, 213n31
Davis, William, 27
Davison, Anna Maria, 132–33, 134, 135, 153, 157–58, 217n1

Degler, Carl N., 18, 188–89n45
Delany, Martin, 135, 217n1
Deslandes, Leopold, *Treatise on the Diseases Produced by Onanism*, 126
Diagnostic and Statistical Manual, 174–75
Dickerson, Martina, 156
Dickerson, Mary Anne, 155, 156
dildos, 30
Dodson, Betty, 2, 173–74, 177
Dolby, John, Jr., 215n51
domestic service: prostitution weighed against, 38; rescue asylums and, 101, 102–3, 106, 132; sexual exploitation during, 24, 65, 66–67, 69–71, 155, 191n69
Dorsey, Sarah, 136
double standards, sexual: adultery and, 171; eliminating, 9–10, 38, 55, 83, 129; false delicacy and, 10; freethinkers and, 39; men challenging, 50–51; passivity and, 72, 75–76, 122; physiological ignorance and, 173–74; protests against, 125–26; racialized dimensions of, 58–62, 64
douching as contraceptive method, 39
Douglass, Frederick, 161
Douglass, Grace Bustill, 59, 72, 75, 135, 136, 205n67
Douglass, Robert, 156, 217n1
Douglass, Sarah Mapps, 59, 72, 75, 96; amativeness concept and, 148–49; antislavery activism, 133; background, 135–37; botanical art, 155–56; elocution taught by, 132, 134, 156–57, 158–59, 162; Sarah Grimké's friendship with, 73, 74, 139, 140, 146, 163, 166, 176; interest in Africa, 217n1; lectures by, 131, 169–70; marriage, 139, 140; in moral reform movement, 11, 73, 149; physiological studies, 139–40, 146–47, 152; protest against Quaker segregation policy, 73, 203–4n59; public lectures by, 140; sex education taught by, 14, 130–31, 132–37, 152–58; virtue advocated over purity by, 11, 74, 133–34, 136, 142–43, 149, 154, 157–58, 176; white abolitionists' critiques of her pedagogy, 132–33, 138, 155–58
Douglass, William, 139, 140
dress, women's intemperance in, 35–36, 91
Drummond, Louisa, 56
Dumond, Dwight, 201n25
Dunbar, Erica Armstrong, 157
Dye, Margaret, 95, 96–97, 101, 129, 147

Earle, Mary, 74
Eastern Lunatic Asylum, 15
Eaton, Rebecca, 88, 90, 94; "Physiological Lecture to Ladies," 103–4
Elders, Joycelyn, 176–77
Elkington, Edith, 140
Ellis, Hannah, 118, 213–14n35, 221n35
Ellis, Havelock: *Autoeroticism*, 171; *Psychology of Sex*, 171–72
Ellis, Susanna, 221n35
Emancipator, 64
Equiano, Olaudah, 65
evangelical Christians: false delicacy and, 72; Graham's support from, 37; missionaries, 103–4; reform physiology and, 5–6, 15, 81–82, 167, 175. *See also* ultras

false delicacy: African American women and, 10–11, 58, 158; amalgamation discourse and, 58; anatomy education and, 111–12, 117, 119, 120, 149, 213n31; arguments against, 94, 134; commercial appropriation of concept, 13; contrasted with true delicacy, 81–82, 119, 122, 198n78; defined, 10; original use in seduction literature, 53, 198n78; physiological ignorance and, 93–94; purity and, 71–72; rioters named in Boston, 84; sexual double standards and, 10, 52–54, 75–76; women's employment and, 138–39
Farnham, Eliza, *Woman and Her Era*, 166–67
Female Benevolent Society, 194n36
Female Literary Association, 135, 136–37
Female Medical College of Pennsylvania, 13, 133, 141–42, 145, 146, 151, 158, 217n2, 221n35
female moral reformers, 4, 10–11, 20, 38, 50, 52–55, 58, 60, 62, 64–66, 69–70, 73, 75–77, 92, 94, 99, 101, 125–26, 129, 150, 166, 168, 172, 176. *See also* moral reform movement; *and individual names*
Female Vigilant Committee, 99
feminism: African American, 2–3, 21, 110, 136, 173, 175–76; early twentieth-century, 172; late nineteenth-century, 166, 167, 171; medical, 140–41, 142–43, 144, 151; mid-nineteenth-century liberal, 146–47, 149, 157, 162; 1970s–80s, 1–4, 105, 173–77; passionlessness and, 20. *See also* moral reform movement; reform physiology movement; women's rights movement; *and individual names*
fertility-control techniques, 17, 18, 22, 39, 80, 112–13, 114, 154, 189n46
Finney, Charles Grandison, 60
Firestone, Shulamith, 174
First Antislavery Convention of American Women (1837), 74–75, 96
Fitz, Susan, 89
flash press, 47, 50
Florence, Col. Thomas B., 125, 215n51
flowers, language of, 158, 217n1, 225n87
Fondey, John, 120
Forten, James, 65, 73, 79, 135
Forten, Margaret, 136
Forten, Sarah, 72, 136
Foucault, Michel, 114
Fowler, Orson Squire, 145–46, 147, 148, 160, 163–64, 166, 222n47
Franklin Institute (Philadelphia), 36
Freedmen's Schools, 15
Free Enquirer, 61
free love movement, 143–44, 176
freethinkers, 18, 37, 39–40, 111, 112, 117, 122–23
Freud, Sigmund, 1, 113, 173
Friend of Virtue, 76, 91–92, 94, 101, 104, 150
Fuller, Lydia, 68–69, 75, 89, 96, 97, 205n67

Gardner, Massachusetts, 80
Gardner, Sylvia, 69
Garrison, Helen, 89
Garrison, William Lloyd, 45, 46, 95
Geneva Medical College, 140
Giddings, Paula, 21
Gilbert Lyceum, 139–40
Ginzberg, Lori, 22
Godey's Lady's Book, 129
Goldman, Emma, 171
gonorrhea, 37, 120, 154, 212n21
Gordon, Linda, 171
Gove, Mary (later Nichols): amativeness concept embraced by, 146; later acceptance of, 107; lectures by, 11–12, 81–82, 87–88, 90, 100, 102, 105, 107, 169–70, 210n1; *Lectures to Ladies*, 92–94; radical individualism, 143–44, 173; *Solitary Vice*, 92, 103, 151; "To Parents, Guardians, and Those Who Have the Care of Children," 92
Grafton Female Moral Reform Society, 91, 92

Graham, George Rex, 115, 121
Graham, Sylvester: Canfield and, 195n41; courses offered by, 35–36; diet of, 6, 12, 40–41, 48–50, 86, 139, 184n13; female testimonials solicited by, 41, 86, 88; Hawaiian translations of works, 104; Hollick's message compared with, 130; ideas on self-restraint for both sexes, 28–29, 49–50, 55, 130; lectures to women suspended by, 52; lecture style, 54; "Lecture to Mothers," 6, 26–28, 29, 34–35, 36–37, 41–42, 54–55, 56–57, 68, 75, 81, 85, 87, 102, 168; *Lecture to Young Men*, 28, 41, 51, 84, 92; medical problems linked to masturbation by, 8–9; "Moral Physiology" lecture, 39–40; portrayed as mass seducer, 50, 68; questionnaire for missionaries, 104; racist elements of advice, 185n17; reform physiology movement, 5–7; retirement of, 11–12, 28, 55; riots against, 6, 8–10, 26–29, 34–35, 37–38, 44–47, 56–58, 68, 75, 84, 117; white southerners' views on, 15
Grahamites, 6, 26–29, 40–41, 48–50, 86, 88–90, 135, 139
Graham Journal, 87
Greene, Charles Gordon, 49–50
Greenfield, William, *The Secret Habits of the Female Sex*, 126
Gregory, Samuel, 151, 152
Grew, Mary, 110, 117–19, 121–23, 125, 126, 127, 142, 213–14n35, 221n35
Grew, Susan, 121–22
Grimké, Angelina (later Weld), 59, 165, 173; diary of, 203n58; family's slaveholding, 72; Graham lecture attended by, 36, 41; marriage, 79, 139; virtue advocated over purity by, 72–73, 76
Grimké, Archibald, 173
Grimké, Henry, 167
Grimké, Sarah M.: amativeness concept embraced by, 146, 148–49; changing ideology of, 166–67; family's slaveholding, 72; friendship with Douglass, 59, 73, 74, 139, 140, 146, 163, 166, 176; Genesis interpretation, 76, 205n74; Longshore and, 141–42; as New York Female Moral Reform Society delegate, 205n67; virtue advocated over purity by, 71–77; withdrawal from lecturing, 79
Grimké, Theodore Weld (Sody), 163–66

Grimké, Thomas Smith, 203n58
group sex, masturbation in, 43–44, 173
Gunn, Thomas Butler, engraving, *49*

Hall, G. Stanley, 16
Hall, Jacqueline Dowd, 21
Hallowell, Rebecca, 221n35
Harrington, Henry F., 28, 47–48, 54
Harris, Leslie, 57
Hawaii, missionaries in, 103–4
heteronormativity, 16–17, 110, 114, 122–23, 145–46, 148–49, 162, 166
heterosexual intercourse: Blackwell's views, 144–45; Ellis's views, 171; Freudian view, 1, 113, 173; Grimké's views, 148–49; Hollick's views, 13, 108–10, 113–14, 116, 119–21, 128, 141; libertine republicans' views, 8; as marital right and duty, 16–17, 32, 55, 143, 148, 157
Higginbotham, Evely Brooks, 24
Hilton, Lavinia, 11, 68–69, 136
Hine, Darlene Clark, 23, 62
Hitchins, Rebecca, 136
Hite, Shere, 1
Hollick, Frederick, 108–31, *109*; amative indulgence philosophy, 108, 110–11, 112, 116–17, 128, 130, 141, 146, 147–48; aphrodisiacs promoted by, 112; career retrospective, 211–12n12; *Diseases of Women*, 152; early career, 110–11; female defenders of, 110, 117–23, 142, 221n35; Friends of, 123–26; *An Inquiry into the Rights, Duties, and Destinies, of the Different Varieties of the Human Race*, 127; lectures by, 108, 112, 115, 117, 124–25, 129–30, 160, 168, 210n2; libel suits against, 109–10, 114–17, 123–26; *The Male Generative Organs in Health and Disease*, 169; *The Marriage Guide*, 108–9, 112–13, 129, 148; *Neuropathy*, 126; notoriety, 108; *The Origin of Life*, 110, 112–13, 115–17, 123, 126, 129, 130, 152, 157; *Outlines of Anatomy and Physiology*, 126, 129; pathologization of African American women's bodies, 128–29, 130; proslavery views, 127, 216n58; reinvention, 111; sexual physiology lectures, 13
Holliston, Massachusetts, 52, 88
Home Guardian, 101
homosexuality, 114, 121, 221n43

Hopkinton, Massachusetts, 103–4
Horowitz, Helen, 184n11
Horton, James Oliver, 191n69
Houses of Industry, 12, 83, 102, 132
Hunt, Harriot Keziah, 140, 141, 143, 144, 146–47, 148–49, 150, 162, 221n39, 223n61
hydrotherapy, 19–20. *See also* water cure
Hysteria (film), 19

Illuminator, 51, 52
Ingraham, Sarah R., 77, 83, 99–100
Institute for Colored Youth (Philadelphia), 14, 25, 132–33, 135, 138, 152–58
interracial sex. *See* amalgamation

Jacobs, Harriet, 23; *Incidents in the Life of a Slave Girl*, 65
Jamaica, 98
Jewett, Helen, 126
"Jezebel" stereotype, 2, 21, 23, 25, 71, 76, 96, 128
Johnson, Mary, 61, 65, 75
Johnson, Mary Ann, 88, 89, 90, 96, 97, 99, 138
Johnson, Oliver, 90
Johnson, Virginia, 2, 174–75
Johnston, David Claypoole, cartoon, *153*
Jones, Margaret, 118
Judd, G. P., 104
Justice, Huldah, 118
Juvenile Reformer, 51

Katz, Jonathan Ned, 16–17
Kelley, Florence, 212–13n26
Kelley, William Darrah, 115–17, 123–24, 212–13n26
Kelly, Hugh, *False Delicacy*, 198n78
Kilton, Catherine, 83, 89, 95
Kilton, John, 87
Kinkelin, Arnold R., 120
Kinsey, Alfred, *Sexual Behavior in the Human Female*, 2
Knight, Ruby, 205n67
Knowlton, Charles, 39
Koedt, Anne, 1

Ladies Moral Reform Association (Providence), 53
Ladies' Phoenix Society, 136
Ladies' Physiological Institute of Boston and Vicinity, 147–48, 152, 154, 206n6

Ladies' Physiological Society of Boston, 11–12, 81–82, 83–90, 95, 105, 206n6
Lallemand, Claude-François, 164, 166
Lane, Mrs. A. J., 205n67
Laqueur, Thomas, 29, 30
Larcombe, Anna, 74
Lasser, Carol, 201n25
Lathrop, Lydia, 89
Leavitt, Clarissa, 89
Lerner, Gerda, 205n74
lesbianism, 3, 31, 34, 42–43, 122, 171, 194n25, 196n52
Letters on the Equality of the Sexes, 76
libertine republicans: amalgamation views, 57–58, 60–62, 127; anti-Graham riots and, 9–10, 45–47, 57–58, 82–83, 125; definition, 7–8, 130; false delicacy claims, 10; fantasies about female masturbators, 43–44; Hollick and, 108–9, 113–14, 125–26, 212n21; masculine rake culture, 46–48; moral guardians' challenges to, 12–13, 28–29, 82–83; in Portland, 45–47; power-sharing ridiculed by, 29; prostitution and, 60, 69
licentiousness: applied to solitary vice, 82, 99–100, 141; applied to women, 77, 79, 81, 92, 93–94, 95, 105–6, 202n32; diet and, 93; moral reform campaign against, 58, 76–77, 92, 95–96; northern, 58–59, 65–71; passive women's collusion, 75–76; race and, 58–62, 136; in rural areas, 81–82; systematized, 38
licentiousness of slavery, concept of, 10–11, 58–59, 62–65, 71, 79, 147
Lincoln, Maria, 92
live model shows, 108
Lombard Street Infant School (Philadelphia), 219n17
Longshore, Hannah, 141–42
Lorde, Audre, 3, 176
love principle concept, 145–49, 154, 157, 164, 222n47
Lowell, Massachusetts, 52
Lynn, Massachusetts, 88
Lyon, Mary, 138

Magdalen Asylums, 38, 101
Maine Anti-slavery Society, 46
Maines, Rachel, 19, 20, 121
male monsters, 7, 48–52, 55, 58
manikins, 6, 117, 118, 138–39, 213n32

Manion, Jen, 17
Mann, Horace, 150–52
marketing of sexual advice and information, 17, 108–9, 120–21, 185n14, 212n21, 213nn30–32, 214n39
marriage: coverture issue and, 143–44; excessive sex during, 37; freethinkers' critique, 39; manuals, 16–17, 32, 108–9, 112–13, 114, 115–17, 119–21; sex as matter of negotiation during, 39–40, 55, 113–14, 141; sex as right and duty during, 16–17, 32, 55, 143, 148
Marten, John: *Onania*, 29–33, 39, 42, 93, 108; "The Supplement to the Onania," 30
Martyn, Grace, 205n67
Martyn, Sarah Towne (née Smith). *See* Smith, Sarah Towne
Massachusetts school system, 150–52
Masters, William, 1–2, 174–75
masturbation, female: abstinence and, 177; African American women and, 157–58; changing discourse on, 174–77; deviance associated with, 16; as erotic right, 168–73; freethinkers' views on, 39; institutionalization of campaign against, 13–14; lesbianism and, 194n25, 196n52; Marten's depictions in *Onania*, 30–31; medicalization of, 134, 142–45, 150–58, 162, 164, 166, 169–70, 171; medical warnings against, 93–94, 109, 113–14, 130, 141, 144–45; mental illness and, 1, 5, 6–7, 13–14, 15, 34, 167; moral guardians' infantilization, 102, 106, 164; 1970s attitudes, 1–3, 17–18; pornographic depictions, 43–44; process of cultural discourse, 14–15; public school discussions, 176–77; racial constructions, 2–3, 44, 110, 128–29, 157, 162; sexual liberalism and, 168–77; as symbol of independence, 173–74; white purity and, 133–34; in women's prisons, 103, 151. *See also specific names, organizations, and topics*
masturbation, male: abstinence and, 177; Alcott's lecture and pamphlet against, 84; British views on, 29–33; conduct manuals, 5; deviance associated with, 16; early American apathy toward subject, 33–34; freethinkers' views on, 39; homosexuality and, 114, 121; medicalization of, 134, 163–64, 166, 169–70; medical warnings against, 30, 34, 109, 113–14, 130, 144–45; mental illness linked to, 6–7, 8, 15, 167; moral guardians' infantilization of, 102, 106, 164; onanism and, 5, 8, 13, 16, 29–33, 105, 126, 130, 166; public school discussions on, 176–77; revolutionary era and, 33. *See also* spermatorrhea
masturbatory insanity, 15, 34, 150–51, 158, 164, 166, 168, 170, 174, 208n27, 223n65; northern versus southern reactions, 15
masturbatory sanity, 173–77
Maternal Association (Hopkinton, Massachusetts), 103–4
Mather, Cotton, 5, 32–33
matrons, 99, 101–2, 103, 105, 107, 151, 170, 172
Matthews, Abby, 136
Maudsley, Henry, 223n65
McDowall, John R., 52, 60, 61, 63–64, 69; Graham and, 37–38, 51, 57; *The Magdalen Report*, 37; *Memoir*, 92
McDowall's Journal, 38, 62
mental health, masturbation and, 1, 171, 172, 173–77, 229n19; birth control and, 229n20
mental illness: asylums, 13, 15, 130, 150–51, 170, 208n27; masturbation linked to, 1, 5, 6–7, 8, 13–14, 15, 33–34, 167, 172–73
Methodist Episcopal church, 96
Millbury, Massachusetts, 88, 92
missionaries, 103–4, 217n1
Mitchell, Michelle, 173
moral guardians: class and, 22; daughters as surveillance targets, 41–42, 170–71; emergence of, 12–13, 80, 83, 101–5, 118; female physiology lecturers as, 107; ideological differences with women's rights movement, 130–31; masturbation infantilized by, 16, 102, 103–4, 105–6, 164; passionlessness and, 25, 83, 102–3, 164; political rights and, 146–47; race and, 167; sex education and, 150–52
moral reform movement: African American women's participation in, 11, 12, 23–25, 55, 56–80, 83, 94–101; amalgamation and, 57–58; antimasturbation lectures and, 10, 81–82; antislavery schism, 95–101, 105; in Boston, 54, 68–69; campaign against licentiousness, 58, 76–77, 78, 79, 202n32; community health and, 135–36; false delicacy and, 10–11, 52–54, 58; fractures in, 12–13, 83; goals, 95–96, 101–2; Hunt

moral reform movement (cont.)
  and, 146–47; ideology, 9; male leaders, 36–37; postbellum racial split, 167, 175; riots targeting, 9–10, 37–38, 44–47; in rural areas, 25, 77, 79, 81–83, 90–94, 95, 106, 168; self-restraint and, 5–7, 9, 37, 55, 82–83, 91–92, 93, 95, 99–100; sexual platform, 65–71; slavery used as metaphor by, 63; split with abolition movement, 95–101, 105, 107, 142; Social Purity movement as distinct from, 167–68, 222n53, 227–28n9; testimonials in, 82, 85–88, 92, 94; turn inward, 80, 83, 95, 106; women outnumbering men in, 38, 54–55, 65, 105. *See also* physiology; reform physiology movement; Social Purity movement
moral reform press, 23–24, 66–67. *See also specific titles*
Moral Reform Retreat, 25, 98–99, 102, 106, 137
Morris, Mary, 118
Morton, Samuel George, *Crania Americana*, 159–60
Mott, Lucretia, 74, 102, 132, 205n67
Mount Holyoke Seminary, 138
Mumford, Janet, 61
Mussey, Charles, 45, 47

National Organization for Women, 1, 3
Neal, John, 47–48, 57
Needles, Edward, 138
Nelson, Dana, 159
New England Anti-slavery Society, 46
New England Female Medical College, 13, 141, 152
New England Galaxy, 47–48, 50
New Haven, Connecticut, 67
New Orleans Charity Hospital, 15
Newton, Massachusetts, 89
New York, New York: amalgamation riots, 59–61; female moral reform societies in, 200n17; First Antislavery Convention of American Women in, 74–75, 96; Graham's lectures in, 36
New York Commercial Advertiser, 57
New York Express, 196n60
New York Female Moral Reform Society, 10, 60–63, 64, 73, 75; auxiliaries, 90–91; delegates, 205n67; formation, 38; Office of Direction for Female Domestics, 66; Philadelphia auxiliary, 74; prevention versus rescue, 70–71, 38, 83, 98, 101–5, 106, 107, 132–33, 206n5; sexual equality and, 77; split with Female Benevolent Society, 194n36
New York Scorpion, 216n58
New York Sun, 127
Nichols, Thomas Low, 143, 144
Nissenbaum, Stephen, 197n62
North American, 115, 117
Nott, Josiah, 159–60
Nudd, Susan A., 129
nymphomania, 16, 128, 129, 157, 170–71, 196n52

Oberlin, Ohio, 89–90
obscenity: charges, 116–17, 119, 123; obscene libel law, 51, 110, 116, 123
onanism, 5, 6, 8, 13, 16, 29–33, 39, 105, 126, 130, 166
Ordway, Abigail, 88, 89, 90, 94
Otis, James F., 45, 46, 196n60
Our Bodies, Ourselves, 2
Owen, Robert, 111, 211n9
Owen, Robert Dale, 211n9; *Moral Physiology*, 39, 111

Painter, Nell Irvin, 21
Parker, Eliza, 89
Parker, Lucy, 89, 205n67
Parker, Mary S., 205n67
Parsons, Anson V., 116, 124, 125
passionlessness, ideology of, 17, 18–20, 214–15n44; false delicacy and, 81, 93–94; Hollick's rejection of, 113, 122; libertinism and, 48; moral guardians and, 25, 83, 102, 105–6; as power-laden concept, 22, 75–77, 95; racial aspects, 20–23, 55, 102–3; as strategy, 18–20
Passion Parties, 177
passivity, female, 2, 8, 18, 52–53, 55, 58, 71, 74, 75–76, 79–80, 122, 173, 176
patriarchal governance, 7–8, 12–13, 17–18, 28–29
Pawtucket, Rhode Island, 52
Pennimen, Mary O. B., 205n67
Pennsylvania Abolition Society, 138
Pennsylvania Society for Discouraging the Use of Ardent Spirits, 35–36
Perry, Sarah, 89
Personal Responsibility and Work Opportunity Act, 177

Peterboro, New York, 79
Peterson, Carla, 56
Peterson, T. B., 126
Philadelphia, Pennsylvania: antislavery activity in, 72–74; Arch Street Society of Friends segregated meeting house, 73, 139, 204n59; Franklin Institute, 36; Graham's lectures in, 36; House of Industry for "Fallen Females," 132; Institute for Colored Youth, 14, 25, 132–33, 135, 138, 152–58; libel suits against Hollick, 114–17, 123–26; Lombard Street Infant School, 219n17; Moral Reform Retreat in, 25, 98–99, 102, 106, 137; Rosine Association, 102–3, 118, 142, 217n2; women's activism, 68, 135–42
Philadelphia Association for Medical Instruction, 159
Philadelphia Female Anti-slavery Society, 58, 65, 72–73, 100, 118, 135, 136, 137–38, 142, 217n2
Philadelphia Female Moral Reform Society, 204n62
Philadelphia Lyceum, 220n25
phrenology, 160–61, 222n47, 226n94
physicians, female, 14, 140–41, 144, 151, 158
physicians, male, 164, 166; condemnation of lecturers on sex, 188n37; Hollick's interactions with, 114–15, 117, 130; lack of authority in 1830s–40s, 15–16
physiological universalism, 7, 42, 128, 161, 185n17
physiology: college curricula, 136, 138, 141, 187n34; depictions of black female bodies, 110, 128–29, 157, 158–61, 162; 1840s studies, 107–31, 139–41; 1850s studies, 133–34, 164; French, 6, 33–34; lectures (*see specific names*); medical profession and, 14, 15–16, 36, 114–15, 134, 159, 164–65, 168; popular, 10, 17, 20, 83–84, 107–14, 124, 128–31, 140–41, 159 60, 185n14, 195n42; public schools and, 14, 132–33, 136, 149–58; racism in, 127–29; sex education for African Americans, 132–37; textbooks, 104, 126, 129, 132, 153–56, 195n41. *See also* reform physiology movement; sex education
Plete, Louisa, 136
Plymouth, Massachusetts, 152
Pollitt, Katha, 176
Pope, Eliza, 205n67

pornography, 43–44, 126, 176–77
Porter, Marcy C., 53–54
Portland, Maine: notes from Graham lecture, 40–41; riots over Graham lectures, 27, 35, 38, 42, 45–47, 53–54, 57
Portland Courier, 53–54
Portland Daily Advertiser, 27, 46
Potts, Anna Longshore, 145, 222n45
Preston, Ann, 141–42, 143, 149, 150, 162, 169–70
Prince, Nancy Gardner, 11, 76, 98; *Narrative*, 69–71; virtue advocated over purity by, 11, 70–71
Prince, Nancy Hobart, 89
Prince, Nero, 69
Prior, Margaret, 205n67
prisons, women's, 103, 151
prostitution: asylums rescuing prostitutes, 38, 101, 102–3, 106, 132; class and, 22, 38; female moral reform movement's crusade against, 60, 61; interracial, 69; McDowall's crusade against, 37; power and, 38, 51, 69–71; in premodern era, 30; prevention of, 10, 37–38, 39, 60, 137, 147; Social Purity movement and, 147; women's suffrage movement and, 222n53
Protestant views on marital restraint, 32
Providence, Rhode Island: McDowall-Graham joint appearances, 37–38, 51, 57; moral reform society, 37, 51–52, 53; prurient interest over Graham lecture attendees, 42–43; reform physiology in, 90; riots over Graham lectures, 26–29, 34–35
Providence Patriot, 34–35, 49
Providence Physiological Society, 90, 148
Purdy, Louisa, 84
purity, white feminine: connotations, 71; false image of, 92–93; Grimké's changing views on, 166–67; moral guardians and, 83, 102–6, 150, 164; notion of, 11, 17, 21, 70–71; racial exclusion in, 21–22, 25, 55, 80, 97, 103, 110, 142, 146–47, 149, 166–67; virtue contrasted with, 11, 21, 70–79, 80, 122, 125, 131, 133–34, 142, 147–48, 149, 154–55, 164, 167, 176
Purvis, Robert, 72

Quincy, Edmund, 9

racial equality issues: Fifteenth Amendment and, 227n9; licentiousness and, 58–62,

racial equality issues (cont.)
  136; moral reform movement and, 12–13, 142, 227–28n9; separatism and, 60; sex and, 7–8; sex education and, 134; skin complexion and, 135, 155; violence against women, 173
racial science, 127–29, 159–62, 185n17
rape: African American women's resistance to, 23; black lasciviousness stereotypes and, 61; coverture and, 143; of domestic servants, 24, 65, 66–67; as racial terror, 21
Ray, Henrietta Cordelia, 137
Ray, Henrietta D., 136–37
Read, Abigail, 91
Real Housewives of Atlanta, The (TV show), 177
Reason, Charles, 152
Reckless, Hetty, 72, 98–99, 137
reform physiology movement: changing messages, 129–30, 164; definition, 5–7, 8–9; divisions within, 88–90; elements, 91–92; female physicians and, 140–41; feminization of, 11–12, 28, 52–55, 84–85; Graham and, 37–55, 82–85; growth, 40, 81–106; ladies' physiology societies, 11–12, 81–82, 83–90, 95, 105, 147–48, 152, 154, 206–7n6; peer education, 85–86, 90, 94; politicization, 138–39, 142–45; principles, 54–55, 82–83; southern views on, 15; unmarried women in, 85, 92; virtue and, 11; white southern women and, 15, 96–97, 101, 147; widows and older women in, 92
respectability, politics of, 24, 42–43, 55, 60–61, 140, 172–73
Restell, Madame, 107
rhythm method, 212n17
Richardson, Hannah White, 217n2
Richardson, Samuel, *Clarissa*, 198n78
Riley, Elizabeth Jackson, 136–37
Rindge, New Hampshire, 79
riots: against amalgamation, 10–11, 57–58, 59–62, 66, 68, 75; against Graham's women-only lectures, 6, 8–10, 12, 26–28, 44–45, 53–55, 56–58, 117
Robinson, H. R., erotic engravings, *43, 44*
Rochester, New York, 65, 102
Rosen, Hannah, 67
Rosenberg, Carroll Smith, 18–19
Rosine Association, 102–3, 118, 142, 217n2

Rousseau, Jean-Jacques, *Émile*, 33
Ruggles, David, 10, 63–64, 77, 79, 201n25
rural areas, moral reform societies in, 25, 77, 79, 81–83, 90–94, 95, 106, 168
Rush, Benjamin, 5, 34; *Medical Inquiries upon Diseases of the Mind*, 51
Ryan, Mary, 22

Salem Female Anti-slavery Society, 65
Sandler, Karen, 174
Sanger, Margaret, 171
Sappol, Michael, 212n21
Sartain, Susanna, 221n35
Scudery, Madeleine de, 194n25
Seaman's Moral Reform Society, 76
Sears, Susan, 84, 88, 89
Sears, Willard, 27
Second Great Awakening, 5, 17
Sedgwick, Eve Kosofsky, 94
self-abuse (as term), 16, 102, 158, 172
self-definition, female: in black feminist thought, 2–3, 4, 175–76; subjectivity and, 2, 4, 22–24, 25, 101–2
self-government: Graham's ideas on, 35–36, 37; peer education and, 137; reform physiology and, 5–7, 9, 55, 82–83, 91–92, 93, 95, 99–100, 114, 142–44, 149, 168; revolutionary era and, 33
self-pollution (as term), 102
sex education: abstinence-only, 177; African American, 14, 25, 130–31, 132–37, 154–58; current, 176–77; early, 15–16, 133–34, 140–58; invention of, 149–58; moral discipline and, 33; in postbellum South, 15
sex toys, 177
sexual exploitation: of colonial women, 104–5; of domestic servants, 24, 65, 66–67, 69–71, 106, 155, 191n69; of enslaved women, 9, 21, 23, 46, 65, 76, 79–80, 96–97; of wives, 16–17, 18, 32, 55, 143, 148
sexuality (as term), 145–46
sexuality, female: 1830s reconsideration of, 11; fertility control and, 189n46; Hollick's lectures on, 108–31; libertine republicans' views on, 8; licentiousness and, 75–76, 77, 79, 81, 92, 93–94, 95, 105–6, 188–89n45, 202n32; 1970s feminist attitudes toward, 1–3, 17–18; orgasmic disorder, 174–75; patriarchal definitions of, 1, 5; premodern views

of, 30; race and, 2–3, 142; sex during pregnancy, 148. *See also* masturbation, female; passionlessness, ideology of
sexuality, male: celibate men as "male monsters," 7, 48–52, 55; hydraulic model of, 7–8, 33–34; licentiousness and, 58–59, 62–71; orgasmic disorder, 230n29; power-sharing and, 28–29; race and, 8. *See also* masturbation, male
sexual liberalism, 167–68
sexually transmitted diseases, 37, 104, 120, 126, 154, 172, 176–77, 212n21
sexual therapeutics, 120–21
sexual trafficking, 98, 147
Shaw, Susan, 118
Sheffield, Ohio, 91
Simmons, Christina, 16
Simmons, J., 220n25
skeletal anatomy, 158–61, 222n47, 226n94
Sklar, Kathryn Kish, 19
slander charges, 119
slavery: churches supporting, 95, 96–97; colonization movement, 160; divided opinion of Hollick's supporters, 125–26, 215n51; exploitation of enslaved women's reproduction, 21; gendered stereotypes rooted in, 212; miscegenation and, 167; resistance through pleasure, 51–52; white men's sexual power and, 58–59, 62–65, 71, 79–80, 167
Smith, Elizabeth Oakes, 53–54
Smith, James McCune, 160
Smith, Mary, 205n67
Smith, Sarah Towne (later Martyn), 66, 77, 79, 99, 100
Smith, Seba, 53–54
Snelling, William J., 47–48
Social Purity movement, 16, 147, 167, 187n34, 222n53, 227–28n9
Society of Friends, 73, 98, 107, 132, 133, 139, 141, 142, 204n59
"solitary vice": as camouflage for discussions, 19–20, 80; commercial appropriation of concept, 13; decline of phrase usage, 102; Gove's use of term, 92–94; Graham's use of term, 8–9, 34, 143; Hollick's use of term, 113–14; licentiousness and, 82, 99–100, 141; Rush's use of term, 34; same-sex desire and, 42–43. *See also* masturbation, female; masturbation, male
Solomon, Samuel, 214n39

southerners, white: reform physiology movement and, 15, 96–97, 147; white women's purity and, 17, 21, 228n9
Spelman College, 187n34
spermatorrhea, 16, 163–64, 166, 167
Spillers, Hortense, 23, 176
Spirit of the Times, 46
Stackhouse, Rebecca, 118
Stackhouse, Susan, 221n35
Stansell, Christine, 22
Sterling, Dorothy, 74
Stewart, Maria W., 65
Stinson, Mary, 151, 170
Stone, William L., 57–58, 59
St. Philips African Episcopal Church (New York), 60
Sturbridge, Massachusetts, 152
sugar, 51
Swedenborg, Emanuel, 222n47
syphilis, 37, 104, 120, 126, 172–73, 212n21

Tappan, Juliana A., 205n67
Tappan, Lewis, 60
teaching profession, 151–52
temperance movement, 6, 36, 77, 79, 91, 227–28n9
Third Free Church (New York), 75
Thomas, William Hannibal, 172–73
Thompson, George, 68
Tissot, Samuel Auguste, *L'Onanisme*, 33–34, 39, 51, 194n25
topless dancing, 108
transatlantic slave trade, ban on, 21
Treadwell, Irena, 205n67
tribadism, 34
Truth, Sojourner, 23, 61

ultras, 54, 130; abolitionism and, 126–27; definition, 9; emergence, 12, 28–29; Graham's views and, 36; masculinity and, 28–29, 37, 52; micropolitics of, 52; moral reform society organized by, 37, 51–52; Otis viewed by, 46; "ultraism" (as term), 9
Una, 138–39, 147
US Sanitary Commission, 15
Utica Female Moral Reform Society, 103
utopian socialism, 111, 211n9

vaginal injections, 19–20
Vainsman, John D., 45

Van Dine, Charlotte, 219n17
vegetarianism, 6, 12, 40–41, 48–50, 86, 174, 184n13
vibrators, 1, 3, 19–20, 177
virgin/whore dichotomy, 8, 44–45, 48, 119
virtue, notion of: chastity contrasted with, 74, 112, 152; class and, 22, 38; connotations, 71; conquering solitary vice and, 8–9, 81–82; defined in terms of activism, 59, 76–77; licentiousness and, 77, 78, 79, 202n32; purity contrasted with, 11, 21, 25, 70–79, 80, 122, 131, 133–34, 142, 147–48, 149, 154–55, 164, 167, 176; race and, 25, 55, 71, 142, 149, 166–67; vice contrasted with, 37; white southern women and, 96–97, 147, 167

Wakefield, Jerome, 230n29
Walker, Alice, 3, 176
water cure, 19–20, 139, 190n53
Waterman, T. T., 37
Webb, Eliza, 118
Webb, Harriet P., 221n35
Webb, James Watson, 57, 59, 61
Webb, Sarah J., 221n35
Weekly Anglo-African, The, 134
Weld, Charles Stuart, 164, 165
Weld, Sarah Grimké ("Sissy"), 165
Weld, Theodore Dwight, 139, 165
Weld, Theodore Grimké ("Sody"), 163–64, 165, 166
Weld Grimké, Angelina. *See* Grimké, Angelina (later Weld)
Wells, Ida B., 228n9
Welter, Barbara, 17
Westborough Asylum, 163
Weston, Deborah, 56
Weston, Lucia, 56
Weston, Nancy, 167
Whipper, William, 72, 73, 76, 79, 160–61
Whipple, Louisa, 205n67
White, Abigail, 84
White, Catherine, 140
White, Deborah Gray, 21
White, Elizabeth, 56
White, Josiah, 217n2
White, Rebecca, 132, 140, 217n2
Whitmarsh, Joseph, 37, 51–52, 92
Whittlesey, Azuba, 205n67
Willard, Francis, 228n9
Willets, Sarah, 61

Williams, A. Wilberforce, 172–73
Williams, Dell, 1, 2, 3
Williams, Julia, 75, 205n68
Williams, Peter, Jr., 60, 75
Wilmot Proviso, 215n51
Winchendon Female Moral Reform Society, 94
Wollstonecraft, Mary, 18
women-only lectures: by female physicians, 141; by Gove, 11–12, 81–82, 87–88, 90, 100, 102, 105, 107; by Hollick, 111–12; by moral guardians, 107; privacy and, 107; reasons for, 35; riots against Graham's, 6, 8–10, 12, 26–28, 44–45, 53–55, 56–58, 117; riots against Whitmarsh's, 52
Women's Christian Temperance Union, 228n9
women's liberation movement, 1–3, 173–77
women's rights movement: abolition movement and, 25, 147; bodily sovereignty, 143–44; coverture issue, 143; fertility control and, 22; Grimké sisters' work, 71–73; ideological differences with moral guardians, 130–31; love principle concept and, 145–49; moral reform movement and, 76–77; postbellum racial split, 167; prostitution and, 222n53; sexual citizenship ideology, 82–83, 110, 113–14, 117–23, 143, 147, 150, 162; sexual liberalism, 167–68; split with abolitionists, 25, 83, 105, 175; white southerners and, 15, 147
women's romantic friendships, 19, 122, 214–15n44
Women's Sexuality Conference (1974), 3
women's suffrage movement, 222n53
Woods, Mary, 136
Woodward, Samuel B., 168, 170, 208n27; *Hints to the Young*, 92, 150–51
Worcester, Massachusetts, 88
Worcester Lunatic Asylum, 150
Worcester State Lunatic Hospital, 151
World Anti-slavery Convention, 118
Wright, Fanny, 18, 39, 40, 111

Yellin, Jean Fagan, 202n32
York, Mrs. Lewis, 56
Young Men's and Women's Christian Associations, 15

Zion Female Moral Reform Society, 59–62, 63–64, 73–74, 96, 97–98, 200n17
Zion's Herald, 87

www.ingramcontent.com/pod-product-compliance
Lightning Source LLC
Chambersburg PA
CBHW021942290426
44108CB00012B/928